Lippincott's Pathophysiology Series

GASTROINTESTINAL PATHOPHYSIOLOGY

Joseph M. Henderson, M.D.
Formerly, Department of Medicine
The University of Michigan Medical Center
Staff Gastroenterologist
Community Hospital of Indianapolis
1400 North Ritter Avenue, Suite 370
Indianapolis, Indiana 46219

D0206923

With 12 additional contributors

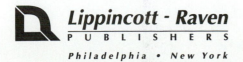

Lippincott - Raven
PUBLISHERS
Philadelphia • New York

Acquisitions Editor: Richard Winters
Developmental Editor: Mary Beth Murphy
Senior Production Editor: Virginia Barishek
Production Service: P. M. Gordon Associates, Inc.
Compositor: Pine Tree Composition
Prepress: Jay's Publishers Services
Printer/Binder: Courier Book Company/Kendallville
Cover Designer: Larry Pezzato
Cover Printer: Lehigh Press

Library of Congress Cataloging-in-Publication Data

Gastrointestinal pathophysiology / [edited by] Joseph M. Henderson :
   with 12 additional contributors.
         p.   cm. — (Lippincott's pathophysiology series)
   Includes bibliographical references and index.
   ISBN 0–397–51403–4
   1. Gastrointestinal system—Pathophysiology.   I. Henderson,
Joseph M.   II. Series.
   [DNLM: 1. Gastrointestinal Diseases—pathophysiology.]
RC802.9.G366   1996
616.3'307—dc20
DNLM/DLC
for Library of Congress   96–23363
                                                                    CIP

Care has been taken to confirm the accuracy of the information presented and to describe generally accepted practices. However, the authors, editors, and publisher are not responsible for errors or omissions or for any consequences from application of the information in this book and make no warranty, express or implied, with respect to the contents of the publication.

The authors, editors, and publisher have exerted every effort to ensure that drug selection and dosage set forth in this text are in accordance with current recommendations and practice at the time of publication. However, in view of ongoing research, changes in government regulations, and the constant flow of information relating to drug therapy and drug reactions, the reader is urged to check the package insert for each drug for any change in indications and dosage and for added warnings and precautions. This is particularly important when the recommended agent is a new or infrequently employed drug.

Some drugs and medical devices presented in this publication have Food and Drug Administration (FDA) clearance for limited use in restricted research settings. It is the responsibility of the health care provider to ascertain the FDA status of each drug or device planned for use in their clinical practice.

9 8 7 6 5 4 3 2 1

To my wife, Lisa, whose love and support keep me aiming high.

To my baby daughter, Lori, who has taught me what is truly important.

To my mother and my late father for their sacrifice and encouragement.

CONTRIBUTORS

C. Richard Boland, M.D.

Professor of Medicine
Division of Gastroenterology
University of California, San Diego,
    School of Medicine
2055 Cellular and Molecular Medicine
    East
9500 Gilman Drive
La Jolla, California 92093–0688

John M. Carethers, M.D.

Assistant Professor of Medicine
Division of Gastroenterology
University of California, San Diego,
    School of Medicine
2054 Cellular and Molecular Medicine
    East
9500 Gilman Drive
La Jolla, California 92093–0688

William D. Chey, M.D.

Lecturer, Division of Gastroenterology
Department of Internal Medicine
The University of Michigan Medical
    Center
3912 Taubman Center
Ann Arbor, Michigan 48109–0362

David C. Dawson, Ph.D.

Department of Physiology
The University of Michigan Medical
    School
1301 East Catherine, Room 7726
    Med Sci 2
Ann Arbor, Michigan 48109–0622

John DelValle, M.D.

Associate Professor of Medicine
The University of Michigan Medical
    Center
6520 MSRB #1, Box 0682
Ann Arbor, Michigan 48109–0682

Grace H. Elta, M.D.

Division of Gastroenterology
Department of Internal Medicine
The University of Michigan Medical
    Center
3912 Taubman Center
Ann Arbor, Michigan 48109–0362

Joseph M. Henderson, M.D., F.A.C.P.

Formerly, Department of Medicine
The University of Michigan Medical
    Center
Staff Gastroenterologist
Community Hospital of Indianapolis
1400 North Ritter Avenue, Suite 370
Indianapolis, Indiana 46219

W. Michael McDonnell, M.D.

Assistant Professor of Medicine
Division of Gastroenterology
The University of Michigan Medical
    Center
IIID, Internal Medicine
Department of Veterans Affairs Medical
    Center
2215 Fuller Road
Ann Arbor, Michigan 48105

CONTRIBUTORS

Richard H. Moseley, M.D.

Associate Professor of Medicine
Division of Gastroenterology
The University of Michigan Medical
  Center
IIID, Internal Medicine
Department of Veterans Affairs Medical
  Center
2215 Fuller Road
Ann Arbor, Michigan 48105

Timothy T. Nostrant, M.D.

Associate Professor of Medicine
Associate Chief, Division of
  Gastroenterology
Department of Internal Medicine
The University of Michigan Medical
  School
3912 Taubman, Box 0362
Ann Arbor, Michigan 48109–0362

James M. Scheiman, M.D.

Associate Professor of Medicine
Division of Gastroenterology
Department of Internal Medicine
The University of Michigan Medical
  Center
3912 Taubman, Box 0362
Ann Arbor, Michigan 48109–0362

D. Kim Turgeon, M.D.

Clinical Assistant Professor of Medicine
Divisions of General Medicine and
  Gastroenterology
The University of Michigan Medical
  Center
3912 Taubman Center
Ann Arbor, Michigan 48109

John W. Wiley, M.D.

Associate Professor of Medicine
Division of Gastroenterology
Attending Physician
The University of Michigan Medical
  Center
6520A MSRB #1
Ann Arbor, Michigan 48109-0682

PREFACE

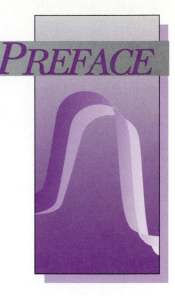

This book has been written in an effort to present the subject of gastrointestinal pathophysiology in a more clinical light than might ordinarily be done in a standard physiology textbook. It is intended primarily for sophomore medical students, but junior and senior students, house staff, and physicians in practice will find its approach useful to the clinical applications of physiology and pathophysiology. The ability to integrate what is seen and discussed on rounds with what is taught in the preclinical sciences underscores the usefulness of a text such as this.

The book's goal is to provide a "bridge" from preclinical science to clinical medicine. Thus it is not intended to serve as an in-depth textbook of physiology or pathology, and it was not written to emphasize diagnosis and therapy of gastrointestinal diseases. The bibliographies at the end of each chapter refer the interested reader to sources with more detailed information. Particularly useful parts of each chapter are found in the discussions of clinical testing and the case summaries. The clinical testing sections explain the physiologic rationale for common clinical tests employed to diagnose or exclude certain gastrointestinal diseases. The case summaries are written to walk the reader through a typical clinical problem and expose him or her to the methods of forming a differential diagnosis list and ultimately narrowing that list to the most likely diagnosis.

The contributors and I have tried to write a text basic enough to allow the student with no clinical exposure to follow along and grasp the important concepts while at the same time keeping enough detail to make the book useful in later years as well. This is not an easy task, and we realize that the level of detail may not please every reader to the same degree. Each author has presented a variety of clinical cases to illustrate certain points. Whether one format is more effective for learning than another is likely a matter of personal preference, but we would appreciate receiving feedback regarding which cases readers find most useful. Further comments are always welcomed and greatly appreciated.

Joseph M. Henderson, M.D.

CONTENTS

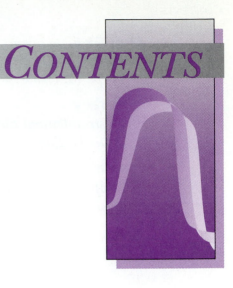

CONTENTS

Lippincott's Pathophysiology Series: Gastrointestinal Pathophysiology, edited by Joseph M. Henderson. Lippincott–Raven Publishers. Philadelphia © 1996.

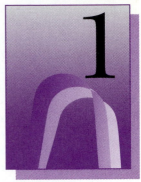

Assessment and Management of Abdominal Pain

John W. Wiley

This chapter covers some general features regarding the mechanisms and assessment of abdominal pain, an understanding of which will help the practitioner manage patients with this common presentation. The perception of pain is a subjective phenomenon resulting from the central transmission of peripherally received noxious stimuli. Abdominal pain is a common reason for patients to seek medical consultation. A careful analysis of the pain, including its location, time of onset, duration, and quality as well as exacerbating and remitting features, often helps the practitioner to determine its cause and to recommend appropriate treatment.

PATIENT PRESENTATION

A 43-year-old male comes to the emergency room with a history of sudden onset abdominal pain of 6 hours' duration. The pain is constant and severe and radiates straight through to the back. The patient lies in the supine position with knees flexed. While in the emergency room he vomits small amounts of greenish liquid on two occasions. During the initial evaluation, he changes position twice, attempting to find a more comfortable position. The patient reports attending a dinner party at which he ate a large amount of food and drank eight or nine beers. He denies gastrointestinal blood loss, diarrhea, dysphagia, cough, chest pain, or shortness of breath and says there have been no previous episodes of similar pain. The patient's wife confides that he has been drinking two cases of beer a week for several months. In the supine position vital signs reveal a blood pressure of 100 mmHg systolic, 60 mmHg diastolic, and a pulse of 82 beats per minute; after sitting for 2 minutes, blood pressure was 90 mmHg systolic, 60 mmHg diastolic, and the pulse was 100 beats per minute. Physical examination indicates that bowel sounds are present but sporadic. The abdomen is distended and tender to deep palpation in the epigastrium. Muscle guarding is present, along with rebound tenderness. Rectal examination is unremarkable. Laboratory results reveal a normal hemoglobin of 16 g/dl, a normal white blood count of 7600/mm^3, an elevated serum amylase level at 860 Us/dl, a normal calcium level of 8.6 mg/dl, and normal serum electrolytes, blood urea nitrogen, creatinine, liver transaminases, and bilirubin levels. The electrocardiogram and chest radiograph are unremarkable. Abdominal x-rays show distended loops of small and large bowel, no air-fluid levels, and no free air under the diaphragm.

This is a typical presentation for acute pancreatitis. The characteristic pattern of the pain as well as other aspects of the history, physical examination, and laboratory findings support the diagnosis of pancreatitis. In the discussion that follows, the reader will be introduced to the anatomic and functional components involved in the transmission of abdominal pain to the central nervous system.

ANATOMY AND PHYSIOLOGY

VISCERAL SENSORY PATHWAYS

The perception of pain is initiated by activation of nociceptors, consisting of free endings of small A-δ and C afferent fibers. Strong mechanical stimulation and extreme heat or cold can activate these receptors. In addition, substances generated at the site of an injury or inflammation, such as bradykinin, histamine, serotonin, and prostaglandin, may either activate pain receptors directly or lower their threshold to other stimuli. A-δ and C fibers transmit distinct sensations. The A-δ fibers innervate skin and muscle and mediate the rapid onset, sharp, well-localized pain that follows an acute injury. The C fibers innervate muscle, periosteum, parietal peritoneum, and viscera and are associated with the transmission of dull, nausea-producing, poorly localized pain that tends to be more gradual in onset and of longer duration.

The extrinsic innervation of the gastrointestinal tract consists of the parasympathetic and sympathetic nerves. These autonomic nerves transmit information to and from the central nervous system via afferent (sensory) and efferent fibers. Sensory information from the gut is carried by vagal and spinal afferent fibers. The central processes of vagal afferents terminate in the nucleus of the solitary tract (NTS) and pass to the periphery in the distribution of the vagi, whereas the central processes of spinal afferents terminate in the dorsal horn of the spinal cord and pass to the periphery in sympathetic nerves. The vagi do not transmit pain from the gut. Visceral pain is transmitted only by the spinal afferents. These neural fibers often travel with the sympathetic neurons. The cell bodies of the visceral afferent neurons are located in the dorsal root ganglia. The visceral afferent neurons synapse with marginal neurons and others at the base of the dorsal horn. The cell bodies in the dorsal horn that mediate visceral pain also receive input from peripheral non-nociceptive fibers. This dual innervation underlies the sensation of referred pain that can accompany visceral pain (see section on Referred Pain).

The spinal afferents contain a variety of neurotransmitter candidates, including the peptides, substance P, calcitonin gene-related peptide, cholecystokinin, somatostatin and dynorphin, and the excitatory amino acid glutamate. It appears that subpopulations of sensory neurons that innervate different sites such as blood vessels, skin, and viscera may demonstrate distinct neurotransmitter coding. The peripheral terminals of sensory neurons also appear to participate in certain so-called "efferent" functions, including vasodilation, smooth muscle contraction and relaxation, and depolarization of efferent neurons in prevertebral ganglia.

At the level of the spinal cord the first-order primary afferent neurons synapse in the dorsal horn with second-order neurons that transmit the nociceptive impulses via fibers that cross through the anterior commissure, ascend in the spinoreticular and lateral spinothalamic tracts, and terminate in the reticular formation of the medulla and pons or the thalamic nuclei (Fig. 1-1). Third-order neurons in the reticular formation terminate in the limbic system and frontal cortex, whereas neurons originating in thalamic nuclei relay pain impulses to the postcentral gyrus of the cerebral cortex, at which point conscious sensation is perceived.

Higher cerebral function can exert a strong inhibitory influence on pain perception. Descending fibers originating in the mesencephalon, periventricular gray matter, and caudate nucleus synapse at various sites in the afferent pathway for pain. These fibers act to inhibit the transmission of painful sensations. The cell bodies of this system possess receptors specific for opiates, and high concentrations of endorphins are present in these areas. The morphine antagonist, naloxone, reverses the inhibition that results from activation of this system. These inhibitory mechanisms allow cerebral activity to modify afferent pain impulses.

Psychologic traits, learning, ethnic and cultural background, personality, and events surrounding the injury are factors that appear to influence an individual's pain experience in response to a specific stimulus. Heightened anxiety decreases the pain threshold, and relief of anxiety or depression generally increases the threshold.

STIMULI FOR ABDOMINAL PAIN

Abdominal viscera are ordinarily insensitive to many stimuli that, when applied to the skin, evoke severe pain. Cutting, tearing, or crushing of viscera does not result in a perceptible sensation. The principal forces to which visceral pain fibers are sensitive are stretching or tension in the wall of the gut. This can be the result of traction on the peritoneum (e.g., neoplasm), distention of a hollow viscus (e.g., biliary colic), or forceful muscular contractions (e.g., intestinal obstruction). The nerve endings of pain fibers in the hollow viscera (gut, gallbladder, and urinary bladder) are located in the muscular walls. Those in the solid viscera, such as the liver and kidneys, supply the capsule and respond to stretching of the capsule from parenchymal swelling. The mesentery, parietal peritoneum, and peritoneal covering of the posterior abdomen are sensitive to pain, but the visceral peritoneum and greater omentum are not. The rate at which tension develops must be fairly rapid for pain to be produced. Gradual distention, such as occurs in malignant biliary obstruction, may be painless.

Inflammation and ischemia may also produce visceral pain. Moreover, inflammation can sensitize the nerve endings and lower the threshold to pain from other stimuli. Tissue hormones such as bradykinin, serotonin, histamine, or prostaglandin appear to participate in the pathway(s) that mediate pain associated with inflammation.

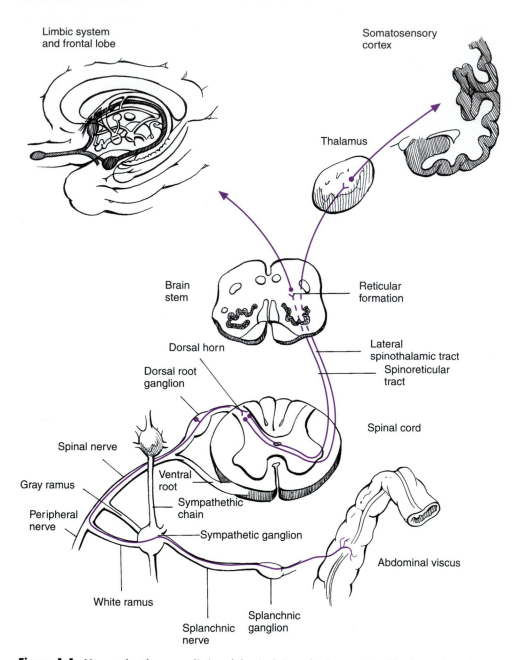

Figure 1-1. Neuronal pathways mediating abdominal visceral pain sensation. The first-order primary afferent neuron travels from the abdominal viscus along the corresponding splanchnic nerve through a ganglion of the sympathetic chain, then by way of the white ramus communicans to the spinal nerve. From there it traverses the dorsal root to enter the dorsal horn of the spinal cord, where it synapses. The second-order neurons leave the dorsal horn, cross the midline, and ascend primarily in two tracts. The spinothalamic tract neurons travel through the brain stem to various nuclei within the thalamus, where they synapse with third-order neurons that go predominantly to the somatosensory cortex. Spino-reticular tract neurons synapse within reticular formation nuclei located primarily in the pons and medulla. Third-order neurons travel predominantly to the limbic system and frontal cortex. (Adapted from Yamada T, Alpers DH, Owyang C, Powell DH, Silverstein FE, eds. Textbook of Gastroenterology, 2nd ed. Philadelphia: JB Lippincott, 1995:752.)

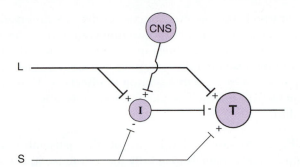

Figure 1-2. The gate control theory of pain. Sensory inputs from the periphery come to the dorsal horn of the spinal cord by way of large (L) myelinated and small (S) unmyelinated nerve fibers. Both fiber types synapse on second-order ("transmission/projection") neurons (T). When the T neurons are activated, they communicate nociceptive information to the brain. The peripheral nerve fibers also synapse on interneurons (I) which when stimulated, inhibit T-neuron firing. The large neurons stimulate and the small neurons inhibit the interneurons, thereby reducing and enhancing, respectively, central transmission of incoming nociceptive signals. In addition, descending inhibitory pathways arising within the central nervous system stimulate the interneuron to inhibit T-neuron firing when activated by a variety of factors. The balance of these excitatory and inhibitory forces determines the degree to which nociceptive information is transmitted to the brain (+ = excitatory signals; − = inhibitory signals). (Adapted from Yamada T, Alpers DH, Owyang C, Powell DW, Silverstein FE, eds. Textbook of Gastroenterology, 2nd ed. Philadelphia: JB Lippincott, 1995:663.)

GATE CONTROL THEORY OF PAIN

Modulation of pain transmission can occur at the level of the spinal cord. One hypothesis to explain this phenomenon is referred to as the gate control model (Fig. 1-2). This model proposes the existence of interneurons in the spinal cord that are spontaneously active and inhibit second-order so-called "projection-transmission" neurons, whose activity results in the sensation of pain. The interneurons are excited by large myelinated non-nociceptive afferents (Aα/Aβ fibers) and inhibited by small unmyelinated nociceptive fibers (C fibers). When the large afferent fibers are stimulated, the activities of the inhibitory interneurons and transmission neurons are increased and decreased, respectively, thereby reducing the perception of pain. Conversely, stimulation of the small afferent fibers suppresses activity of the inhibitory interneurons, resulting in an increased perception of pain. Descending inhibitory pathways from the central nervous system also appear to stimulate the interneurons, resulting in inhibition of transmission cell firing. Therefore, enhancement or inhibition of the pain impulses before they reach consciousness in the cerebral cortex is possible. The perception of pain reflects the balance of these inhibitory and excitatory pathways.

CLINICAL CORRELATES

Abdominal pain can be separated into three categories: visceral pain, parietal pain, and referred pain. The distinctions can be useful for understanding the patterns of clinical pain.

Visceral Pain. Visceral pain is experienced when noxious stimuli affect an abdominal viscus. Typically, the pain is dull and poorly localized in the epigastrium, periumbilical region, or lower midabdomen. Visceral pain is often localized near the midline because the abdominal organs receive sensory input from both sides of the spinal cord. The site where the pain is felt corresponds roughly to the dermatomes from which the involved organ receives its innervation. The pain is poorly localized because most viscera receive innervation from several segments. In addition, the number of nerve endings in viscera are fewer than the number in skin. The quality of pain is generally cramping, burning, or gnawing. Visceral pain is often accompanied by secondary autonomic effects such as sweating, restlessness, nausea, emesis, and pallor. The patient may move about in an attempt to relieve the discomfort.

Parietal Pain. Noxious stimulation of the parietal peritoneum elicits parietal-type pain. Parietal pain is generally more intense and localized than visceral pain. A frequently cited example is the localized pain associated with acute appendicitis produced by inflammatory involvement of the peritoneum at McBurney's point. This pain is often made worse by movement or coughing; therefore, patients often avoid any unnecessary movements. Lateralization of parietal pain can be observed because at any given point the parietal peritoneum obtains innervation from only one side of the nervous system.

Referred Pain. Referred pain is experienced in remote areas supplied by the same neurosegment as the involved organ and is thought to result from the existence of shared central pathways for afferent neurons from different sites. For example, visceral afferents from the capsule of the liver, the splenic capsule, and the pericardium are derived from dermatomes C3 to C5 and reach the central nervous system via the phrenic nerve. Afferents from the gallbladder, stomach, pancreas, and small intestine travel through the celiac plexus and the greater splanchnic nerves and enter the spinal cord from T6 to T9. Stimuli from the appendix, colon, and pelvic viscera enter the spinal cord at the level of T10–T11 by way of the mesenteric plexus and lesser splanchnic nerves. The sigmoid colon, rectum, renal pelvis and capsule, ureter, and testes are innervated by fibers that reach the T11 to L1 segments through the lowest splanchnic nerve. The rectosigmoid colon and bladder send afferents through the hypogastric plexus to enter the spinal cord from S2 to S4. Referred pain may be perceived in skin or deeper tissues. It is usually fairly well localized. Frequently cited examples are the perception of pain in the shoulder region after a liver biopsy and in the neck area during a myocardial infarction. In general, referred pain is experienced when the noxious visceral stimulus becomes more intense. For example, balloon distention–generated pain in the intestine is initially experienced as visceral pain but can be accompanied by referred pain in the back as the level of distention is increased. Hyperesthesia of skin and hyperalgesia of muscle may develop in the distribution of the referred pain.

CLINICAL ASSESSMENT AND MANAGEMENT

The patient who presents with abdominal pain requires a thorough history, physical examination, and often some screening laboratory studies. This information usually suggests the diagnosis or guides further diagnostic strategies. The acuteness of the illness is a major factor in determining the clinical approach to abdominal pain. Acute abdominal pain generally requires the practitioner to make a decision regarding the urgency of additional diagnostic testing, e.g., laboratory or x-ray studies or both to determine if an immediate laparotomy is indicated. If symptoms have been present for weeks or months without recent exacerbation, the work-up can proceed more slowly.

HISTORY

The patient should be questioned carefully regarding the following aspects of the abdominal pain:

Location. The site of the pain and the extent to which it is localized must be determined. Significant radiation of the pain to other areas may be present, such as the sensation of pain in the thigh with disease in the ureter or testicle. Pain in the shoulder may signify diaphragmatic involvement. The pain in biliary, duodenal, or pancreatic disease is often referred to the back. Visceral pain tends to be poorly localized, but pain produced by irritation of the parietal peritoneum is confined to the area involved by disease.

Intensity and Character. The severity of the pain is loosely related to the magnitude of the noxious stimulus. For example, acute perforated duodenal ulcer can evoke excruciating pain, and the intensity of the pain is of diagnostic value. However, estimates of the severity of pain can be unreliable because of the interaction of the various factors that influence pain perception. It can be helpful to inquire about the patient's most severe pain in the past and to compare the intensity of the current pain. Certain diseases produce pain with distinct qualities. The gnawing pain of duodenal ulcer and the cramping pain of intestinal obstruction are examples. The pain in biliary colic may be constricting; in ruptured aneurysm, tearing; in pancreatitis, stabbing; and in acute appendicitis, aching.

Quality and Quantity. The quality and quantity of pain in relationship to time can help guide the practitioner to the cause. Acute abdominal pain that has persisted for longer than 6 hours usually indicates a surgical problem. The chronic pain of duodenal ulcer does not typically occur before breakfast but appears later in the interprandial period. Pain associated with acute appendicitis usually progresses steadily over 12 hours without remission. Intestinal obstruction is associated with cramping pain, separated by pain-free intervals. Steady pain is produced by ischemia whether solely caused by vascular disease or secondary to strangulation obstruction.

Aggravating or Alleviating Factors. A number of important diagnostic clues are included in this category, such as pain initiated on swallowing, which implicates the esophagus. Peptic ulcer pain tends to improve with taking of antacids. Duodenal ulcer pain can improve with ingestion of food. Movement typically aggravates the pain associated with peritonitis, whereas patients with obstruction of a hollow viscus tend to seek different positions to decrease the pain but to no avail. The pain experienced with disorders such as pancreatic cancer that involve the retroperitoneum can be aggravated in the supine position and improved by sitting up or bending forward. In the appropriate clinical setting, therapeutic trials of antacids, antispasmodics, or special diets are sometimes prescribed with the aim of obtaining diagnostic data as well as relieving the patient's discomfort.

Associated Signs and Symptoms. Information should be sought regarding changes in gastric function (nausea, emesis, anorexia), defecation (diarrhea, constipation), weight, renal function, and gynecologic function. Diarrhea may signify pain from gastroenteritis, whereas obstipation suggests intestinal obstruction. Bloody urine may be seen with ureteral colic caused by a ureteral stone. Jaundice can direct attention to the biliary tree in cases of upper abdominal pain.

Setting. What are the circumstances in which the pain appears? Heartburn may be experienced only when abdominal pressure is increased. Emotional tension may aggravate peptic ulcer pain or that associated with the irritable colon syndrome.

PHYSICAL EXAMINATION

The clinical history is often nonspecific regarding the etiology of abdominal pain. A thorough physical examination should be carried out because it will often suggest a probable diagnosis or reduce the group of potential diagnoses.

The patient's general appearance may provide clues regarding the etiology of the pain. Tachycardia, fever, and perspiration suggest sepsis from peritonitis, cholangitis, pyelonephritis, or severe bacterial enteritis. The patient with pure visceral pain may change position frequently, but if localized or general peritonitis is present he or she will avoid movement.

The abdomen should be inspected for distention from intestinal obstruction or ascites. All potential hernia sites should be carefully examined. Incarceration of a segment of bowel in a small femoral hernia can easily be missed if not specifically looked for. Hyperperistalsis may be audible with the stethoscope in intestinal obstruction or enteritis. Generalized peritonitis usually causes decreased or absent peristalsis. Auscultatory evidence of vascular bruits may indicate an aortic or splenic artery aneurysm. Palpation of the abdomen should be gentle at first and initiated at a distance from the painful area so that the patient does not become so guarded that an accurate examination is impossible.

Abdominal rigidity or involuntary guarding may indicate the presence of adjacent peritonitis. The most classic example is the board-like upper abdominal rigidity that occurs early in perforated peptic ulcer. Lesser degrees of guarding or rigidity develop over the area of an acutely inflamed gallbladder or appendix or in acute diverticulitis. If the patient's knees are drawn up, this may provide just enough relaxation to allow an examination that was otherwise impossible because of guarding. An abnormal mass may be caused by enlargement of a diseased organ, a malignancy, or inflammatory processes.

Pure visceral pain is usually not accompanied by tenderness. When tenderness is present, the most important question is the extent of its localization. Generalized peritonitis is suggested by severe diffuse tenderness with rigidity and clinical toxicity. However, mild general tenderness without toxicity is more compatible with acute gastroenteritis, salpingitis, or some other nonsurgical condition. The early uncomplicated stage of acute cholecystitis, appendicitis, or diverticulitis is characterized by tenderness that can usually be well localized to a small area. The key to determining localization is gentle palpation with one finger until the tender area has been thoroughly mapped out. Localized tenderness over McBurney's point is a useful finding when making the diagnosis of acute appendicitis. Rebound pain is produced by pressing slowly and deeply over a tender area and then suddenly releasing the hand. Rebound tenderness supports the presence of peritonitis of the parietal peritoneum. Hyperesthesia in response to gently touching the skin may be present in the dermatome affected by intraperitoneal parietal pain.

Genital, rectal, and pelvic examinations are part of the evaluation of every patient with abdominal pain. Acute pelvic inflammation or a twisted ovarian cyst or a uterine fibroid may be noted, or rectal examination may reveal a tumor or an abscess or occult blood in the feces.

LABORATORY FINDINGS

Routine hematologic studies should include a complete blood count and a serum creatinine concentration. The presence of leukocytosis supports an inflammatory condition. The presence of an anemia may indicate that gastrointestinal blood loss has occurred. Urine analysis can be helpful to rule out renal calculi, renal malignancy, and urinary tract infection. The presence of elevated amylase and lipase levels supports the diagnosis of pancreatitis. Elevated alkaline phosphatase and bilirubin levels suggest that a problem may be present in the pancreas or biliary tree, whereas elevated transaminases support the presence of hepatocellular injury. Other tests should be ordered according to clinical clues derived from the history and physical examination. For example, the diagnosis of acute porphyria requires specific laboratory testing.

Gastrointestinal x-ray examination with barium sulfate and/or endoscopic evaluation of the upper gastrointestinal tract, small bowel, or colon can be very useful to establish the correct diagnosis of disorders affecting these regions. Oral cholecystography, ultrasonography, hepato-iminodiacetic acid (HIDA) scans, and endoscopic retrograde cholangiopancreatopathy can be very helpful to confirm pancreatic or biliary disease. Selective mesenteric angiography can reveal mesenteric arterial stenosis in patients suspected of suffering from intestinal angina. Esophageal manometry is clinically useful in the differential diagnosis of substernal pain, and gastroduodenal manometry is gaining acceptance in the evaluation of motility disorders affecting this region.

DIFFERENTIAL DIAGNOSIS

The history, physical examination, and laboratory findings will generally guide the practitioner to the correct diagnosis. Occasionally, the cause of recurrent abdominal pain cannot be identified on the basis of this information and a long list of uncommon etiologies must be considered. The pain patterns of several disorders—including biliary tract disease, duodenal and gastric ulcer, gastritis, esophagitis, and cancer—can overlap. Therefore, accurate identification of the etiology of recurrent or persistent upper abdominal pain often necessitates obtaining x-ray studies (barium studies and/or computed tomographic [CT] scanning) or upper endoscopic examination.

Chronic, undiagnosed abdominal pain is a significant clinical problem that can lead to repeated laparotomies. Patients report a history of recurrent attacks for years without experiencing weight loss or developing morbidity other than the pain. Barium x-ray studies or endoscopic examination of the upper and lower gastrointestinal tracts may be normal or reveal minimal changes in the duodenal bulb, culminating in a partial gastrectomy. Other individuals may present with abdominal pain after having undergone an appendectomy for suspected appendicitis, repair of a hiatal hernia for poorly documented esophageal reflux, or cholecystectomy for postprandial pain, although no objective evidence was found supporting the linkage of these disorders to the pain.

Examination of psychologic profiles suggest that patients with undiagnosed chronic abdominal pain demonstrate a higher than normal incidence of depression and anxiety disorders. In some cases, functional disturbances characterized by spasm of the gut are responsible for pain. For example, increased intraluminal pressures coincident with pain have been found in patients with the irritable colon syndrome. This population appears to have a lower threshold for detecting abdominal discomfort associated with balloon distention. Repetitive evaluations of patients with chronic abdominal pain in the absence of objective findings are generally not fruitful. In unresolved cases with no objective findings (e.g., fever, jaundice, mass, radiographic abnormality, or laboratory abnormalities), laparotomy usually yields negative findings.

TREATMENT

Treatment of abdominal pain should be guided by the diagnosis and influenced by the severity and chronicity of the presentation. In patients with acute abdominal pain, the practitioner may not be able to define the condition more precisely than an "acute surgical abdomen." In such cases, laparotomy is indicated because of the protean nature of common problems such as acute appendicitis and the increased morbidity if perforation occurs.

Medications are frequently employed with success in the treatment of abdominal pain. Drugs tend to be more effective in the treatment of acute pain then of chronic pain syndromes. Frequently used agents include nonsteroidal anti-inflammatory agents and opiates. Antidepressants and anxiolytics have also been employed with some success in the treatment of appropriate cases of chronic abdominal pain. Transcutaneous electrical nerve stimulation (TENS) also has been employed in the treatment of chronic pain. This technique appears to work by stimulating the descending pathways in the dorsal columns which, in turn, activate the inhibitory interneurons and thereby reduce the transmission of nociceptive impulses.

The care of patients with chronic pain can be very challenging. Numerous multidisciplinary treatment centers devoted to the management of chronic pain have evolved in recent years where various specialists jointly contribute to the management plan. Therapy generally is tailored to the patient's life expectancy, e.g., patients with terminal illnesses and a limited life expectancy should be treated with narcotics and mood-altering drugs without concern for the potential of addiction. The therapy of patients with benign disease is more complex. In these individuals the use of addicting drugs must be carefully monitored. A treatment goal is to help the patient adapt to the problem. In carefully selected cases, ablative or other neurosurgical techniques may play a role in pain management. Some patients meet the criteria for chronic intractable abdominal pain, which is defined as persistent abdominal pain that has been present for at least 6 months without evidence of a pathophysiologic diagnosis. Optimal management of the pain in this population typically requires a number of therapeutic approaches centering on adjustment to the illness and establishing realistic goals. In general, narcotic analgesics should be avoided in this group because of the potential for addiction. Relaxation training, physical therapy, biofeedback, and hypnosis can be useful in the management of pain in these individuals.

Patients recovering from surgery can experience substantial pain relief in response to administration of a placebo. The effectiveness of placebo analgesia seems to be directly related to the intensity of the pain stimulus. The placebo response is blocked by naloxone, which suggests that it is probably mediated by the central opioid inhibitory system. The biology of placebo analgesia remains poorly understood and therefore it is not well utilized by the medical profession.

SELECTED READING

Cervero F. Neurophysiology of gastrointestinal pain. Baillieres Clin Gastroenterol 2:183, 1988.

Fields HL. Pain from deep tissues and referred pain. In: Melzack R, Wall PD, eds. The Challenge of Pain, 2nd ed. London: Penguin Books, 1988:122.

Klein KB, Mellinkoff SM. Approach to the patient with abdominal pain. In: Yamada T, Alpers DH, Owyang C, Powell DH, Silverstein FE, eds. Textbook of Gastroenterology. Philadelphia: JB Lippincott, 1991:660.

Levine JD, Fields HL, Basbaum AI. Peptides and the primary afferent nociceptor. J Neurosci 13:2273, 1993.

Meller ST, Gebhart GF. Nitric oxide (NO) and nociceptive processing in the spinal cord. Pain 52:127, 1993.

Melzack R, Wall PD. Pain mechanisms: A new theory. Science 150:971, 1965.

Selzer M, Spencer WA. Interactions between visceral and cutaneous afferents in the spinal cord: Reciprocal primary afferent fiber depolarization. Brain Res 14:349, 1969.

Willis WD Jr. Visceral inputs to sensory pathways in the spinal cord. In: Cervero F, Morrison JFB, eds. Visceral Sensation. Amsterdam: Elsevier, 1986:207.

Lippincott's Pathophysiology Series: Gastrointestinal Pathophysiology, edited by Joseph M. Henderson. Lippincott–Raven Publishers. Philadelphia © 1996.

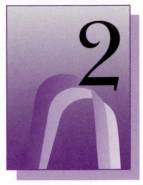

Dysphagia, Chest Pain, and Gastroesophageal Reflux

Timothy T. Nostrant

Dysphagia and chest pain are common clinical problems that can significantly reduce quality of life and frequently require extensive evaluation to diagnose. The purpose of this chapter is to introduce the reader to the physiology of normal esophageal function and to use this as a framework to evaluate patients with dysphagia and chest pain. Pathophysiologic correlates of esophageal dysfunction and an illustrative case to point out the diagnostic approach are presented.

PHYSIOLOGY OF SWALLOWING

The esophagus is a simple hollow organ designed to keep itself empty despite acid reflux and food ingestion. The oral cavity, pharynx, and larynx are involved in food transfer into the esophagus, while passage of food into the airway is avoided (Fig. 2-1). The walls of the oropharynx are composed of three sets of constrictors—superior, middle, and inferior. These constrictors, in conjunction with the laryngeal strap muscles, are designed to elevate the larynx away from the esophageal inlet during swallowing while contracting the oropharynx and hypopharynx in a posteroanterior direction. These muscles have dense innervation with ratios of nerve fibers to muscles consistent with those seen with extraocular muscles (1:2 to 1:6), suggesting exquisitely fine motor control. Central control and programmed triggering of neurons determine the sequence of muscle contraction and the swallow response.

Swallowing is a neuromuscular response with voluntary and involuntary com-

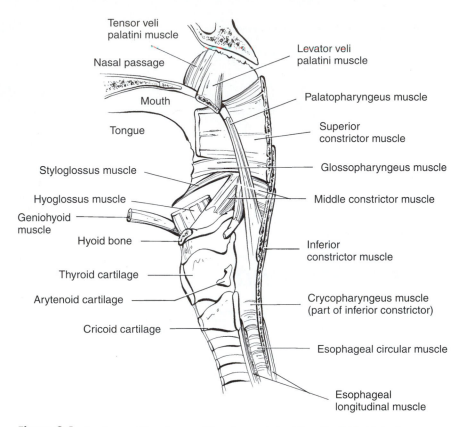

Figure 2-1. Anatomy of the pharynx. The pharynx is traditionally divided into three segments. The nasopharynx is not part of the alimentary canal and the levator and tensor veli palatini muscles close the nasopharynx during swallowing to prevent regurgitation. The oropharynx is where the respiratory and alimentary tracts pass. Its major purposes are to elevate and displace the larynx anteriorly and superiorly. The hypopharynx is most important in bolus propulsion and movement through the UES (cricopharyngeus and inferior constrictors). (Adapted from Yamada T, Alpers DH, Owyang C, Powell DW, Silverstein FE, eds. Textbook of Gastroenterology, 2nd ed. Philadelphia: JB Lippincott, 1995:160.)

ponents (Fig. 2-2). A typical individual swallows 600 times/day (350 times while awake, 200 times while eating, and 50 times while asleep), most of the time unconsciously. Liquid or solid food is important in beginning and sustaining the response, since it is difficult to swallow with a completely empty oral cavity. Swallowing can be divided into the oral and pharyngeal phases. The oral phase is primarily voluntary. The minimal response is lip sealing anteriorly, molding the food into a solid bolus on the central groove of the tongue and propelling the bolus backward by pushing the tongue up against the hard palate. The tongue supplies 80% of the total energy needed for bolus transport into the esophagus. The pharyngeal response is triggered by the bolus on the posterior surface of the tongue, and subsequent movement is largely involuntary. The pharyngeal response is composed of five stages and is accomplished in one second. The first stage is closure of the nasopharynx with contraction of the soft palate. This prevents passage of the bolus back out through the nose and promotes effective energy passage to the hypopharynx. The second phase is anterosuperior displacement of the larynx to prevent food aspiration. To further prevent laryngeal penetration of food, the larynx is

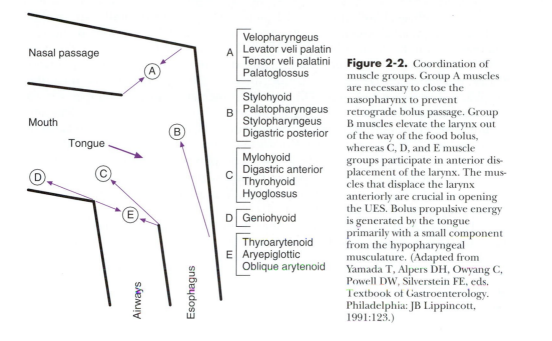

Figure 2-2. Coordination of muscle groups. Group A muscles are necessary to close the nasopharynx to prevent retrograde bolus passage. Group B muscles elevate the larynx out of the way of the food bolus, whereas C, D, and E muscle groups participate in anterior displacement of the larynx. The muscles that displace the larynx anteriorly are crucial in opening the UES. Bolus propulsive energy is generated by the tongue primarily with a small component from the hypopharyngeal musculature. (Adapted from Yamada T, Alpers DH, Owyang C, Powell DW, Silverstein FE, eds. Textbook of Gastroenterology. Philadelphia: JB Lippincott, 1991:123.)

closed by the epiglottis, true vocal cords, and false vocal cords, forming a closed cup configuration (phase three). Relaxation of the upper esophageal sphincter occurs after closure and displacement of the larynx and constitutes phase four. The upper esophageal sphincter is composed of the inferior margin of the inferior constrictor and the cricopharyngeal muscles. These muscles are constantly contracted actively by continuous neural activity. Cessation of neural activity signals the onset of relaxation with 90% of muscle tone secondary to neural input and 10% produced by intrinsic muscle tone. The last phase of swallowing is the initiation of pharyngeal contraction with subsequent passage of the bolus into an open esophagus. The sphincter contracts predominantly in an anteroposterior direction and produces a slit-like "C" configuration around the cricoid cartilage. Upper esophageal sphincter (UES) pressure decreases with sleep and during sleep maintains only intrinsic muscle tone to keep it closed. However, the UES is rapidly responsive to respiration, phonation, head position, intraluminal distention, stimulation, and stress, and therefore protection of the esophagus and airway can be produced instantly. All of the swallow responses, but particularly opening of the UES and pharyngeal contraction, are influenced by the consistency of the food or liquid bolus. Solid boluses require greater UES opening and stronger pharyngeal contraction. Smaller UES opening and lower pharyngeal contraction amplitudes are needed for mushy or liquid boluses. In addition to UES opening and pharyngeal contraction amplitudes, the duration of UES opening depends on the consistency and size of the bolus. Longer durations of opening are needed to pass large or solid boluses. Sphincter closure coincides with the arrival of the propagated pharyngeal contraction, and postbolus passage UES pressures greater than baseline pressure prevent retrograde bolus passage. During retrograde air passage (belching), UES relaxation is triggered by distention of a long length of esophageal body by gas reflux, and relaxation is prolonged to permit full gas passage. Gas or balloon distention of the esophageal body produces a UES relaxation in a fashion similar to that for natural retrograde gas passage.

The esophageal body is a 20- to 22-cm muscular tube with a wall composed of skeletal and smooth muscles. In humans, the proximal 5% is striated muscle, whereas the middle 35 to 40% is mixed smooth and striated muscle. The distal 50 to 60% of esophageal body musculature, including the lower esophageal sphincter (LES), is smooth muscle entirely. Unlike the rest of the gastrointestinal tract, the esophagus has no serosal layer. The extrinsic innervation to the esophagus is via the vagus nerve. Striated esophageal motor neurons originate in the nucleus ambiguus, whereas smooth muscle neurons originate in the dorsal motor nucleus of the vagus nerve. These neurons have relays to the myenteric plexi between the longitudinal and circular muscles. These myenteric plexi are more numerous in the smooth muscle compared to the striated muscle regions of the esophagus but are less dense than in other regions of the gut. The submucosal plexi (Meissner's plexus) are exceedingly sparse.

Esophageal peristalsis is evident shortly after pharyngeal contraction passes the UES. The average speed of peristalsis is between 2 and 4 cm/sec. Primary peristalsis is initiated by swallowing, whereas secondary peristalsis is initiated by esophageal distention and begins distal to the area of distention. Peristalsis in the absence of extrinsic innervation is termed autonomous peristalsis, suggesting that peristalsis can be initiated totally at the esophageal intramural level.

Another property of the peristaltic mechanism is deglutitive inhibition. A second swallow completely inhibits the contraction of a first swallow if the second swallow begins before the first swallow has traversed the striated portion of the esophagus. The first swallow is partially inhibited with decreasing contraction amplitudes in the distal esophagus if the esophageal wave is passing through the smooth muscle esophageal body at the beginning of a second swallow. Repetitive short interval swallowing produces total esophageal inhibition with a relaxed LES. A normal peristaltic contraction will follow the last swallow of such a series and clear the esophagus completely.

The mechanical equivalent of peristalsis is the stripping wave seen on barium studies of the esophagus. The inverted "V" of the stripping wave corresponds to the upstroke of the esophageal pressure wave and travels at a speed similar to the manometrically determined velocity of contraction. The level of esophageal body pressure needed to clear the esophagus effectively increases as one proceeds distally in the esophagus. In addition, solid boluses require higher pressures for effective clearance. Although liquids pass predominantly by gravity to the distal esophagus, effective clearance still requires intact peristaltic function.

The physiologic control mechanisms for striated muscle of the esophagus receive excitatory vagal input preferentially; sequential innervation produces the characteristic peristaltic complex (Fig. 2-3). Experimental proof using vagal nerve transection and reanastomosis of the distal nerve segment to skeletal muscle efferents has demonstrated sequential vagal spike discharges during striated esophageal body peristalsis. Afferent fiber input from the esophageal body modulates this vagal input with increased vagal tone if large or solid boluses pass through the esophagus. These data demonstrate that striated esophageal body peristalsis is mediated by central input in a fashion similar to the oropharyngeal musculature.

Esophageal smooth muscle peristalsis differs from striated muscle peristalsis because of the roles of vagal and intramural ganglion input to each muscle group. The major innervation to the striated muscle group is from the vagus nerve with no intramural nerve input. Programming of response for striated muscle is central in origin. Although central input is present in the esophageal smooth muscle, com-

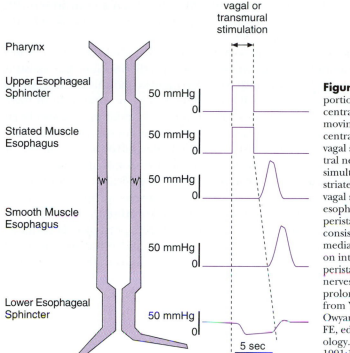

Figure 2-3. The striated muscle portion of the esophagus has a central programmed response moving proximally to distally. This central response is shown when vagal stimulation outside the central nervous system produces simultaneous contraction in all striated esophageal muscles. After vagal stimulation stops, esophageal smooth muscle peristalsis occurs. This finding is consistent with initial inhibition mediated by central vagal input on intramural neuron followed by peristalsis initiated by either nerves or muscles with distally prolonged latencies. (Adapted from Yamada T, Alpers DH, Owyang C, Powell DW, Silverstein FE, eds. Textbook of Gastroenterology. Philadelphia: JB Lippincott, 1991:129.)

plete central denervation does not stop peristalsis. Vagal input is important in modulating response through sensory vagal afferents producing stronger peristaltic waves with larger or more solid boluses. Secondary peristalsis produced by esophageal distention is mediated by vagal afferent input and is abolished with nerve transection.

The intrinsic control of smooth muscle peristalsis is mediated by a rich intramural nerve network. The persistence of peristalsis after vagal deinnervation highlights the role of this intramural network in generating peristalsis. This network contains both excitatory and inhibitory components. Excitatory neurons mediate contraction in both the longitudinal and circular muscle layers via cholinergic M_2 receptors. Inhibitory neurons predominate in the circular muscle layer and inhibit contraction via a noncholinergic, nonadrenergic neurotransmitter. Both vasoactive intestinal polypeptide and nitric oxide have been implicated as the primary inhibitory neurotransmitters. Cholinergic excitation of the excitatory neurons is nicotinic, whereas the excitation of the noncholinergic, nonadrenergic neurotransmitter can be both nicotinic and muscarinic (M_1). Both types of neurons innervate the esophageal body and lower esophageal sphincter. The precise mechanisms responsible for generating esophageal peristalsis are still unknown, although electrical stimulation of the esophagus produces an initial inhibition of the entire esophagus with a resultant contraction wave simulating peristalsis after electrical stimulation is stopped. Peristalsis is produced by sequential depolarization of intramural neurons, which occurs because of longer latent periods of hyperpolarization as one progresses down the esophagus. The electric stimulation model of peristalsis in the esophagus is not identical to that of spontaneous swallow–induced peristalsis because it does not take into account the sequential nature of central vagal tone on the smooth muscle of the esophagus, which has been shown to sequentially activate from the proximal to the distal esophagus at a rate consistent with primary peristalsis.

To date the predominant view of esophageal peristalsis is that it is determined in large part by neurally dependent esophageal gradients, since peristalsis is abolished by tetrodotoxin (a potent neural inhibitor) and is aborally contracted no matter where the stimulus is applied in the esophagus. The possible role of myogenic gradients in the esophagus independent of neural stimulation has also been proposed, and muscle contraction latencies similar to spontaneous peristalsis have been demonstrated in muscle preparations rendered devoid of neural input by tetrodotoxin. However, high frequency stimuli known only to stimulate muscles directly tend to propagate muscle contractions both orally and aborally and therefore do not mimic swallow-induced peristalsis. These instrinsic properties of muscle include resting membrane potentials, potassium concentrations, and calcium permeability. It is likely that spontaneous swallow-induced peristalsis is induced and maintained by a combination of both central and intramural neural input modulated by intrinsic myogenic properties. Like the neural input these properties induce more prolonged muscle contraction latencies proceeding from the proximal to the distal smooth muscle of the esophagus.

The LES represents the major barrier between the acid-filled stomach and the predominantly more alkaline empty esophageal lumen. Although the LES was initially thought to be a functional barrier without an anatomic correlate, recent meticulous studies have identified a ring of maximal thickness that runs obliquely upward from the lesser to the greater curvature of the stomach. The average length of the ring is 31 mm and corresponds to the manometrically determined high-pressure zone. In addition, the physiologic lower esophageal barrier receives components from the right crus of the diaphragm. Recent studies have demonstrated that compression of the LES by the diaphragmatic crus is the major factor determining competency of the LES barrier during abdominal compression and other stress maneuvers aimed at breaching the lower esophageal antireflux barrier.

Physiologically, the LES is a 3- to 4-cm long segment of tonically contracted smooth muscle at the distal end of the esophagus. Resting tone varies from 10 to 30 mmHg in normal individuals. LES pressure is lowest postprandially and highest at night. The LES pressure is predominantly myogenic because it is not affected by the use of tetrodotoxin. However, in humans, atropine does decrease tonic LES pressure and therefore neural modulation is present. In addition, hormones and other agents may modulate the myogenic properties of LES smooth muscle during fasting and feeding.

Basal LES tone is inhibited with swallowing concurrently with the deglutitive inhibition that traverses the smooth muscle esophagus. LES relaxation is vagally mediated by preganglionic cholinergic nerves and postganglionic noncholinergic, nonadrenergic nerves. The process mediating relaxation of the LES is identical to that mediating the inhibitory front along the smooth muscle esophageal body. The noncholinergic, nonadrenergic neurotransmitter is still unknown but candidates include vasoactive intestinal polypeptide, peptide histidine isoleucine, and nitric oxide. Since all three have potential interactions in many species, one or more combinations may be important in humans. The role of the diaphragm in LES relaxation has been suggested by the fact that crural fibers are electrically silent during times of LES relaxation, whereas the dome of the diaphragm is active. Reflex inhibition of the crura disappears with vagotomy.

Another complex phenomenon was discovered during investigations into the mechanism of gastroesophageal reflux. Dent and colleagues found that normal individuals demonstrated gastroesophageal reflux through a mechanism of transient nonswallow–induced LES relaxation despite a normal basal LES pressure. In patients with esophagitis, the percentage of transient lower esophageal sphincter relaxations that are accompanied by acid reflux increases above the percentage seen in normal individuals. Transient lower esophageal sphincter relaxation is the major mechanism of air venting during belching, and this may represent the physiologic role for transient LES relaxations. Distention of the stomach is associated with a marked increase in LES relaxations. Although some investigators believe that transient LES relaxations are just manifestations of incomplete swallowing responses, the evidence points primarily to the role of transient nonswallow–induced LES relaxation in gas venting after meals.

CLINICAL CORRELATES OF ESOPHAGEAL DYSFUNCTION

OROPHARYNGEAL DYSFUNCTION

Virtually any disease of the central nervous system can cause dysphagia. Since the neural circuitry responsible for the pharyngeal swallow is located in the brain stem, it follows that impairment of swallowing is worse with brain stem cerebrovascular infarcts. Either extreme difficulty in initiating swallowing or complete loss of the swallow response can be observed in such cases. Bilateral infarcts produce worse and more irreversible deficits. Observed abnormalities with cortical infarcts include significant delays in triggering of the pharyngeal swallow response, poor lingual control of the bolus because of the loss of tongue musculature or loss of coordinated propulsion, poor pharyngeal clearance, and aspiration (Fig. 2-4). Chest infections, dehydration, weight loss, and death can be consequences of dysphagia that is related to cerebrovascular disease. Other diseases that can affect the swallowing mechanism include poliomyelitis (viral damage to brain stem nuclei and axons), which can produce dysarthria and dysphagia because of pharyngeal muscle weakness, and amyotrophic lateral sclerosis (degeneration of motor neurons in the brain, brain stem, and spinal cord), with recurrent aspiration during and after swallowing caused by poor pharyngeal clearance. Weakness of the tongue is common and separates amyotrophic lateral sclerosis from more localized brain stem abnormalities and from Parkinson's disease, which can mimic both poliomyelitis and amyotrophic lateral sclerosis but has characteristic extrabulbar findings such as rigidity and cogwheeling of the extremities.

Muscular disorders such as muscular dystrophy can produce significant dysphagia owing to involvement of both tongue and pharyngeal musculature. Voice nasality and nasopharyngeal regurgitation are common. Aspiration occurs because of weakness of the laryngeal elevators. Patients eat more slowly at first and then change their diets to more mushy foods that are more easily handled by weak swallowing muscles. Aspiration of more than 10% of a food consistency usually makes individuals eliminate that food from the diet. Speech and swallowing pathologists can be extremely helpful in localizing the specific defects and planning swallowing maneuvers to optimize food intake and minimize aspiration. As swallowing worsens, nasogastric and gastrostomy tube feeding may be the only means available to sustain nutrition. Other conditions mimicking muscular dystrophy include myasthenia gravis (destruction of acetylcholine receptors at the neuromuscular junc-

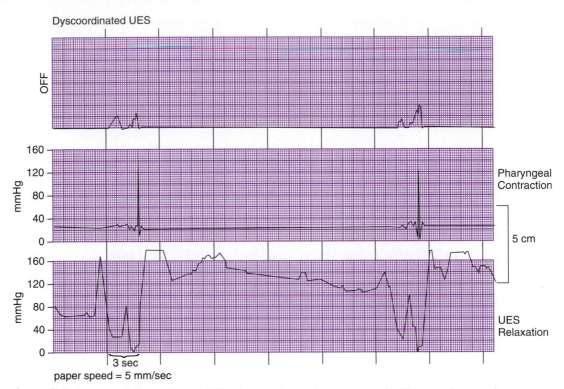

Figure 2-4. Example of discoordinated UES relaxation in a patient after a stroke. Pharyngeal contractions are shown in the proximal two leads and UES pressure in the last lead. Intermittently (first but not second sequence), pharyngeal contraction occurs after UES pressure has returned to baseline rather than at the nadir of sphincter relaxation. Symptoms improved after a cricopharyngeal myotomy. (Adapted from Yamada T, Alpers DH, Owyang C, Powell DW, Silverstein FE, eds. Textbook of Gastroenterology. Philadelphia: JB Lippincott, 1992:125.)

tion) and those causing drying of the mouth (xerostomia) such as primary xerostomia or medication-induced xerostomia (caused by anticholinergics).

Disorders affecting the upper esophageal sphincter (UES) and proximal striated muscles of the esophagus include diseases that affect the muscles (dermatomyositis) and those causing progressive narrowing of the UES (following laryngectomy and nemataline rod disease). Progressive muscular destruction of the striated esophageal muscles leads to upper esophageal dysphagia mimicking oropharyngeal-pharyngeal dysphagia. Characteristic rashes on the face simulating raccoon eyes (heliotropic rash), proximal muscle weakness including the upper and lower extremities, and biochemical evidence of muscle inflammation (increased aldolase, lactate dehydrogenase, and creatine phosphokinase muscle enzyme levels) usually confirm the diagnosis of dermatomyositis.

The diagnosis of UES narrowing is much more difficult to make. This narrowing causes progressive dysphagia with solids and large liquid boluses. Progressive UES narrowing should be suspected if there is no evidence of oropharyngeal-pharyngeal dysfunction and a prominent cricopharygeus muscle is found. This progressive narrowing can cause a posteriorly directed outpouching in the hypopharynx called a Zenker's diverticulum, which produces progressive food stasis and dysphagia (Fig. 2-5). Poor relaxation of the UES may be found but is detected in only the most severe cases. UES dilation or cricopharyngeal myotomy may improve the symptoms.

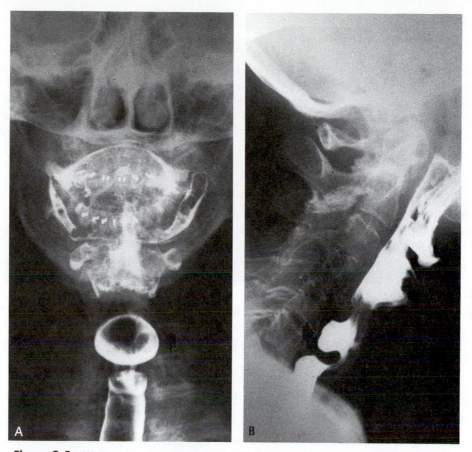

Figure 2-5. (**A**) Anterior view of barium-filled Zenker's diverticulum (*arrow*). The narrowed segment just distal is the lumen of the cricopharyngeus muscle. (**B**) Lateral view of Zenker's diverticulum (*arrow*) in the same patient. The prominent closure of the cricopharyngeus muscle (UES) is shown just distal to this diverticulum. (From Yamada T, Alpers DH, Owyang C, Powell DW, Silverstein FE, eds. Textbook of Gastroenterology, 2nd ed. Philadelphia: JB Lippincott, 1995:1168.)

ESOPHAGEAL BODY DYSFUNCTION

The major motor disorders affecting the esophageal body include achalasia, diffuse esophageal spasm, and scleroderma. Achalasia is characterized by loss of inhibitory neural input to the smooth muscle of the esophageal body and LES. The cholinergic input is still intact. Complete loss of peristasis coupled with poor relaxation of the lower esophageal sphincter is a requirement for the diagnosis. Patients present first with solid food sticking in the mid- or distal esophagus. Liquids that pass predominantly by gravity are used to push solids through. Dysphagia is usually progressive but can be slow enough so that the patient changes his or her diet to accommodate it and does not seek medical help. Weight loss and aspiration symptoms usually predict a dilated esophagus full of food and are the common presenting symptoms. Treatment includes medications such as calcium blocking agents that reduce LES pressure, forceful dilatation of the LES (to decrease basal tone), and cutting of the LES and esophageal smooth muscle surgically to allow easier food passage. A novel treatment involving injection of botulinum toxin into the

LES (to decrease cholinergic input and reduce LES pressure) has recently produced promising results.

Diffuse esophageal spasm such as achalasia shares a loss of inhibitory input to the smooth muscle esophageal body while normal LES function is retained. Chest pain is the major symptom and is caused by simultaneous contractions in the esophageal body. Dysphagia can also be seen but is a secondary phenomenon. Diffuse esophageal spasm is an uncommon cause of chest pain that mimics coronary artery disease. Treatment choices are limited to calcium blocking agents or nitrates, which reduce pressure.

Scleroderma is one of the primary collagen vascular diseases and primarily affects the skin and internal organs. The most common area of gastrointestinal involvement is the esophagus. Progressive loss of esophageal and LES smooth muscle and replacement with dense fibrous tissue produce progressive loss of esophageal body peristalsis and markedly decreased LES pressure. Symptoms include dysphagia and acid gastroesophageal reflux (heartburn and regurgitation). Since acid is not cleared adequately in a nonperistaltic poorly contracting esophagus, mucosal damage (esophagitis) is almost universal and is frequently progressive. Stricture formation, intestinal/gastric metaplasia (Barrett's esophagus), and resultant adenocarcinoma of the esophagus have been reported. Treatment to reduce acid (H_2 receptor antagonists, proton pump inhibitors) and prokinetic agents (cisapride, metoclopramide, domperidone) are commonly used but become less effective as fibrosis and dysfunction progress.

LOWER ESOPHAGEAL SPHINCTER DYSFUNCTION

The major correlate of LES dysfunction is gastroesophageal reflux. Lack of an effective esophagogastric barrier is manifested by a low LES pressure, an LES pressure easily overcome by abdominal pressure, or a sphincter that relaxes inappropriately (Fig. 2-6). Symptoms of heartburn and regurgitation are seen intermittently in everyone, but daily symptoms can be seen in up to 7% of patients. In addition to heartburn and regurgitation, noncardiac chest pain, including exercise-induced chest pain, cervical dysphagia, cough, and bronchospasm, may be seen. Esophageal inflammation including erosions, ulcers, and stricture formation are common in the acid reflux group with low LES pressure but are not common in the group with normal LES pressure despite a similar frequency of reflux episodes, degree of acid exposure, and severity of symptoms. A diagnosis is usually made clinically but can be substantiated if necessary by endoscopic examination, 24-hour pH monitoring, or both. Treatment aimed at decreasing acid production (H_2 receptor antagonists, proton pump inhibitors) or decreasing acid exposure (cisapride, metoclopramide) is usually necessary and may have to be used continuously. Surgical correction of the antireflux barrier by fundoplication (wrapping the stomach around the distal esophagus to increase LES pressure) may be necessary for long-term control in young patients or patients not responding to medical treatment. Surgical failure and long-term breakdown of the stomach wrap occur in 20% of these patients.

CLINICAL TESTING

Patients with dysphagia and chest pain should be evaluated in a systematic way to minimize cost and maximize ease of diagnosis and treatment. In most cases, a series of three or four questions allows accurate diagnosis and a focused evalua-

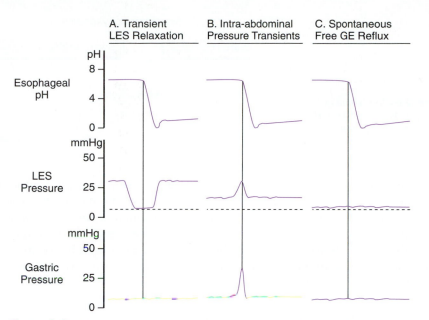

Figure 2-6. Schematic representation of three different mechanisms of gastroesophageal (GE) reflux. GE reflux events (*vertical lines*) may (**A**), accompany a transient LES relaxation; (**B**), develop as stress reflux during a transient increase in intra-abdominal pressure that overcomes LES resistance; or (**C**), occur as spontaneous free reflux across an atonic sphincter. (From Dodds WJ, Dent J, Hogan WJ, et al. Mechanisms of gastroesophageal reflux in patients with reflux esophagitis. N Engl J Med 307:1547, 1982.)

tion. The first step is to differentiate oropharyngeal dysphagia from esophageal dysphagia (Fig. 2-7). Food stopping in the throat usually means an oropharyngeal source, whereas food sticking in the chest signifies an esophageal source. Food sticking in the suprasternal notch can come from both areas, and further questioning of the patient is necessary. The timing of food sticking is also helpful. Times from swallow initiation to dysphagia longer than 2 seconds usually denote

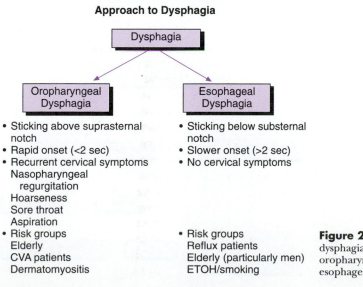

Figure 2-7. Evaluation of dysphagia: differentiate oropharyngeal dysphagia from esophageal dysphagia.

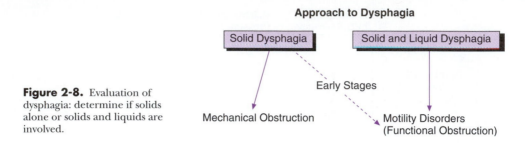

Figure 2-8. Evaluation of dysphagia: determine if solids alone or solids and liquids are involved.

esophageal dysfunction. The presence of cough, hoarseness, nasal regurgitation, or a history of significant central nervous system disease should signify an oropharyngeal source. If an oropharyngeal source is determined, a barium swallow study with multiple food forms under the direction of a speech pathologist and a radiologist is the test of choice. Specific deficits can be best appraised by barium radiography, and techniques to improve swallowing and minimize aspiration can be tested immediately. Objective re-evaluation over time is facilitated by this approach. If dysphagia is esophageal in origin, the next stage is to determine if solids alone or solids and liquids are involved (Fig. 2-8). Solid food dysphagia usually signifies a mechanical obstruction to flow, whereas solid and liquid dysphagia usually means a motility disorder. Solid food dysphagia is common, however, in the early stages of dysphagia from any cause, and therefore exclusion of a mechanical obstruction should not end the evaluation.

Intermittent solid dysphagia usually indicates either a congenital problem such as a proximal esophageal web or a distal esophageal ring or the beginning of a more serious problem (Fig. 2-9). Longstanding symptoms point to a congenital source. Progressive symptoms point to either acid reflux or cancer. Older age, lack of heartburn, and rapid weight loss often point to cancer. Longstanding reflux symptoms could mean either reflux stricture or reflux-induced adenocarcinoma arising from intestinal metaplasia in the esophagus. Endoscopic evaluation with mucosal biopsies is necessary in most if not all cases.

Solid and liquid dysphagia point to an esophageal motility disorder (Fig. 2-10). Patients with achalasia present with dysphagia (food sticking) that is progres-

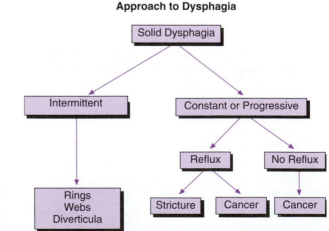

Figure 2-9. Evaluation of solid dysphagia.

Approach to Dysphagia

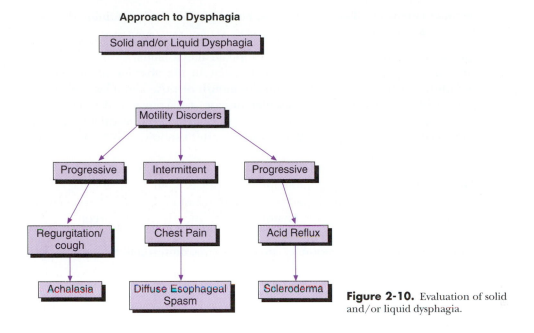

Figure 2-10. Evaluation of solid and/or liquid dysphagia.

sive, but progression can be slow. Chest pain can be present but is usually a secondary symptom. Nocturnal cough, regurgitation, or aspiration are accompanying symptoms and are consistent with retained food in the esophagus. Marked phlegm production can also be present. Diffuse esophageal spasm is primarily an intermittent painful condition with dysphagia occurring only during times of pain. Scleroderma may be accompanied by dysphagia early on, but concurrent gastroesophageal reflux is common and is usually seen at the time of initial presentation. Skin thickening with prominent subepithelial vessels, finger or toe ischemic changes, and shortness of breath are common accompanying symptoms.

CASE PRESENTATION

A 32-year-old man comes to his physician with a 4-year history of increasing difficulty with eating. After swallowing any solid food, he notes a feeling of pressure in the suprasternal notch occurring 2 to 3 seconds after swallowing. This sensation began intermittently, but in the last year it has become continuous with every meal. In addition, over the last year, the patient wakes up with "gurgling in the chest" and coughing. Both the pressure and coughing can be relieved with liquids, although liquids at times result in coughing too. The patient denies choking on food, fatigue with eating, regurgitation back through the mouth or nose, hoarseness, sore throat, weight loss, or evidence of gastrointestinal bleeding (no blood in stools or black and tarry stools). He also does not have muscle pain, muscle tenderness, a family or personal history of collagen vascular disease or cancer, and heartburn or acid regurgitation. His past medical history is completely negative. The physical examination and routine laboratory work, including a complete blood count, sedimentation rate, liver chemistries, blood glucose and creatinine determinations, are normal.

Question 1. Is this oropharyngeal or esophageal dysphagia?

Answer. Oropharyngeal dysphagia is unlikely in the absence of pharyngeal symptoms such as regurgitation into the mouth or nose and a lack of predisposing illness such as cerebrovascular disease, collagen vascular disease or neurologic complaints (fatigue with eating would suggest myasthenis gravis). The occurrence of symptoms 2 to 3 seconds after swallowing is a positive clue to esophageal dysphagia.

Question 2. Is this solid food dysphagia or solid and liquid food dysphagia?

Answer. Although the predominant symptom is solid food dysphagia, the presence of difficulty with liquids in the absence of cachexia makes mechanical causes less likely. However, anatomic verification is still required.

Based on the above symptoms, an upper gastrointestinal radiograph was done (Fig. 2-11).

Question 3. What does the x-ray film show?

Answer. Obvious dilation and abundant food particles are seen (top of figure). In addition, smooth narrowing of the distal esophagus is noted without

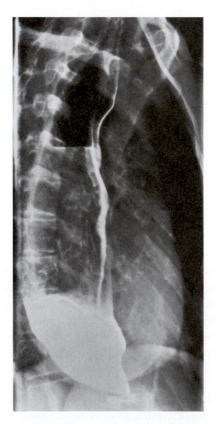

Figure 2-11. Classic radiographic features of achalasia showing a dilated esophagus, smooth tapering at the esophagogastric junction ("bird beaking"), and retained barium. (From Yamada T, Alpers DH, Owyang C, Powell DW, Silverstein FE, eds. Atlas of Gastroenterology. Philadelphia: JB Lippincott, 1992:126.)

evidence of an intraluminal mass in the esophagus or stomach. An air-fluid level is also seen.

Question 4. What would you do next?

Answer. Esophageal manometry should be the next test because it allows documentation of esophageal motility disturbance and predicts response to treatment (dilation or surgery).

Esophageal manometry was performed next and showed complete absence of peristalsis and failure of relaxation of the LES (Fig. 2-12).

Question 5. What is the diagnosis?

Answer. Achalasia is the diagnosis. The x-ray findings and the manometric

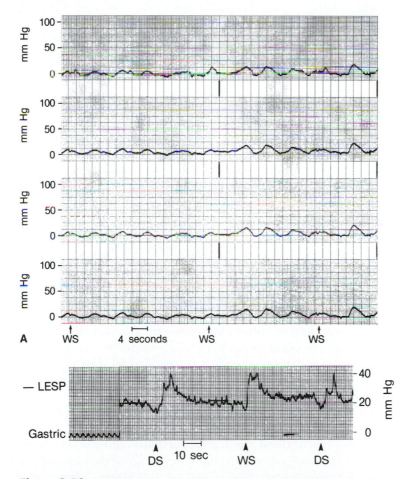

Figure 2-12. Typical manometric findings in the esophageal body (**A**) and LES (**B**) in achalasia. In the body, recording sites from the proximal to distal portion of the esophagus (*top to bottom of figure*) with spacings at 5-cm intervals reveal a total absence of peristaltic activity during a series of wet swallows (*WS*). When the esophagus is extremely dilated, no contractions will be measured and the minor changes simply result from the water bolus entering the esophagus. *LES* tracing reveals normal basal pressure (20 mmHg) with incomplete relaxation to gastric baseline after both dry (*DS*) and wet (*WS*) swallows. (From Yamada T, Alpers DH, Owyang C, Powell DW, Silverstein FE, eds. Atlas of Gastroenterology. Philadelphia: JB Lippincott, 1992:126.)

tracings are classic for achalasia. Achalasia was the first motor disorder of the esophagus to be described. Sir Thomas Willis described the first patient with achalasia and the first dilation treatment with a whalebone with a sponge at the end. Achalasia usually occurs in patients between 25 and 60 years of age, is most likely an acquired condition, and has a prevalence of 10 to 15 cases/100,000 patients. The primary deficit appears to be neurologic, with abnormalities in the brain stem, vagal nuclei, intramural ganglion cells, and distal esophageal smooth muscle. The absence of the neurotransmitter for muscle relaxation is the major factor. This neurotransmitter is noncholinergic and nonadrenergic and is purported to be vasoactive intestinal polypeptide. The role of vasoactive intestinal polypeptide loss as the cause for achalasia is supported by the fact that vasoactive intestinal polypeptide levels and vasoactive intestinal polypeptide–containing neurons are decreased in patients with achalasia when compared with normal subjects. Nitric oxide, a potent vasodilator, is also a potent smooth muscle relaxant and is decreased in distal smooth muscle in achalasia patients. Nitric oxide may be the final neurotransmitter, since it is released by vasoactive intestinal polypeptide from esophageal neurons.

The clinical features of achalasia include dysphagia, regurgitation, heartburn, and chest pain. Solid food dysphagia is the hallmark, with a variable percentage of patients having liquid dysphagia. The duration of symptoms is usually longer than 2 years at presentation but can be more rapid. A feeling of fullness and pressure in the chest is the earliest symptom, and this progresses to overflow of food and airway symptoms. Emotional stress and rapid eating often worsen symptoms of dysphagia. Symptoms of dysphagia always progress, but progression can be slow. Food retention can lead to food aversion and subsequent weight loss.

Regurgitation occurs in 60 to 90% of patients. Material brought back up is frequently recognized as nondigested food eaten several hours earlier. Eating increases regurgitation. Regurgitation can lead to pulmonary soilage with pneumonia, and aspiration is a frequent cause of death in patients with achalasia. This regurgitation can be mistaken for an eating disorder, and achalasia can mimic anorexia nervosa in young women.

Chest pain and heartburn are common secondary symptoms in achalasia. Chest pain can occur secondary to high amplitude contraction waves and mucosal irritation can be secondary to retained food or esophageal cancer. Heartburn is acid-induced, but the acid is lactic acid and comes from food fermentation and not gastroesophageal acid reflux.

Diagnosis is confirmed by radiologic examination, esophageal manometry, and endoscopic evaluation of the esophagus. A barium esophagogram usually shows loss of distal esophageal peristalsis and smooth tapering of the LES zone. Dilation occurs in the later stages. Esophageal cancer and esophageal stricture from acid reflux are the major differential diagnoses. Mucosal abnormalities or a mass favors a diagnosis of cancer whereas a longstanding history of acid reflux favors a diagnosis of stricture. Upper gastrointestinal endoscopic examination is required in all patients over the age of 40, all those who have a history suspicious for cancer (rapid onset of symptoms with a significant weight loss), and in those who do not respond to medical treatment.

Esophageal manometry is the definitive diagnostic test. Absence of peristalsis is a diagnostic requirement, and poor LES relaxation should be seen. High LES pressures are seen in 60% of patients with achalasia and are not required for the diagnosis. Patients who do not have all these features have a lower response to treatment with medication, pneumatic dilation, or surgery.

Based on the findings of x-ray studies, the patient was treated with calcium blocking agents and nitrates but did not respond favorably.

Question 6. Why were these agents chosen?
Answer. Both calcium blockers and nitrates reduce LES pressure and distal esophageal pressure, thus potentially increasing bolus clearance. These medications should be taken just before meals and at bedtime (to decrease nocturnal regurgitation). Treatment response is only about 40%, is best with oral agents compared with sublingual agents, and produces the best results with a nondilated esophagus.

Because the patient did not respond to medication, surgery or pneumatic dilation was offered.

Question 7. How do these modalities work?
Answer. Both pneumatic dilation and surgery work by markedly reducing LES pressure by forcefully disrupting LES fibers. Surgery cuts the LES and circular smooth muscle of the distal esophagus to the level of the aortic arch. Surgery is effective in 80 to 90% of patients with morbidity and mortality rates of less than 1%. Gastroesophageal reflux is the only long-term complication, and many surgeons do a loose antireflux procedure at the time of myotomy to decrease this complication.

Pneumatic dilation involves forceful balloon dilatation of the LES (Fig.

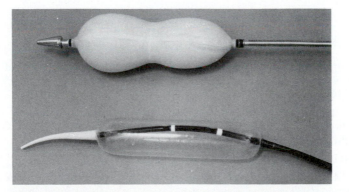

Figure 2-13. Two types of currently available pneumatic dilators for the treatment of achalasia. The Rider-Moeller balloon (*top*) is dumbbell-shaped and attached to a semirigid metal post. A flanged tip on the dilator can be passed over a guidewire. Three balloon sizes are available: 2.9, 3.8, and 4.8 cm at maximum distention. The Rigiflex dilator (*bottom*) has a cylindrical balloon and a double-lumen catheter that allows placement of the entire dilator over a guidewire. Balloons are available in 3.0-, 3.5-, and 4.0-cm sizes at maximum distention. (From Yamada T, Alpers DH, Owyang C, Powell DW, Silverstein FE, eds. Textbook of Gastroenterology. Philadelphia: JB Lippincott, 1995:1191.)

2-13). It reduces LES pressure by 50 to 70%, with the best predictor of positive response being a LES pressure after dilation of less than 10 mmHg. Pneumatic dilation is not a permanent cure in many patients and has to be repeated in up to 50% of patients. Surgery is a more permanent solution and requires repeat treatment in only 10%. If the patient does not respond to two dilation procedures, then surgery is indicated. However, if the patient does respond to initial dilation, repeat dilations are also likely to be successful and usually result in a longer symptom-free period after each subsequent dilation. Most physicians consider pneumatic dilation as first-line therapy and surgery for dilation failures. Pneumatic dilation does carry a 4 to 6% risk for esophageal perforation, but patients with perforation followed by reparative surgery do as well as patients with achalasia initially treated with surgery.

The patient chose pneumatic dilation, and two treatment sessions failed to produce a positive response. Endoscopic examination was negative for cancer; surgery was performed.

Question 8. What do you think was found at surgery?
Answer. A 3-cm intramural adenocarcinoma of the proximal stomach was found and removed. The intraluminal component was only 1 to 2 mm in size.

Cancer should always be considered in the differential diagnosis of patients with achalasia. This patient's age and duration of symptoms as well as a normal gastrointestinal x-ray and negative endoscopic findings were against this diagnosis. Esophageal and proximal gastric tumors are the most common cancers, although small cell lung cancer, lymphoma, hepatoma, and prostatic cancer can produce symptoms without esophageal involvement, presumably by a paraneoplastic mechanism.

The patient is alive and well and without recurrent cancer 7 years after surgery.

SELECTED READING

Biancani P, Behar J. Esophageal motor function. In: Yamada T, Alpers DH, Owyang C, Powell DW, Silverstein FE, eds. Textbook of Gastroenterology. Philadelphia: JB Lippincott, 1991:119.

Castell DO. Approach to the patient with dysphagia. In: Yamada T, Alpers DH, Owyang C, Powell DW, Silverstein FE, eds. Textbook of Gastroenterology. Philadelphia: JB Lippincott, 1991:562.

Castell DO, ed. The Esophagus. Boston: Little, Brown, 1992.

Gelfand DW, Richter JE, eds. Dysphagia: Diagnosis and treatment. New York: Igaku-Shoin, 1989.

Nostrant TT. Approach to the patient with chest pain. In: Yamada T, Alpers DH, Owyang C, Powell DW, Silverstein FE, eds. Textbook of Gastroenterology. Philadelphia: JB Lippincott, 1991:573.

Richter JE. Motility disorders of the esophagus. In: Yamada T, Alpers DH, Owyang C, Powell DW, Silverstein FE, eds. Textbook of Gastroenterology. Philadelphia: JB Lippincott, 1991:1083.

Lippincott's Pathophysiology Series: Gastrointestinal Pathophysiology, edited by Joseph M. Henderson. Lippincott–Raven Publishers. Philadelphia © 1996.

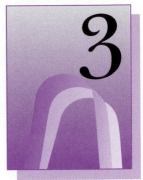

Peptic Ulcer Disease

John DelValle

Peptic ulcer disease (PUD) represents a heterogeneous group of disorders that has as a common denominator a local defect or excavation in the mucosal surface of the stomach or duodenum or both. Accounting for approximately 10% of the cost of gastrointestinal disease in the United States, PUD is a very common disorder affecting 10% of American men and 5% of American women during their lifetimes. Its pathogenesis is multifactorial, stemming from an imbalance between a series of protective (mucus, microcirculation, hormones, reconstitution, mucosal bicarbonate) and aggressive (acid, pepsin, *Helicobacter pylori*) factors. Major efforts have been aimed at elucidating the pathophysiology of PUD over the past two decades. These efforts have led to important developments in the diagnosis and therapy of this commonly encountered disorder. This chapter reviews the pathophysiologic basis of common peptic ulcer disease and Zollinger-Ellison syndrome (gastric acid hypersecretion and PUD secondary to an endocrine tumor). In addition, a brief summary of the diagnostic tests and therapeutic options related to acid peptic disorders is presented. Finally, a representative case history is examined, highlighting the important concepts outlined in the chapter.

PATHOPHYSIOLOGY

PUD is the product of an imbalance between a series of protective (mucus secretion, prostaglandins, bicarbonate secretion, blood flow, and cell renewal) and aggressive (acid, pepsin, bile acids, pancreatic enzymes, and bacteria) factors. The old dictum by Schwartz, "no acid, no ulcer," seems to hold true in most cases of duodenal ulcer disease, but this is not necessarily the case in gastric ulcer disease. Factors such as bacterial infection (with *Helicobacter pylori*), drugs (nonsteroidal anti-inflammatory drugs), cigarette smoking, heredity, and gastric emptying disorders create an imbalance between aggressive and defensive factors within the stomach and duodenum, resulting in ulcer formation. With this in mind, it is essential to review the physiologic basis for gastric mucosal protection when attempting to understand the pathophysiologic basis of acid peptic disorders.

GASTRIC MUCOSAL DEFENSE

The gastric mucosa is under continuous attack by acid and pepsin (see below). The gastric pH can fall below 2.0 for significant periods of time throughout the day. Therefore effective mechanisms for maintaining mucosal integrity in view of this noxious environment must be in place.

Recognition of the anatomic constituents within the gastric mucosa provides a basis for understanding the elements involved in both the aggressive and protective aspects of acid peptic disease. Figure 3-1 illustrates the cells that constitute an oxyntic gastric gland. From the mucosal defense standpoint, the mucus cell provides the first line of protection against aggressive factors. The surface mucus cells line the luminal surface of the stomach and secrete mucus and bicarbonate, forming a physicochemical barrier for the gastric epithelium (Fig. 3-2). This barrier is in the form of a gel containing a pH gradient that provides a neutral pH at the cell surface. The gel consists of an unstirred layer of mucus, bicarbonate, surface phospholipids, and water. It appears that many of the factors that lead to stimulation of acid and pepsin also regulate mucus and bicarbonate secretion in a parallel fashion.

Mucosal bicarbonate is essential in maintaining the pH adjacent to the surface epithelium close to neutral. The epithelial cells lining the stomach and duo-

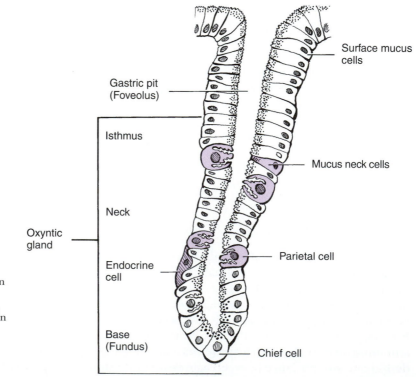

Figure 3-1. Oxyntic gastric gland. (Adapted from Ito S, Winchester, RJ. The final structure of the gastric mucosa in the bat. J Cell Biol 16:541, 1963; and from Yamada T, Alpers DH, Owyang C, Powell DW, Silverstein FE, eds. Textbook of Gastroenterology, 2nd ed. Philadelphia: JB Lippincott, 1995:297.)

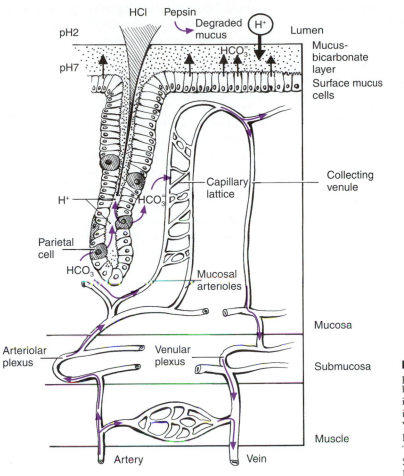

HCl   Pepsin
pH2   Degraded   H⁺   Lumen
             mucus

pH7   Mucus-
                                 bicarbonate
                                 layer
                                 Surface mucus
                                 cells

H⁺   HCO₃⁼   Capillary   Collecting
                               lattice   venule

Parietal
cell
HCO₃   Mucosal
                               arterioles
                                                  Mucosa

Arteriolar   Venular
plexus   plexus   Submucosa

                                                  Muscle

Artery   Vein

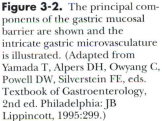

Figure 3-2. The principal components of the gastric mucosal barrier are shown and the intricate gastric microvasculature is illustrated. (Adapted from Yamada T, Alpers DH, Owyang C, Powell DW, Silverstein FE, eds. Textbook of Gastroenterology, 2nd ed. Philadelphia: JB Lippincott, 1995:299.)

denum synthesize and secrete bicarbonate. The mucosa in the proximal duodenum secretes approximately twice the amount of bicarbonate secreted in the entire stomach. Endogenous prostaglandins (see below) play an important role in maintaining basal levels of bicarbonate secretion. Of interest, patients with active duodenal ulcers have a marked decrease in proximal duodenal bicarbonate production as compared with normal subjects. The mechanism for decreased bicarbonate secretion is not clear, but recent studies suggest that *Helicobacter pylori* infection may play a role in this process.

Additional factors important in maintaining gastroduodenal mucosal integrity in response to injury include cell restitution, abundant microcirculation, and the secretion of several chemical mediators of protection, including prostaglandins and growth factors (epidermal growth factor or EGF and transforming growth factor alpha or TGFα). Both the gastric and duodenal mucosa can undergo rapid (15 to 30 minutes) *reconstitution* or *restitution* after injury. This process does not require cell division but involves movement of epithelial cells from the crypt of the gland upward along the basement membrane, eventually covering the damaged epithelium. *Prostaglandins* are present in the gastric mucosa and can be secreted by mucus, chief, and parietal cells. In addition to their antisecretory effect on parietal cells (prostaglandin E_2), prostaglandins mediate gastric protection by stimulating mucus and bicarbonate secretion, enhancing mucosal blood flow, reducing mucosal H^+ ion back-diffusion, and enhancing cell turnover.

Aggressive Factors

Gastric Acid. As mentioned earlier, the dictum by Schwartz, "no acid, no ulcer," seems to be true in most cases of peptic-related disorders. Because of this, there has been an enormous effort to understand the physiology of gastric acid secretion. Although a detailed review of the factors involved in regulating gastric acid secretion is beyond the scope of this chapter, it is important to outline a few of the fundamental pathways that orchestrate this complex secretory process.

Basal acid secretion follows a circadian pattern, with the lowest rates of secretion occurring in the morning and the highest occurring at night. It appears that cholinergic input via the vagus nerve and histaminergic input from locally released histamine are the main determinants of basal gastric acid output. The principal physiologic stimulant of acid production is food. Meal-stimulated acid secretion is typically described as occurring in three phases. These refer to the site of origin of the stimuli and include the cephalic, gastric, and intestinal phases. The principal determinants of the cephalic phase include sight, smell, and taste of food. Each of these leads to stimulation of gastric acid secretion via cholinergic input through the vagus nerve. Once food enters the stomach, the gastric phase of acid secretion is activated. Gastric distention leads to an increase in acid secretion through neural and hormonal pathways. Nutrients (amino acids and amines) directly stimulate gastrin release (see below), which in turn increases the secretory response. As nutrients enter the intestine the last phase of meal-stimulated gastric acid secretion is initiated. The principal stimulatory factors during this phase include distention and proteins and their breakdown products. The exact mediators responsible for this later phase have not been fully elucidated. As is the case with most biologic systems, there are a series of inhibitory pathways that are activated during the different phases of gastric secretion and that serve as a counterbalance for the secretory process. Reviewing each of these is beyond the scope of this chapter, but the gastrointestinal hormone somatostatin seems to be an important element in this inhibitory process.

The cell responsible for formation and secretion of gastric acid is the parietal cell (see Fig. 3-1), which is located in the gastric fundus. The three primary stimulants of acid secretion are histamine, gastrin, and acetylcholine. Various factors inhibit acid secretion, with prostaglandins and somatostatin being the most important ones. Both inhibitory and stimulatory factors regulate the gastric secretory process via specific receptors located on the parietal cell. Histamine, which is released primarily from gastric mucosal enterochromaffin cells, stimulates acid secretion via an H_2 receptor linked to cyclic adenosine monophosphate. Gastrin and acetylcholine activate specific receptors linked to the calcium/protein kinase–C pathway. After activation of their respective pathways, the hydrogen-potassium (H^+/K^+) adenosine triphosphatase (ATPase) pump is stimulated, leading to the production and extrusion of hydrogen ions. Elucidation of these fundamental physiologic concepts has led to major advances in the therapy of peptic ulcer disease. A summary of the factors important in regulating gastric acid secretion is shown in Figure 3-3.

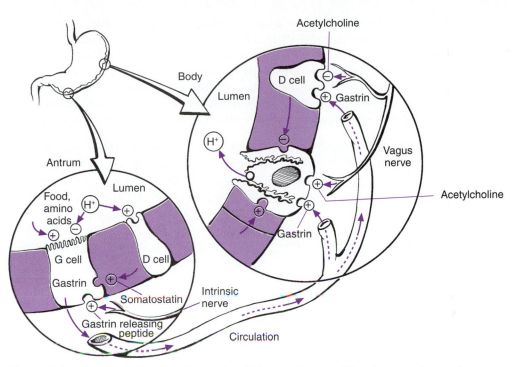

Figure 3-3. Regulation of gastric acid secretion. Major gastric mucosal ligand receptor interactions regulating parietal cell hydrochloric acid secretion are shown. D cell, somatostatin cell; G cell, gastrin cell. (Adapted from Feldman M. Acid and gastric secretion in duodenal ulcer disease. Regul Pept Lett 1:1, 1989 and Yamada T, Alpers DH, Owyang C, Powell DW, Silverstein FE, eds. Textbook of Gastroenterology, 2nd ed. Philadelphia: JB Lippincott, 1995:308.)

Basal acid secretion is normal or high normal in the majority of patients with duodenal ulcer disease. Although maximal acid secretion tends to be elevated in duodenal ulcer patients, there is a significant degree of overlap with normal individuals. A small group of ulcer disease patients have very high basal acid secretion ratio (see below).

Pepsin. Pepsinogen, the inactive precursor of the proteolytic enzyme pepsin, is produced by the chief cell, which is found primarily in the gastric fundus. The pathogenetic importance of derangements in pepsinogen secretion in peptic ulcer disease remains to be established.

Helicobacter pylori. An exciting development in the field of gastroenterology has been the recent observation that *Helicobacter pylori* infection of the stomach is related to the development of peptic ulcer disease. *H. pylori* is a gram-negative microaerophilic flagellated urease-producing rod, found to be a frequent resident of the gastric mucosa. It is sometimes found in asymptomatic healthy individuals but is much more commonly associated with active gastritis and duodenal ulcer disease (> 95%). Treatment of both gastritis and duodenal ulcers with anti-*H. pylori* regimens such as bismuth compounds and antibiotics has led to symptomatic and morphologic resolution of these entities. Although the presence of this organism is clearly associated with active gastritis and duodenal ulcer disease, the mechanism by which it contributes to PUD remains to be established. Initial studies suggest that *H. pylori* can induce mucosal damage via both direct and indirect mechanisms (Fig. 3-4). The bacteria produces urease, lipopolysaccharides, and cytotoxin, which in turn can lead to recruitment and activation of inflammatory cells. In addition, recent *in vitro* and *in vivo* studies demonstrate that patients infected with *H. pylori* may have mild hypergastrinemia associated with the local inflammatory response.

Other. Nonsteroidal anti-inflammatory drugs are important aggressive factors that frequently lead to gastroduodenal mucosal damage. The ability of these drugs to inhibit prostaglandin synthesis (an important factor for mucosal protection) predisposes the stomach and duodenum to mucosal injury. Cigarette smoking also predisposes to recurrent duodenal ulcers that are often more difficult to treat. Other factors that have been implicated in the ulcerogenic process, such as stress, diet and corticosteroids, have not been clearly proved to be causative.

CLINICAL CORRELATES

PEPTIC ULCER DISEASE

Epidemiology

Definitive data regarding the prevalence and incidence of PUD are difficult to assess. Estimates based on various studies suggest that approximately 10% of American men and 5% of American women will have PUD during their lifetimes. The overall trend in its frequency is also unsettled, but it appears that the incidence and prevalence are decreasing. Previously, PUD was found more commonly

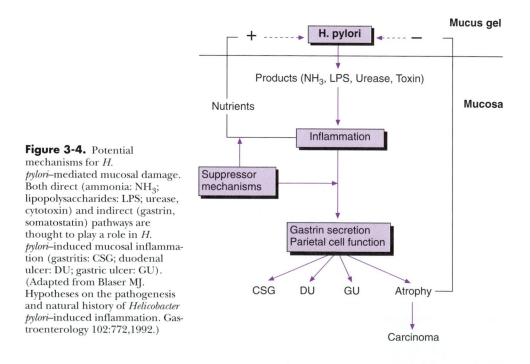

Figure 3-4. Potential mechanisms for *H. pylori*–mediated mucosal damage. Both direct (ammonia: NH$_3$; lipopolysaccharides: LPS; urease, cytotoxin) and indirect (gastrin, somatostatin) pathways are thought to play a role in *H. pylori*–induced mucosal inflammation (gastritis: CSG; duodenal ulcer: DU; gastric ulcer: GU). (Adapted from Blaser MJ. Hypotheses on the pathogenesis and natural history of *Helicobacter pylori*–induced inflammation. Gastroenterology 102:772,1992.)

in men (ratio 4:1). It now appears that a decreasing incidence in men with a stable incidence in women has changed this ratio to 2:1. Rates of hospitalization for gastric ulcer disease have not changed, whereas there has been a dramatic decrease in hospitalization for uncomplicated duodenal ulcer. The rates of ulcer complications, i.e., perforation and bleeding, have remained unchanged. Mortality related to duodenal and gastric ulcers has decreased by approximately 60 to 75% in men, with a less profound drop in mortality among women with gastric ulcers. Bleeding continues to be the most common cause of death.

Several chronic disorders have been associated with an increased incidence of PUD: of these chronic obstructive pulmonary disease, cirrhosis, and renal disease are the most commonly encountered.

Signs and Symptoms

Burning epigastric pain starting 1 to 3 hours after a meal, frequently relieved by antacids or food, is the classic symptom associated with duodenal ulcer disease. In reality, symptoms related to PUD can vary widely from the absence of symptoms to the classic symptom complex described above.

Physical examination is not helpful in establishing the presence or absence of an uncomplicated ulcer but is important in ruling out other possible sources of abdominal pain (masses, neuropathic pain, or musculoskeletal pain) and in detecting complications of peptic disease (bleeding, perforation, obstruction).

Differential Diagnosis

Dyspeptic symptoms are among the most frequent complaints that bring a patient to his or her physician. Numerous disorders can manifest with dyspepsia; thus every attempt should be made to distinguish among this extensive differential diagnosis. The diagnostic evaluation for PUD is reviewed in the Clinical Testing section (see below).

Medical Therapy

The goals of medical therapy for uncomplicated PUD include resolution of pain, induction of ulcer healing, and elimination of ulcer recurrence and complications. Specific antiulcer drug therapy should be supplemented by measures such as cessation of cigarette smoking and avoidance of nonsteroidal anti-inflammatory drugs. There is no proven benefit to dietary restrictions or manipulations.

During the last decade there has been a dramatic increase in the number of antiulcer medications available. Extensive basic science research aimed at understanding the regulation of acid secretion has led to the development of tailor-made drugs aimed at inhibiting this aggressive factor. The recent understanding of the protective elements of the stomach has led to the development of drugs aimed at enhancing gastric protection without altering acid secretion. In addition, the importance of *H. pylori* in the pathogenesis of PUD has led to the development of multiple antibiotic regimens useful for eradicating this organism.

Acid Inhibitory/Neutralizing Agents

Antacids. The first therapeutic regimen that showed ulcer healing rates higher than those achieved with placebo included antacids. Antacids act by neutralizing luminal acid. They have numerous disadvantages, including the requirement of frequent administration, production of altered bowel habits (magnesium-induced diarrhea and aluminum-induced constipation), and aluminum-induced phosphate depletion. Since the advent of H_2 antagonists, antacids have played a secondary role in the treatment of peptic disease of the stomach.

H_2 Antagonists. As mentioned earlier, there are three primary stimulants of the parietal cell: gastrin, acetylcholine, and histamine. Specific antagonists for these three secretagogues have been developed, with blockers of the histamine (H_2) receptor being the most effective ones for the treatment of PUD. H_2 blockers inhibit both basal and stimulated acid secretion. Preparations available at present include cimetidine, ranitidine, famotidine, and nizatidine. It appears that nocturnal acid secretion is of major importance in the pathogenesis of duodenal ulcers. Thus therapy has been modified from multiple daily doses to a single nocturnal dose. Approximately 80% of duodenal ulcers heal after 4 weeks of administration of H_2 blockers compared with 40% treated with placebo. Minimal side effects have been reported with these agents when used at the proper dosing schedules. The most commonly encountered problems with high-dose H_2 blockers (predominantly cimetidine) include alteration in drug metabolism due to inhibition of hepatic cytochrome P450, gynecomastia, and confusion, the last especially in older patients with liver or renal insufficiency.

Prostaglandins. Misoprostol, the prostaglandin E_1 analogue, is commercially available and is as effective as cimetidine in promoting duodenal ulcer healing. Early studies suggest that prostaglandins are superior to H_2 blockers in healing gastroduodenal inflammation related to the use of nonsteroidal anti-inflammatory drugs. Major side effects include diarrhea and uterine contraction, which can lead to the induction of abortion.

Inhibition of H^+-K^+-ATPase. As noted earlier, the enzyme responsible for the generation of hydrogen ions in the parietal cell is H^+-K^+-ATPase. Omeprazole is a substituted benzimidazole that prevents activation of this enzyme by binding to it covalently through a disulfide bond. It is the most effective inhibitor of acid secretion available at present. Pronounced hypochlorhydria produced by this agent is associated with hypergastrinemia. The clinical significance of drug-induced hypergastrinemia in humans remains to be established. Initially, this drug was reserved for treatment of patients with PUD refractory to H_2 blockers or to individuals with Zollinger-Ellison syndrome (see below), but more recently it has been approved by the Food and Drug Administration for short-term treatment of duodenal ulcers.

Anticholinergic Agents. Nonselective anticholinergic agents are of limited value in the treatment of acid peptic disease when used as single agents because of their weak acid inhibitory action and their association with significant side effects.

Nonacid Inhibitory Agents

Sucralfate. This sulfated disaccharide compound induces ulcer healing rates comparable to those obtained with H_2 blockers. The exact mechanism of action for this drug is unknown, but it appears to enhance the gastroduodenal protective barrier.

Colloidal Bismuth. Colloidal bismuth preparations induce ulcer healing rates superior to those of placebo and comparable to rates obtained with H_2 antagonists. The observed antibacterial effect of this compound on *H. pylori* may in fact lead to periods of remission that are higher than those obtained with H_2 blockers.

Antibiotics. Effective therapy against *H. pylori* requires eradication of the bacteria (absence of the organism 4 weeks after therapy). Eradication of the organism is associated with a dramatic decrease in the incidence of recurrent peptic ulcers. Standard therapy requires the combination of three agents, including metronidazole, amoxicillin or tetracycline, and a bismuth preparation for 7 to 10 days. This combination leads to an eradication rate of over 85%. The complexity of this regimen, coupled with the potential adverse effects of antibiotics (nausea, diarrhea, *Clostridium difficile* colitis), has led to interest in developing a simpler treatment plan. Other regimens being examined include high-dose omeprazole in combination with a single antibiotic (amoxicillin). Definitive studies using this new therapeutic approach are not yet available.

Surgical Therapy of Peptic Ulcer Disease

Definitive indications for surgery include gastrointestinal bleeding unresponsive to medical therapy, refractory gastric outlet obstruction, perforation, and malignancy. Other potential indications are recurrent bouts of self-limited hemorrhage, penetrating ulcer, or refractoriness to medical therapy. Surgical procedures include antral resection combined with vagotomy, truncal vagotomy with a drainage procedure (pyloroplasty), and highly selective vagotomy. All of these are aimed at decreasing the primary stimulants of acid secretion. Vagotomy decreases cholinergic drive to the stomach and reduces parietal cell sensitivity to gastrin. Antrectomy removes the principal source of gastrin. The type of operation performed is in part determined by the specific indication and the local expertise.

ZOLLINGER-ELLISON SYNDROME

Gastric acid hypersecretion and severe peptic ulcer diathesis secondary to unbridled release of gastrin from a non–β cell endocrine neoplasm (gastrinoma) constitute the Zollinger-Ellison syndrome. In addition to its stimulatory effect on gastric acid secretion, gastrin also has a well-established trophic effect on gastrointestinal tissues. Gastrin increases protein and DNA synthesis and total DNA content of gastric mucosa and other tissues. In Zollinger-Ellison syndrome, the hypergastrinemia that results from the release of peptide from an endocrine neoplasm free of the usual regulatory restraints has two synergistic effects: (1) overstimulation of gastric parietal cells to secrete acid, and (2) increased mass of parietal cells susceptible to overstimulation. The potentiated gastric acid hypersecretion that results is presumably the cause of the clinical manifestations (i.e., acid peptic disease and diarrhea) of the gastrinoma syndrome.

Clinical Manifestations

Symptoms and signs in patients with Zollinger-Ellison syndrome are primarily related to gastric acid hypersecretion and its consequences. More than 90% of gastrinoma patients develop ulcers in the upper gastrointestinal tract at some point during their disease. Presenting ulcer symptoms are indistinguishable from those associated with benign PUD but frequently are less responsive to standard therapy. As in benign PUD, ulcers in Zollinger-Ellison syndrome patients occur most often in the first portion of the duodenum (75%) and are usually solitary. However, ulcers in gastrinoma patients may also occur in the second, third, and fourth portions of the duodenum (14%) and in the jejunum (11%). PUD refractory to standard medical therapy, recurrent ulcers after prior gastric surgery, diarrhea in patients with ulcers, or peptic disease occurring with complications such as obstruction, perforation, or bleeding should lead to the suspicion of Zollinger-Ellison syndrome. Esophageal symptoms caused by acid reflux are seen in as many as two thirds of patients with Zollinger-Ellison syndrome.

Aside from peptic ulcers, the other common feature of Zollinger-Ellison syndrome is diarrhea. Diarrhea can be present in over half the patients with gastrinoma and can occur in the absence of peptic ulcer symptoms. Diarrhea may also precede the diagnosis of Zollinger-Ellison syndrome by many years. The pathogenesis of diarrhea is felt to be multifactorial, but its dependence on acid hypersecretion is demonstrated by amelioration of symptoms upon continuous nasogastric suction or inhibition of acid secretion. Thus, the severe volume load represented by the acid, which can be secreted at the rate of several liters per day, can account for some of the diarrhea. An added feature of the diarrhea is steatorrhea and maldigestion, which result from the inactivity of pancreatic enzymes at the low pH of the duodenum caused by the excessive acid load. The acidic pH of the small bowel may also lead to damage of the intestinal mucosa, resulting in a sprue-like state with flattened intestinal villi and accompanying malabsorption. Bile acids are poorly soluble in an acid milieu; thus Zollinger-Ellison syndrome may result in decrease micelle formation and subsequent malabsorption of vitamin B_{12} and other lipid-soluble nutrients and vitamins. It is possible that in the presence of markedly high serum gastrin levels, gastrin itself may increase secretion of potassium and reduce absorption of sodium and water by the small intestine, thus potentially leading to a secretory diarrhea. Secretory diarrhea may also occur in Zollinger-Ellison syndrome in association with the secretion of another hormone besides gastrin, such as vasoactive intestinal polypeptide.

Twenty-five percent of gastrinoma patients have multiple endocrine neoplasia type I (MEN I) syndrome. The primary sites of organ involvement in this autosomal dominant genetic disorder include the parathyroid, pancreas, pituitary, and less commonly, the adrenal cortex and thyroid. The consequences of Zollinger-Ellison syndrome (ulcer complications, gastric or pancreatic surgery) account for the major morbidity and mortality related to MEN I.

Hyperparathyroidism and its associated hypercalcemia have a direct bearing on the gastric acid hypersecretory state found in patients with Zollinger-Ellison syndrome and MEN I. Intravenous infusion of calcium in healthy human volunteers induces gastric acid hypersecretion. In addition, calcium has been shown both *in vivo* and *in vitro* to stimulate gastrin release directly from gastrinomas. Indeed, previous reports have demonstrated that resolution of hypercalcemia by parathyroidectomy reduces basal acid output and fasting serum gastrin concentrations in gastrinoma patients with MEN I. Thus, resolution of hypercalcemia may play an important role in the therapy of this subgroup of gastrinoma patients.

Tumor Distribution

Although initial studies observed that the majority of gastrinomas occur within the pancreas, modern diagnostic tools coupled with aggressive surgical intervention have revealed that a large number are extrapancreatic and extraintestinal. More than 80% of gastrinomas have been localized in the anatomic area known as the gastrinoma triangle. The boundaries of this triangle include the confluence of the cystic and common bile ducts superiorly, the junction of the second and third portions of the duodenum inferiorly, and the junction of the neck and body of the pancreas medially. The most common extrapancreatic site is the duodenum, where up to 40% of gastrinomas arise.

Differential Diagnosis

The hallmark of Zollinger-Ellison syndrome is the presence of circulating hypergastrinemia. The various clinical circumstances in which a serum gastrin reading should be obtained because of a suspected gastrinoma are outlined in Table 3-1. Fasting serum gastrin levels in normal subjects and in patients with routine PUD are usually less than 150 pg/ml. The degree of hypergastrinemia in patients with Zollinger-Ellison syndrome varies greatly. Elevated serum gastrin levels are seen in a number of other clinical conditions as well (Table 3-2). The most common cause of hypergastrinemia is gastric atrophy. Gastric acid is the primary inhibitor of gastrin release; therefore its absence leads to uninhibited secretion of the hormone with concomitant hyperplasia of antral G cells and hypergastrinemia, as observed in pernicious anemia. Up to 75% of patients with pernicious anemia have substantial hypergastrinemia. The gastrin levels in these patients can approximate those found in gastrinoma patients, reaching values higher than 1000 pg/ml. Chronic atrophic gastritis and gastric carcinoma are two other conditions associated with hypo- or achlorhydria and hypergastrinemia.

Therapy

There are two objectives in the therapy of patients with Zollinger-Ellison syndrome: control of gastric acid hypersecretion and treatment of the malignant neoplasm. The emphasis placed upon each of these objectives has shifted over the past three decades. Initially, total gastrectomy appeared to be the only option for effective treatment of the potentially lethal ulcer disease, and less attention was directed at tumor excision because many of the patients died from ulcer complications long before their tumors became problematic. The availability of highly effective antisecretory therapy such as H_2 blockers and H^+,K^+-ATPase antagonists has led to a significant reduction in mortality related to the complication of acid peptic disease. Under these circumstances, it has become increasingly apparent that the major cause of morbidity and mortality in Zollinger-Ellison syndrome is widespread

---

TABLE 3-1. *WHEN TO OBTAIN A SERUM GASTRIN DETERMINATION IN PATIENTS WITH PEPTIC ULCER*

Multiple ulcers
Ulcers in unusual locations
Ulcers associated with severe esophagitis
Ulcers resistant to therapy with frequent recurrences
Ulcer patients awaiting surgery
Extensive family history for PUD
Postoperative ulcer recurrence
Basal hyperchlorhydria
Unexplained diarrhea or steatorrhea
Hypercalcemia
Family history of pancreatic islet, pituitary, or parathyroid tumor
Prominent gastric or duodenal folds

TABLE 3-2. *HYPERGASTRINEMIA: DIFFERENTIAL DIAGNOSIS*

Hypochlorhydria or achlorhydria with or without pernicious anemia

Retained gastric antrum

G cell hyperplasia

Renal insufficiency

Massive small bowel resection

Gastric outlet obstruction

Others: rheumatoid arthritis, vitiligo, diabetes, pheochromocytoma

---

metastatic disease. Thus early tumor detection and excision have assumed primary importance (see the later section on clinical testing).

Medical Therapy. The primary aim of medical therapy in Zollinger-Ellison syndrome is control of gastric acid hypersecretion. The development of histamine (H_2) receptor antagonists was a major breakthrough in achieving this goal. Cimetidine, the first of these agents, proved to be very efficacious in controlling acid hypersecretion and prompted ulcer healing and symptom improvement in over 80% of Zollinger-Ellison syndrome patients treated on a short-term basis. However, over a longer term, these patients often required progressive increases in the frequency and dose of medication. To correct this problem, anticholinergic agents were used as adjunctive therapy, but significant adverse effects were noted. H_2 receptor antagonists with greater potency and duration of action, such as ranitidine and famotidine, have since been developed and have proved efficacious in relieving symptoms and promoting ulcer healing in gastrinoma patients.

An important new class of drugs made available for the treatment of Zollinger-Ellison syndrome is the substituted benzimidazoles, of which omeprazole is the first. As mentioned earlier, these compounds are the most potent acid inhibitory agents because they covalently bind to H^+,K^+-ATPase, the enzyme responsible for the generation of H^+ in the parietal cell. Their efficacy in inhibiting acid secretion, relieving dyspeptic symptoms, and promoting ulcer healing in gastrinoma patients has been established. Their marked potency, prolonged duration of action, and safety profile make substituted benzimidazoles the treatment of choice for peptic disease in Zollinger-Ellison syndrome patients.

Somatostatin is a known peptide inhibitor of gastric acid secretion and gastrin release. The biochemically stable analogue of somatostatin, octreotide, has been utilized with varying success in gastrinoma patients; thus it is rarely used as a first-line agent in the treatment of Zollinger-Ellison syndrome.

Surgical Therapy. Prior to the advent of potent antisecretory agents, total gastrectomy was the treatment of choice in Zollinger-Ellison syndrome. Nevertheless, the new gastric antisecretory agents have obviated the need for total gastrectomy, and at present this procedure should be considered only in the rare patient with nonresectable gastrinoma in whom aggressive medical therapy has failed or in those individuals who cannot take oral medications.

Clearly, the appropriate surgical approach for therapy of Zollinger-Ellison syndrome today is curative resection of neoplasm. Although initial series reported less than 10% chance of total cure following tumor resection, present data indicate that this may be possible in as many as 30% of the cases. Improved diagnostic capabilities have led not only to a reduction in unnecessary surgery in patients with metastatic disease but also to the identification of extrapancreatic neoplasms with increasing frequency.

Operative management of Zollinger-Ellison syndrome should be undertaken by a surgeon with expertise in the treatment of islet cell tumors. Careful and detailed mobilization and exploration of the entire pancreas and surrounding areas should be performed. Meticulous evaluation of the duodenal mucosa by either duodenotomy or intraoperative endoscopic transillumination is essential. Any tumors that are found in the region of the pancreatic head should be enucleated, and tumors located elsewhere should be resected with great care.

Gastrinoma patients with MEN I represent a particularly difficult problem for the surgeon. Because of the multicentric nature and extrapancreatic location of tumors in MEN I syndrome, curative resection is virtually impossible. Although this is a controversial area, many would argue that the diagnosis of MEN I syndrome precludes surgical exploration unless a single resectable lesion can be identified. Some advocate an aggressive approach whereby all patients without evidence of hepatic metastasis are surgically explored, with removal of all duodenal lesions found by duodenotomy, enucleation of all tumors found in the head of the pancreas, and distal pancreatectomy. The rationale for this approach is to effect a potential cure and, failing that, to prevent the development of future pancreatic neoplasms. The long-term benefit of such an aggressive approach remains to be established.

Therapy of Metastatic Gastrinoma. Although major advances have been made in the diagnosis and medical and surgical treatment of Zollinger-Ellison syndrome, an effective approach to the management of patients with metastatic disease has yet to be developed. Metastatic disease occurs in 25 to 40% of patients with gastrinoma and at present is the most common source of morbidity and mortality in this disease. Antineoplastic chemotherapy has been of limited usefulness in Zollinger-Ellison syndrome and the question as to when to treat patients having metastatic gastrinoma with chemotherapy remains unanswered. Although an occasional patient with metastatic disease may survive up to 20 years, it appears that the majority die within 5 years.

CLINICAL TESTING

TESTING IN PEPTIC ULCER DISEASE

Laboratory Studies

Although routine laboratory studies are of limited value in the evaluation of a PUD patient, one should obtain a complete blood count and serum calcium and serum creatinine determinations to exclude blood loss, hypercalcemia, or renal insufficiency. Specialized laboratory studies are helpful in a subgroup of patients in whom peptic disease related to a hypersecretory state is suspected (see below). The specialized studies include serum fasting gastrin level, provocative gastrin testing (secretin stimulation, meal stimulation), serum pepsinogen I levels, and gastric acid secretory studies.

In view of the importance of *H. pylori* in the pathogenesis and treatment of peptic ulcer disease, it is essential to be cognizant of the methods employed to establish its presence in patients with PUD. The methods utilized for diagnosing *H. pylori* can be divided into those requiring tissue samples obtained via endoscopy (invasive) and those that do not require this procedure (noninvasive). These are briefly summarized in Table 3-3. At present, the gold standard for diagnosing *H. pylori* is histologic examination of antral mucosal biopsies. A rapid slide test that capitalizes on the ability of this organism to produce urease is very sensitive and specific but requires an antral mucosal biopsy. More recently, noninvasive tests such as *H. pylori* serology and the urea breath test (^{13}C, ^{14}C) are showing considerable promise.

Ulcer Visualization

Radiographic Evaluation. Barium studies of the upper gastrointestinal tract can be utilized for the detection of gastric and duodenal ulcers (Fig. 3-5). Barium found within a round ulcer crater surrounded by edematous folds of mucosa constitutes the classic radiographic finding of gastric and duodenal ulcers. Utilization of double-contrast barium in addition to abdominal compression and multiple spot films can lead to detection of 80 to 90% of ulcers. A scarred bulb and postoperative changes make the diagnosis more difficult, as does the presence of lesions smaller than 0.5 cm. Radiographic studies continue to be especially useful in the identification of infiltrative disorders and extrinsic compression of the gastroduodenal area.

Endoscopy. The advent of fiberoptic endoscopy has facilitated the direct visualization of gastric and duodenal peptic lesions (Fig. 3-6). This procedure allows detection of small ulcers, diffuse erosive mucosal changes, evaluation of anatomically altered areas (scarred pylorus), and allows one to biopsy and brush abnormal lesions when this is clinically indicated. Experienced endoscopists detect approximately 90% of gastroduodenal lesions, with a specificity in excess of 90%.

TABLE 3-3.   *METHOD OF DIAGNOSIS:* **HELICOBACTER PYLORI**

Invasive (endoscopic biopsy required)
A. Rapid diagnosis
    1. Gram's stain of biopsy touch preparation
    2. Urease test (broth, gel [CLOtest])
B. Delayed diagnosis
    1. Histologic study (stains: Giemsa, Warthin-Starry silver, hemotoxylin and eosin, acridine orange, Gimenez; immunohistochemical arrays)
    2. Bacterial culture

Noninvasive
A. Urea breath test (^{13}C or ^{14}C)
B. Serologic testing for antibioties to *Helicobacter pylori*
    1. Enzyme-linked immunosorbent array (ELISA)
       a. Vs. pooled whole extracts of *Helicobacter pylori*
       b. Vs. high-molecular-weight cell-associated protein (urease)
    2. Other tests (immunoblot, complement fixation, passive hemagglutination)

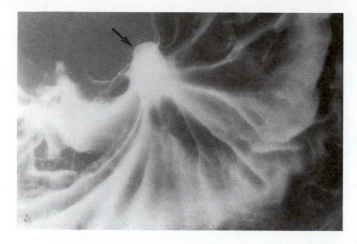

Figure 3-5. Upper gastrointestinal barium study of a benign lesser curvature gastric ulcer. There is a well-demarcated ulcer crater with smooth radiating folds and no mass effect. (From Yamada T, Alpers DH, Owyang C, Powell DW, Silverstein FE, eds. Atlas of Gastroenterology. Philadelphia: JB Lippincott, 1992:480.)

TESTING IN ZOLLINGER-ELLISON SYNDROME

Provocative Testing

To differentiate among the many causes of hypergastrinemia, a variety of provocative tests have been developed (Table 3-4). The secretin test has proved to be the easiest and most reliable study to perform. The mechanism by which secretin stimulates release of gastrin from this endocrine neoplasm involves direct activation of a secretin receptor expressed on gastrinoma cells. This receptor has not been found on antral G cells. Secretin is infused by intravenous bolus and serum for gastrin measurement is obtained 10 minutes and 1 minute before, and at 2, 5, 10, 15, 20, and 30 minutes after secretin injection. Over 90% of gastrinoma patients exhibit a rise in serum gastrin levels within 15 minutes of secretin administration. An increase in gastrin of 200 pg/ml or more constitutes a positive test.

The less commonly employed provocative test is the calcium infusion study. Calcium directly stimulates gastrin release from these tumor cells. Calcium gluconate is administered intravenously for 3 hours with simultaneous measurement

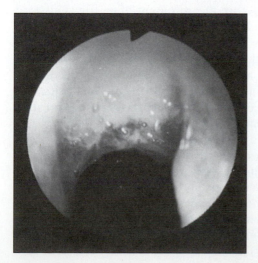

Figure 3-6. Benign gastric ulcer at the angle. The margin is smooth, and there is no evidence of surrounding mucosal discoloration or nodularity. Multiple four-quadrant biopsies are indicated to rule out tumor. (From Yamada T, Alpers DH, Owyang C, Powell DW, Silverstein FE, eds. Atlas of Gastroenterology. Philadelphia: JB Lippincott, 1992:443.)

TABLE 3-4. *GASTRIN PROVOCATIVE TESTING*

DISORDER	CALCIUM INFUSION	SECRETIN INJECTION	TEST MEAL
Gastrinoma	Increase serum gastrin by more than 400 pg/ml	Increase is usually greater than 200 pg/ml	Increase is less than 50%
Antral G cell hyperfunction	May or may not have increase in serum gastrin greater than 400 pg/ml	Decrease, no change, or slight increase in serum gastrin	Increase by more than 200%
Common duodenal ulcer	Small increase in serum gastrin	Increase is less than 200 pg/ml	Moderate increase in serum gastrin

of serum gastrin levels at 30-minute intervals. Over 80% of gastrinoma patients demonstrate an increase in gastrin levels of more than 400 pg/ml during the third hour of calcium infusion. This study is less sensitive and specific than secretin stimulation for identifying patients with Zollinger-Ellison syndrome. The lack of specificity, diminished sensitivity, and the potential adverse effects of administering intravenous calcium have made this provocative test less useful than the secretin test in diagnosing Zollinger-Ellison syndrome. It is usually reserved for patients with a negative secretin test in the presence of gastric acid hypersecretion and a strong clinical suspicion of gastrinoma.

Standard meal studies have been employed to distinguish hypergastrinemia of gastric origin (as in G cell hyperplasia/hyperfunction) from that of pancreatic origin (gastrinoma). In this study the gastric G cells release gastrin in response to a physiologic stimulus (nutrients), whereas the gastrinoma cells are not affected by meal ingestion.

Acid Secretory Studies

As reviewed earlier, hypergastrinemia can be either primary, in which case gastric acid output is elevated, or secondary to hypo- or achlorhydria, in which case acid secretion is reduced or absent. Therefore measurement of gastric acid secretion plays an important role in distinguishing between these possibilities. Gastric acid secretion is measured by analyzing volume and H^+ ion output in gastric contents obtained via a nasogastric tube. Both basal and stimulated (pentagastrin, synthetic gastrin analogue) secretion can be assessed in this manner. The net effect of hypergastrinemia is increased gastric acid secretion. Thus it is not surprising that basal acid output of 15 mEq/hr (normal <5 mEq/hr) or greater is found in as many as 90% of patients with gastrinoma. It is important to note, however, that 12% of patients with common duodenal ulcer disease can manifest similar levels of acid secretion. To enhance the sensitivity of gastric secretory studies, maximal acid output values may also be measured. Since gastrinoma patients are presumed to have near maximal secretion of gastric acid even under basal conditions, the acid secretory response to exogenously administered secretagogue (pentagastrin) is diminished. Accordingly, basal acid output-maximal acid output ratio of greater than 0.6 is highly suggestive of Zollinger-Ellison syndrome, although a ratio of less than 0.6 does not exclude the diagnosis.

Tumor Localization in Zollinger-Ellison Syndrome

Gastrinomas are notoriously difficult to localize. The tumor is not found in approximately 30 to 50% of Zollinger-Ellison syndrome patients who eventually undergo surgery, and more than 20% are found to have metastatic disease at surgery. The availability of potent antisecretory drugs has significantly decreased the morbidity and mortality associated with uncontrollable acid hypersecretion. Thus emergency or urgent total gastrectomy is rarely if ever needed. However, recent studies indicate that the tumor itself, rather than the acid hypersecretion, is responsible for the majority of the adverse sequelae associated with Zollinger-Ellison syndrome. Early intervention with resection of a localized tumor presents the only opportunity to cure this disease. In addition, detection of metastatic disease prevents unnecessary surgery. Accordingly, every effort should be made to localize the tumor preoperatively. A diagnostic plan for localizing gastrinomas in Zollinger-Ellison patients is depicted in Figure 3-7.

The approach to patients with gastrinomas as part of the MEN I syndrome differs from that taken in individuals with sporadic gastrinoma. Once a secretory endocrine tumor is diagnosed, MEN I patients should be evaluated carefully for the presence of other endocrinopathies. A thorough medical and family history

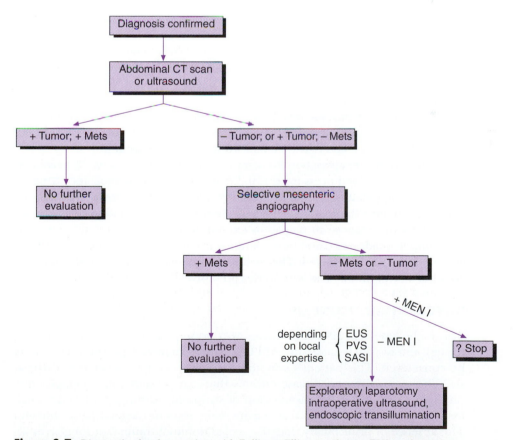

Figure 3-7. Diagnostic plan for a patient with Zollinger-Ellison syndrome. EUS: endoscopic ultrasound; PVS: portal venous sampling; SASI: selective arterial injection of secretin. (Adapted from Yamada T, Alpers DH, Owyang C, Powell DW, Silverstein FE, eds. Textbook of Gastroenterology, 2nd ed. Philadelphia: JB Lippincott, 1995:1436.)

must be obtained. MEN I is an autosomal dominant disorder with a high degree of penetrance. Offspring of these patients have an approximately 50% of developing this disorder by 20 years of age; thus genetic counseling and screening of family members are mandatory.

CASE PRESENTATION

A 39-year-old male comes to your office complaining of burning epigastric pain of 4 months' duration.

The patient was in his usual state of good health until approximately 6 months ago, when he noticed burning discomfort in the epigastric region. The pain occurred two to three times per week and 1 to 2 hours after meals. The discomfort lasted approximately 30 to 60 minutes and occasionally radiated to his right upper abdominal quadrant. The pain was somewhat relieved by intake of food. The patient denied having nausea, vomiting, melena, or blood per rectum. He was seen by his family physician, who prescribed two antacid tablets four times per day. He noted improvement in his symptoms and stopped taking antacids after 3 weeks of therapy. He remained asymptomatic until 1 month ago, when he again noted recurrent epigastric pain. The discomfort was lessened but not completely relieved by antacids. He now reports that the pain occurs daily, at times awakens him from sleep, and is associated with nausea. He does not have fever, chills, vomiting, melena, hematemesis, hematochezia, or weight loss. He smokes one to two packs of cigarettes per day and drinks one to two beers per week. He does not use nonsteroidal anti-inflammatory drugs.

The patient's past medical history is noncontributory, and he is not taking any medications. The family medical history is significant for PUD in his father. He is single, heterosexual, and works as an accountant.

On physical examination his temperature is 37°F, pulse is 72 beats per minute, and his blood pressure is 110/70 mmHg without orthostatic changes. His general appearance is that of a healthy male in mild distress. Head, neck, heart, and lungs examination is normal. Abdominal examination reveals mild tenderness in response to palpation extending from the epigastrium to the right upper quadrant. Good bowel sounds are heard, and no masses or hepatosplenomegaly is detected. The rectal examination reveals brown stool negative for occult blood. The extremities are normal.

DIFFERENTIAL DIAGNOSIS

This is the case of a 39-year-old male who presents with abdominal pain. Although the history is suggestive of PUD, other diagnostic possibilities should be considered. This patient's symptom complex can be classified as dyspepsia. The most common disease entities that can present with dyspepsia are outlined in Table 3-5. The association of symptoms with meal intake and the lack of association with physical activity make musculoskeletal pain unlikely. The absence of prior biliary tract disease, abdominal trauma, or long-term alcohol use in combination with the location and nature of the pain make pancreatic and biliary pain less likely. Pain from pancreatitis is persistent, severe, and frequently radiates to the back. Biliary-type pain is colicky in nature and

---

TABLE 3-5.	*DIFFERENTIAL DIAGNOSIS OF DYSPEPSIA*

Duodenal ulcer

Gastric ulcer

Gastritis, duodenitis

Drug-induced dyspepsia

Nonulcer dyspepsia

Reflux esophagitis

Gastroduodenal neoplasm

Gastroduodenal Crohn's disease

Biliary tract disease

Pancreatic disease

Musculoskeletal disorders

---

is usually localized to the right upper abdominal quadrant. The patient does not have diarrhea, nausea, vomiting, or weight loss, making gastroduodenal Crohn's disease less likely. His relatively young age and lack of constitutional signs and symptoms are not typical of gastroduodenal neoplasms. The lack of pyrosis, chest pain, and hoarse voice goes somewhat against but does not exclude esophageal reflux. His age, symptom complex, and history of cigarette smoking may be consistent with duodenal or gastric ulcers, gastritis, duodenitis, and nonulcer dyspepsia. The physical examination does not reveal overt evidence of an ulcer complication such as bleeding, perforation, or gastric outlet obstruction.

DIAGNOSTIC PLAN

In an effort to determine whether the patient's signs and symptoms are evidence of pancreatic-biliary tract disease or whether there is evidence of slow blood loss from an ulcer, a complete blood count and a liver chemistry profile including total bilirubin and alkaline phosphatase, amylase, and lipase levels were obtained. The findings were all within normal limits.

In view of the persistent symptoms, the patient underwent an upper endoscopic examination to rule out gastroduodenal disease. The results of the upper endoscopic study are shown in Figure 3-8. A 0.5-cm ulcer was noted in the duodenal bulb. The base of the ulcer is clean, and the margins are sharp. Antral biopsies were taken for a urease rapid slide test and histologic analysis. The slide test was negative, and the results of hematoxylin and eosin and silver staining are shown in Figure 3-9. Seen best in the silver-stained material are the small curved rods, which represent *H. pylori*.

TREATMENT PLAN

The patient returns to your office after completing these studies for your recommendations.

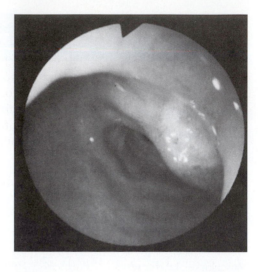

Figure 3-8. Endoscopic view of a duodenal bulb ulcer. The ulcer has a clean base with smooth margins indicative of a benign ulcer. (From Yamada T, Alpers DH, Owyang C, Powell DW, Silverstein FE, eds. Textbook of Gastroenterology, 2nd ed. Philadelphia: JB Lippincott, 1995:448.)

The initial approach must include cessation of cigarette smoking, since smoking has been shown to render ulcers refractory to medical therapy. Although the likelihood of healing this ulcer with standard H_2 blockers alone is over 80% in 8 weeks, the probability of recurrence within 1 year (in view of the infection with *H. pylori*) is virtually 100%. With this in mind, you recommend a 2-week course of metronidazole, amoxicillin, and bismuth subsalicylate. In addition, you recommend ranitidine for 4 weeks.

The patient returns for a follow-up visit in 8 weeks feeling dramatically improved. He has completed his treatment and stopped smoking.

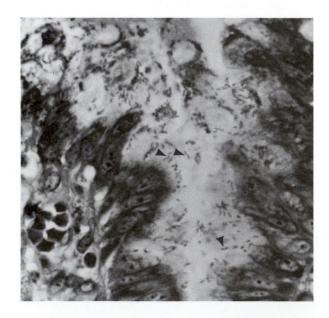

Figure 3-9. Histologic appearance of *H. pylori* in an antral biopsy specimen. Examination of the surface foveolar epithelium at high power microscopy discloses numerous curved bacilli that are *Helicobacter pylori* (arrowheads). (From Yamada T, Alpers DH, Owyang C, Powell DW, Silverstein FE, eds. Atlas of Gastroenterology. Philadelphia: JB Lippincott, 1992:595.)

SUMMARY

In summary, PUD is the product of an imbalance between a series of protective and aggressive factors in the stomach and duodenum. By understanding the factors important in protecting the gastroduodenal mucosa, insight regarding the pathogenesis of PUD can be gained. Inroads into the therapy of this common disorder have been achieved by understanding the factors involved in regulating gastric acid secretion. In addition, the identification of *H. pylori* as an important factor in the pathogenesis of PUD has revolutionalized the manner in which we approach this common disorder.

Acknowledgments. I am grateful to Carolyn Pivirotto and Marcia Barrett for typing this manuscript.

SELECTED READING

Blaser MJ. Hypotheses on the pathogenesis and natural history of *Helicobacter pyrlori*-induced inflammation. Gastroenterology 102:720, 1992.

Debas HT, Orloff SL. Surgery for peptic ulcer disease. In: Yamada T, Alpers DH, Owyang C, Powell DW, Silverstein FE, eds. Atlas of Gastroenterology. Philadelphia: JB Lippincott, 1992:176–182.

DelValle J, Lucey MR, Yamada T. Gastric secretion. In: Yamada T, Alpers DH, Owyang C, Powell DW, Silverstein FE, eds. Textbook of Gastroenterology, 2nd ed. Philadelphia: JB Lippincott, vol 2, 1995.

DelValle J, Yamada T. Zollinger-Ellison syndrome. In: Yamada T, Alpers DH, Owyang C, Powell DW, Silverstein FE, eds. Textbook of Gastroenterology, 2nd ed. Philadelphia: JB Lippincott, vol 2, 1995:1340–1352.

Isenberg JI, McQuaid KR, Laine L, Rubin W. Acid-peptic disorders. In: Yamada T, Alpers DH, Owyang C, Powell DW, Silverstein FE, eds. Textbook of Gastroenterology. Philadelphia: JB Lippincott, vol. 1, 1991:1241–1339.

Lippincott's Pathophysiology Series: Gastrointestinal Pathophysiology, edited by Joseph M. Henderson. Lippincott–Raven Publishers. Philadelphia © 1996.

The Pathophysiology of Nausea and Vomiting

William D. Chey

The sensation of nausea and the act of vomiting represent nonspecific responses to complex interactions between central and peripheral sites. A wide variety of conditions, both physiologic and pathologic, can lead to nausea and vomiting. These responses ideally serve a physiologic purpose, that is, to protect the body from ingested substances that are potentially harmful. However, pathologic nausea and vomiting that are unrelated to this purpose also occur. In this chapter we discuss terminology, pathophysiology, the act of vomiting and its consequences, a number of clinical scenarios, and clinical testing as they pertain to nausea and vomiting.

TERMINOLOGY

A clear understanding of pertinent terminology is important. *Nausea* is the unpleasant, painless, subjective feeling that one will imminently vomit. Nausea is sometimes associated with *anorexia,* which refers to the absence of the urge to eat. Anorexia should not be confused with *sitophobia* or the fear of eating because of associated or consequent pain. Sitophobia is classically seen in conjunction with disorders such as gastric ulcer or intestinal ischemia. *Vomiting* refers to the forceful expulsion of gastric contents through the mouth. As discussed in the following chapter, vomiting is the culmination of a characteristic set of physiologic actions involving the somatic and autonomic nervous systems, the oropharynx, the gastrointestinal tract, and the skeletal muscles of the thorax and abdomen. Vomiting should be differentiated from *retching* and *regurgitation*. Retching refers to the labored, rhythmic respiratory activity and abdominal musculature contractions that often but not always precede vomiting. Retching, also known as the "dry heaves," does not lead to the oral expulsion of gastric contents. Regurgitation refers to the bringing up of food into the mouth in the absence of the characteristic motor and autonomic changes seen with vomiting. Regurgitation is commonly seen in conjunction with free gastroesophageal reflux or in the presence of a mechanical (benign or malignant) or functional (achalasia) esophageal narrowing. *Rumination* refers to repeated, involuntary postprandial regurgitation of recently ingested food. The food is expectorated or chewed and reswallowed. This cycle can recur repeatedly for up to an hour after a meal. It typically ceases when food begins to take on an acid taste.

PATHOPHYSIOLOGY

The pathophysiology of vomiting was elegantly studied by Borison and Wang in 1953. Utilizing ablative techniques as well as electrical stimulation in cats, they identified two sites in the brain stem that are important in the generation of the emetic response. One site served to receive emetogenic information, whereas the other initiated the motor aspects of the emetic response. They proposed a "vomiting center" that was localized to the dorsal aspect of the lateral reticular formation in the medulla. Electrical stimulation of this area led to the initiation of vomiting. This vomiting center was not directly stimulated by humoral substances. Rather, the vomiting center coordinated input from other neural structures to produce a preprogrammed emetic response.

The second site they found to be important in the emetic response was the area postrema or so-called "chemoreceptor trigger zone" (CTZ) located in the floor of the fourth ventricle of the brain. Anatomically, the CTZ was located outside of the blood-brain barrier. Unlike the vomiting center, the CTZ was directly stimulated by circulating humoral factors and not responsive to electrical stimulation. The CTZ did not independently initiate emesis but acted through stimulation of the vomiting center. This observation was made utilizing the opiate and dopamine agonist apomorphine, which reliably induced emesis in animals. The emetic response was nearly eliminated by ablation of the area postrema or the vomiting center, suggesting that both of these areas are necessary for the initiation of vomiting in response to apomorphine. However, in the absence of an intact CTZ, apomorphine did not induce emesis. This suggested that apomorphine acted on the CTZ, which relayed information to the vomiting center to induce the emetic response.

The vagus and splanchnic nerves, which provide afferent innervation (to the central nervous system) and efferent innervation (away from the central nervous system) to the abdominal viscera, are important in relaying information regarding noxious peripheral stimuli to central sites for processing. This relay of information can be dependent or independent of the CTZ. Oral ingestion of copper sulfate reliably induces emesis. This response can be markedly attenuated by disruption of the abdominal vagus nerve. Ablation of the CTZ has no effect on the emetic response induced by oral copper sulfate. This suggests that the CTZ is not involved in the emesis induced by oral copper sulfate. Rather, afferent input from the vagus and splanchnic nerves can directly stimulate the vomiting center in response to specific peripheral stimuli such as copper sulfate. Other stimuli, such as various gastrointestinal mucosal irritants (e.g, radiation therapy, chemotherapeutic agents, ingested toxins), activate vagal or splanchnic afferent pathways that do involve the

CTZ. In addition to chemical agents and mucosal irritants, distention of hollow viscera and visceral pain can induce emesis, which is eliminated by vagotomy. Regardless of the emetogenic stimuli, afferent neurons are likely to be activated by the production of neuroactive agents such as 5-hydroxytryptamine, prostaglandins, and various free radicals.

Emetogenic afferent input can arise from areas other than the gastrointestinal tract (Fig. 4-1). The vestibular system can induce vomiting in susceptible individuals. In motion sickness, variable types of motion stimulate the vestibular system, which in turn activates the vomiting center. Involvement of the CTZ in motion sickness is not well defined and may be species-specific. Higher brain stem and cortical centers can also induce the emetic response. Electrical stimulation of the cerebral cortex, hypothalamus, and thalamus can induce emesis. Certain smells, tastes, and sights can stimulate corticobulbar afferents, which in turn stimulate the vomiting center. However, these higher centers are not absolutely necessary for the emetic response, as vomiting can occur even in decerebrate animals. Afferent emetogenic input can also arise from a number of peripheral sites, includ-

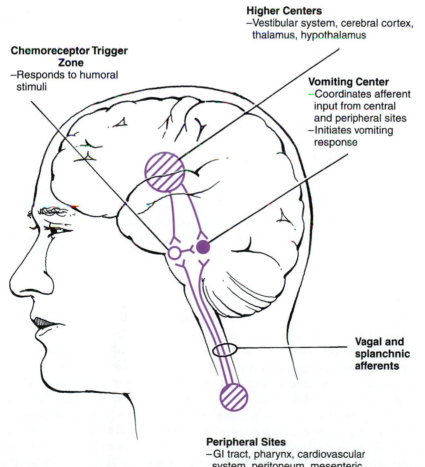

Figure 4-1. Interactions of the vomiting center with central and peripheral sources of afferent neural input.

ing the pharynx, heart, peritoneum, mesenteric vasculature, and bile ducts. These peripheral sites probably communicate directly with the vomiting center to induce emesis.

Regardless of how the central centers are stimulated, a number of brain neurotransmitters are important to the emetic response. These include dopamine, histamine, acetylcholine, endogenous opiates, serotonin, γ-aminobutyric acid, and substance P. Pharmacologic manipulation of these final common mediators and their receptors forms the basis for many of today's therapies for nausea and vomiting.

THE ACT OF VOMITING

The act of vomiting is a highly preprogrammed response that involves both the autonomic and somatic nervous systems. Vomiting is usually preceded by nausea. However, nausea does not always lead to vomiting. The neural pathways responsible for nausea are poorly defined but may be the same as those responsible for vomiting. Some investigators have suggested that varying degrees of activation of these pathways might explain why some develop nausea and others go on to develop vomiting. Alternatively, nausea and vomiting may be initiated by more than one set of neural pathways. This remains a difficult question to resolve, as animal models do not lend themselves to the study of subjective sensations such as nausea.

Retching is the mechanical precursor of vomiting and consists of rhythmic, simultaneous contraction of the diaphragm, external intercostal muscles, and abdominal musculature against a closed glottis. This results in forceful inspiratory movements of the chest wall and diaphragm with concurrent expiratory contraction of the abdominal vasculature. The mouth remains closed during retching. These changes cause retropulsion of gastric contents into the esophagus during retching. However, since the glottis is closed and negative pressure exists in the chest, gastric contents are not expelled through the mouth.

During vomiting, the diaphragm, abdominal musculature, and external oblique muscles contract, creating positive pressure in both the abdomen and the chest. In conjunction with a relaxed upper esophageal sphincter, ablation of the intra-abdominal portion of the esophagus, and contraction of the pylorus, gastric contents are forcefully expelled through the mouth (Fig. 4-2). A characteristic posture can be seen with both retching and vomiting.

A number of physiologic changes accompany nausea and vomiting. Hypersalivation occurs and is probably attributable to the close proximity of the facial and glossopharyngeal nerve cell bodies (which innervate the salivary glands) to the vomiting center. Tachycardia also typically accompanies nausea. It is unclear if changes in cardiac rhythm are caused by the stress of nausea or represent part of a preprogrammed response. Gastric acid production is suppressed with nausea and vomiting. Defecation can also accompany vomiting. This may be related to the close proximity of the vomiting and defecation pathways in the area postrema (Fig. 4-3).

A number of alterations in gastrointestinal motility occur in response to nausea and vomiting. In the stomach, tone in the fundus and generalized peristaltic activity are decreased. Tone of the duodenum and proximal jejunum are increased with associated reflux of duodenal contents into the stomach. In addition to changes in small intestinal tone, reverse peristalsis has been observed during retching and vomiting. A role for reverse peristalsis in vomiting is supported by experiments in dogs and cats given emetogenic agents intracerebroventricularly. In these

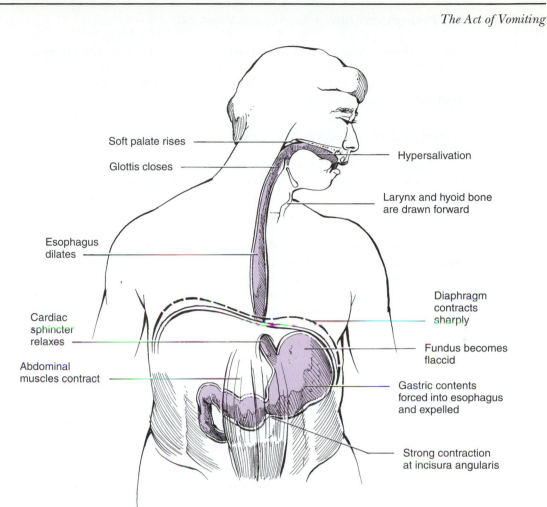

Soft palate rises

Glottis closes

Hypersalivation

Larynx and hyoid bone are drawn forward

Esophagus dilates

Diaphragm contracts sharply

Cardiac sphincter relaxes

Fundus becomes flaccid

Abdominal muscles contract

Gastric contents forced into esophagus and expelled

Strong contraction at incisura angularis

Figure 4-2. The act of vomiting. (Adapted from Searle. Research in the service of medicine. 44:2, 1956.)

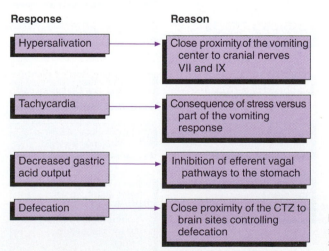

Response

Hypersalivation

Tachycardia

Decreased gastric acid output

Defecation

Reason

Close proximity of the vomiting center to cranial nerves VII and IX

Consequence of stress versus part of the vomiting response

Inhibition of efferent vagal pathways to the stomach

Close proximity of the CTZ to brain sites controlling defecation

Figure 4-3. Physiologic responses associated with nausea and vomiting.

studies, a characteristic myoelectrical pattern consisting of intense bursts of electrical activity or spike potentials migrating in an orad direction precedes emesis. The clinical importance of reverse peristalsis is supported by the frequent presence of intestinal contents in vomitus.

METABOLIC CONSEQUENCES OF VOMITING

Nausea and vomiting can result in a number of important clinical and metabolic consequences (Fig. 4-4). In this section, we focus on the metabolic sequelae of nausea and vomiting. In the vast majority of cases, nausea and vomiting are not severe enough to induce measurable metabolic abnormalities. However, protracted emesis can result in a number of metabolic derangements. The best understood metabolic consequences of chronic emesis include metabolic alkalosis, hypokalemia, and hyponatremia.

Emesis can result in the development of a hypochloremic, metabolic alkalosis. Metabolic alkalosis is a systemic disorder resulting from an increase in plasma bicarbonate concentration. In general, metabolic alkalosis can occur in three ways: (1) the net loss of H^+ from the extracellular fluid (ECF) space; (2) the loss of fluid containing chloride in a concentration disproportionately greater than that of bicarbonate in the ECF; and (3) the net addition of bicarbonate or substances that lead to bicarbonate formation in the ECF.

The gastric parietal cell generates H^+ and HCO_3^- from CO_2 and H_2O. H^+ is secreted into the gastric lumen in the form of hydrochloric acid. Emesis leads to the loss of hydrochloric acid in the vomitus without an equivalent loss of bicarbon-

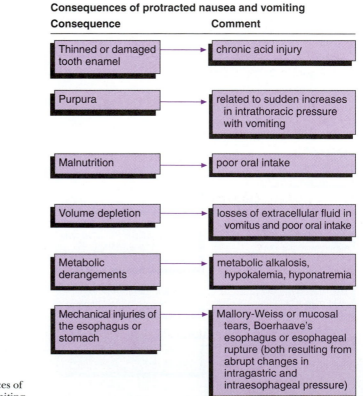

Consequences of protracted nausea and vomiting

Consequence	Comment
Thinned or damaged tooth enamel	chronic acid injury
Purpura	related to sudden increases in intrathoracic pressure with vomiting
Malnutrition	poor oral intake
Volume depletion	losses of extracellular fluid in vomitus and poor oral intake
Metabolic derangements	metabolic alkalosis, hypokalemia, hyponatremia
Mechanical injuries of the esophagus or stomach	Mallory-Weiss or mucosal tears, Boerhaave's esophagus or esophageal rupture (both resulting from abrupt changes in intragastric and intraesophageal pressure)

Figure 4-4. Consequences of protracted nausea and vomiting.

ate. This preferential loss of H^+ allows the *generation* of a metabolic alkalosis. In addition to the loss of both H^+ and Cl^-, contraction of the ECF space occurs. This volume depletion allows the *maintenance* of the metabolic alkalosis by stimulating active sodium reabsorption in kidney. Antidiuretic hormone–dependent sodium and bicarbonate reabsorption occurs in the proximal tubule. Mineralocorticoid-dependent sodium reabsorption also occurs in the distal tubule. This reabsorption is electrically balanced by cation (H^+ or K^+) secretion. With the secretion of H^+, the net generation of bicarbonate occurs.

Hypokalemia, or an abnormally low serum potassium concentration, occurs with protracted emesis both on the basis of decreased intake and increased wasting. With persistent nausea or vomiting, potassium intake can be decreased. Recurrent emesis leads to potassium wasting in the vomitus. Perhaps the most important factor in the development of hypokalemia is wasting by the kidney, which occurs only in the setting of volume depletion and metabolic alkalosis. As discussed above, to maintain the ECF space, the distal nephron reabsorbs sodium at the expense of potassium secretion. This leads to significant renal potassium wasting despite the presence of whole body potassium depletion. Potassium depletion further aggravates the metabolic alkalosis described above by causing the intracellular shift of H^+.

Hyponatremia, or decreased serum sodium concentration, occurs because of losses in the vomitus and, in some cases of marked metabolic alkalosis, because of renal wasting. In patients with normal renal function and the absence of significant metabolic alkalosis, the kidney efficiently compensates for gastrointestinal sodium losses and hyponatremia does not occur. However, when metabolic alkalosis is severe enough to exceed the kidney's ability to reabsorb bicarbonate, bicarbonaturia occurs. This obligates the concomitant secretion of cations such as sodium or potassium to maintain electroneutrality. The net result is inappropriate renal sodium wasting despite whole body sodium depletion.

CLINICAL CORRELATES

In this section, a number of etiologies of nausea and vomiting are briefly discussed. These examples are intended to provide a clinical basis for several of the pathophysiologic concepts discussed earlier. The following group of disorders is not intended to provide a complete differential diagnosis of nausea and vomiting. A more complete differential diagnosis is provided in Table 4-1.

MECHANICAL OBSTRUCTION

Mechanical obstruction can cause either acute or chronic nausea and vomiting. Whether onset is acute or chronic, it is useful to divide the etiologies of mechanical obstruction into three categories: intraluminal lesions, intrinsic bowel wall lesions, and extrinsic lesions. Disorders such as intussusception, pyloric channel ulceration, volvulus involving the small intestine, or an incarcerated hernia are causes of acute symptoms. In addition to the acute obstruction induced by these disorders, associated pain often exacerbates the nausea and emesis. Recall that pain from both gastrointestinal sources (e.g., perforation of a viscus, acute inflammatory conditions such as appendicitis) and nongastrointestinal sources (e.g., nephrolithiasis and myocardial infarction, particularly of the posterior wall) can induce nausea and vomiting.

The most common obstructive cause of protracted nausea and emesis is

TABLE 4-1. *DIFFERENTIAL DIAGNOSIS OF NAUSEA AND VOMITING*

1. Infections
   A. Viral (Norwalk agent, Hawaii agent, hepatitis A and B)
   B. Bacterial (*Staphylococcus aureus* toxin, *Bacillus cereus* toxin, *Clostridium perfringens* toxin, *Salmonella*)
2. Drugs (chemotherapeutic agents, antibiotics, narcotics, cardiac glycosides, aminophylline)
3. Gastric outlet obstruction
   A. Mechanical (peptic ulcer disease, gastric, duodenal, or pancreatic malignancy, Crohn's disease)
   B. Functional (gastroparesis, drug-induced, postviral, postsurgical)
4. Small intestinal obstruction
   A. Mechanical (hernia, adhesions, volvulus, intussusception, space-occupying lesions, Crohn's disease, foreign body ingestion)
   B. Functional (intestinal pseudo-obstruction syndromes)
5. Psychogenic
6. Central nervous system (vestibular disorders, increased intracranial pressure, infections)
7. Pregnancy
8. Metabolic/endocrine (hyperthyroidism, Addison's disease)
9. Visceral pain (peritonitis, pancreatitis, cholecystitis, myocardial infarction)
10. Miscellaneous (radiation therapy/exposure)

chronic peptic ulcer disease with deformity and fibrosis of the antrum, pylorus, or duodenum. A better understanding of the pathophysiology and treatment of *Helicobacter pylori* infection may make chronic peptic ulcer disease a less common scenario in the future. Other causes of chronic symptoms include intraluminal narrowing from gastric or small intestinal malignancy, stricturing at a previous surgical anastomosis or as the result of Crohn's disease, and extraluminal compression such as from adhesions or a pancreatic mass lesion.

Several clinical features are characteristic of mechanical obstruction. Patients usually describe the onset of vomiting more than an hour after ingestion of a meal. Onset of vomiting can be seen promptly after eating in some patients with an ulcer of the pyloric channel. In general, vomiting of undigested food suggests a gastric outlet obstruction. The presence of bile in the vomitus effectively rules out a mechanical gastric outlet obstruction. Patients with a more distal obstruction have feculent vomitus. Unlike gastric outlet obstruction or functional small bowel obstruction, mechanical small bowel obstruction typically manifests with associated abdominal pain. Pain is often transiently improved after vomiting. Other causes of feculent vomitus include ileus, gastrocolonic fistula, intestinal ischemia, small bowel bacterial overgrowth, and longstanding gastric outlet obstruction with bacterial overgrowth in the stomach. On physical examination, the presence of a succussion splash suggests delayed gastric emptying. Clues can be gleaned not only from the presence or absence of bowel sounds but also from their quality and pitch. High-pitched, tinkling bowel sounds occur in the setting of mechanical small bowel obstruction. Unfortunately, the above clinical features are not unique to mechanical obstruction but can also be seen with functional obstruction, which is the subject of the following section.

FUNCTIONAL OBSTRUCTION

Functional obstruction occurs as a consequence of abnormalities in gastric or small intestinal motility. Abnormalities of upper gastrointestinal motor function have been closely linked to nausea and vomiting in diseases such as gastroparesis and intestinal pseudo-obstruction. In addition, a number of alterations in gastrointestinal motility occur in response to vomiting.

Disorders of Gastric Emptying

The term "gastroparesis" refers to the delayed emptying of contents from the stomach. Abnormalities in the neurohormonal regulation, smooth muscle function, or perhaps the pacemaker of the stomach can lead to gastroparesis. For example, surgical disruption of the vagus nerve alters gastric emptying. "Truncal" vagotomy or severing of the vagal trunks typically results in increased tone of the proximal stomach as well as decreased phasic activity of the distal stomach. The functional consequences are accelerated liquid and delayed solid emptying.

A potential complication of longstanding diabetes mellitus is delayed gastric emptying. Gastroparesis typically occurs in diabetics with evidence of other complications such as peripheral neuropathy, autonomic neuropathy (bladder dysfunction, impotence, orthostatic hypotension, anhydrosis), nephropathy, or retinopathy. The etiology of gastroparesis is probably linked to the underlying autonomic neuropathy in these patients. Hyperglycemia may also play a primary etiologic role. Although nausea and emesis in a chronic diabetic are commonly attributable to gastroparesis, other etiologies, including drug-induced and psychogenic vomiting, should also be considered. In addition, not all diabetics with delayed gastric emptying experience nausea or vomiting.

Gastroparesis can also occur as the result of primary or secondary gastric smooth muscle dysfunction. Diseases such as scleroderma, polymyositis, and dermatomyositis affect the gastric smooth muscle primarily. Surgical procedures such as antrectomy or partial gastrectomy delay the emptying of solids by removal or alteration of the antrum and pylorus.

Both the heart and the stomach have a pacemaker. The gastric pacemaker is located in the body of the stomach and normally generates a gastric slow wave frequency of 3 to 4 cycles/minute. Disturbances in gastric slow wave activity have been linked to the development of gastroparesis. "Tachygastria," or an accelerated gastric slow wave rhythm (>5 cycles per minute), has been described in a subset of patients with nausea and vomiting. "Bradygastria," or a slow gastric slow wave rhythm (<2 cycles per minute), has also been described. Delayed gastric emptying is sometimes associated with these rhythm disturbances. Whether tachygastria and bradygastria are the causes or results of nausea, vomiting, and delayed gastric emptying remains the subject of some debate. The observation that tachygastria precedes the onset of nausea and emesis supports a primary role for gastric dysrhythmias in the pathogenesis of these problems.

Other etiologies of delayed gastric emptying include drugs (e.g., opiates, antidepressants, anticholinergics, levodopa), metabolic abnormalities (e.g., diabetic ketoacidosis, hypothyroidism, electrolyte abnormalities), psychiatric diseases (e.g., anorexia nervosa), central nervous system processes (e.g., brain tumor), infections (e.g., acute viral gastroenteritis), and idiopathic. The pathophysiology of gastroparesis in each of these disorders probably involves multiple factors, including effects on neural and hormonal input, gastric electrical rhythm, and smooth muscle function.

Disorders of Small Intestinal Motility

Disorders of small intestinal motility can lead to a clinical scenario compatible with bowel obstruction. In the absence of gastroparesis, nausea and vomiting are less prominent features of these diseases. Reversible abnormalities in small intestinal motility are termed paralytic ileus. Paralytic ileus is commonly seen following abdominal surgery or in conjunction with severe infections (e.g., gram-negative sepsis) or electrolyte disturbances (e.g., hypokalemia).

When abnormalities are irreversible and progressive, the disorders are collectively known as the chronic intestinal pseudo-obstruction syndromes. Chronic pseudo-obstruction syndromes may be of primary or secondary etiology. Primary etiologies are quite rare and include familial and nonfamilial forms. The familial forms consist of familial visceral myopathy and familial visceral neuropathy. In familial visceral myopathy, there is progressive degeneration and fibrous replacement of the smooth muscle of the gastrointestinal tract. This process has also involved the urinary tract in several families. In familial visceral neuropathy, there is degeneration of the myenteric plexus with concomitant hypertrophy of the smooth muscle layers. The several families described in the literature had varying degrees of extraintestinal involvement (various neurologic abnormalities, small bowel malrotation). Rare, nonfamilial cases of visceral myopathy and neuropathy have also been described in the literature.

The differential diagnosis of secondary intestinal pseudo-obstruction is extensive. It is useful to place the many causes into categories: (1) diseases affecting intestinal smooth muscle function (scleroderma, dermatomyositis/polymyositis, amyloidosis, myotonic dystrophy); (2) neurologic diseases (Chagas' disease, visceral neuropathy associated with carcinomatosis, Parkinson's disease); (3) endocrine disorders (myxedema, hypoparathyroidism); (4) drug-related disorders (phenothiazines, tricyclics, antiparkinsonian medications, narcotics); and (5) miscellaneous causes (jejunoileal bypass, porphyria, radiation enteritis, celiac sprue, systemic lupus erythematosus).

DRUGS AND CHEMICALS

Patients presenting with nausea and vomiting should always be carefully questioned about the medications they are taking. Drugs may induce nausea and vomiting by acting directly on the CTZ. Examples include dopamine agonists, opiates, digitalis, and certain chemotherapeutic agents. Other drugs induce nausea and vomiting by stimulation of the vomiting center via vagal afferent neurons. Drugs such as nonsteroidal anti-inflammatory agents probably cause local gastric irritation and consequent stimulation of vagal afferent nerve fibers. As mentioned earlier, medications may also induce nausea and vomiting by their effects on the motor function of the stomach or small intestine.

ACUTE SYSTEMIC INFECTIONS

Nausea and vomiting are commonly associated with many febrile illnesses. Viral, bacterial, and parasitic infections that primarily affect not only the gastrointestinal tract (viral gastroenteritis, food poisoning) but other sites (viral hepatitis, meningitis) cause nausea and vomiting by mechanisms that are as yet poorly defined. Possibilities include effects on gastrointestinal motility or central sites either by the release of endotoxin or endogenous mediators.

DISORDERS OF THE CENTRAL NERVOUS SYSTEM

Processes that lead to increased intracranial pressure such as inflammation, space-occupying lesions, hydrocephalus, and intracranial hemorrhage often cause nausea and vomiting. As discussed earlier, this likely results from activation of sites in the cerebral cortex, hypothalamus, and thalamus. Projectile vomiting is said to occur more commonly in the setting of increased intracranial pressure.

Disorders of the vestibular system, such as Meniere's disease and infectious labyrinthitis, can lead to nausea and vomiting. Motion sickness is also the consequence of pathologic stimulation of the vestibular system.

PREGNANCY-ASSOCIATED NAUSEA AND VOMITING

Nausea and vomiting accompany 50 to 90% of pregnancies. Onset is usually after the first missed menstrual period. They tend to be more common in primigravid, younger, nonsmoking, obese, less educated women and in women who experienced nausea while taking oral contraceptives. Although nausea and vomiting typically occur in the morning, they can happen at any time during the day. In uncomplicated cases, termed the nausea and vomiting of pregnancy, symptoms usually cease by the fourth month of gestation. Women who suffer with the nausea and vomiting of pregnancy tend to have recurrent symptoms with subsequent pregnancies.

The cause of the nausea and vomiting of pregnancy remains ill defined. Hormonal and psychologic causes have been suggested. Possible hormonal etiologies have included human chorionic gonadotropin, progesterone, and androgens. However, studies of plasma levels during pregnancy and response to exogenous administration of these hormones have been variable. Whether high levels of these circulating hormones might stimulate the CTZ or neural elements communicating with the vomiting center remains the subject of investigation. Psychologic testing reveals that women afflicted with the nausea and vomiting of pregnancy tend to have a higher incidence of unwanted pregnancies and negative relationships with their mothers than those not so afflicted.

When fluid, electrolyte, or nutritional disturbances accompany intractable nausea and vomiting during pregnancy, it is called hyperemesis gravidarum. Hyperemesis occurs in less than 0.5% of pregnancies. Like uncomplicated cases of nausea in pregnancy, hyperemesis usually begins soon after the first missed menstrual period and ceases by the third or fourth month of gestation. The incidence of hyperemesis is not affected by parity, race, or desire for an abortion. The likelihood of birth defects or pre-eclampsia is not increased in these patients.

The precise pathogenesis of hyperemesis remains unclear. As for the nausea and vomiting of pregnancy, hormonal and psychologic etiologies have been proposed. Molar pregnancies, which are associated with much greater levels of human chorionic gonadotropin, have a higher incidence of hyperemesis. Women afflicted with hyperemesis are more commonly emotionally immature and sexually maladjusted. The importance of psychosocial factors in hyperemesis is underscored by its occurrence only in humans, its successful treatment by hypnosis, and a very low incidence of the disorder in underdeveloped countries and during wartime.

Another rare cause of nausea and vomiting during pregnancy is acute fatty liver of pregnancy. This disorder typically occurs after week 35 of gestation and is often associated with pre-eclampsia. Its etiology is unknown. Clinically, patients present with nausea, vomiting, headache, and malaise. Liver enzyme levels are elevated. Histologic examination of the liver reveals microvesicular fat deposition. Liver injury can progress to fulminant liver failure. Treatment includes aggressive supportive measures and termination of pregnancy.

PSYCHOGENIC DISORDERS

Nausea and vomiting can sometimes serve as the physiologic expression of emotional distress. The neuroendocrine pathways responsible for this problem have not been elucidated, but a number of clinical observations have been made. Psychogenic vomiting is more common in women and often associated with marital or unresolved sexual conflict, severe emotional turmoil such as seen with the recent loss of a loved one, and depression. A longstanding history of vomiting, typically exacerbated by stressful situations, is common in these patients. A family history of unexplained vomiting is common. Vomiting is sometimes not associated with nausea and characteristically occurs while eating or shortly after the completion of a meal. Patients commonly seem unconcerned about the problem, and appetite is usually normal. The degree of weight loss in these patients is quite variable. Eating disorders such as anorexia nervosa and bulimia are sometimes associated.

CLINICAL TESTING

RADIOGRAPHIC STUDIES

Abdominal radiographs in the flat and upright positions can reveal gaseous dilatation of the intestinal lumen suggestive of obstruction. Air-fluid levels can also be seen in the upright or decubitus position. Pathologic air-fluid levels are typically seen at different levels in the abdomen and have a stepladder appearance (Fig. 4-5A). Mechanical obstruction can be difficult to distinguish from functional obstruction on plain films. Mechanical obstruction tends to cause greater bowel dilatation from accumulated fluid and gas. When gaseous dilatation is present in the stomach, small intestine, and colon, the diagnosis is more likely to be a functional obstruction.

Intraperitoneal free air can be seen in the upright or decubitus position and suggests visceral perforation. In the setting of intestinal strangulation, the bowel wall loses its normal contour. Edema and air in the bowel wall can result in "thumb-printing" (Fig. 4-5B). Pancreatic calcification is seen in some patients with chronic pancreatitis. In the appropriate clinical setting, foreign body ingestion can be confirmed by standard abdominal radiographs.

Barium studies are helpful in demonstrating intraluminal lesions (ulcers), space-occupying lesions (malignancy), strictures, or the level of mechanical obstruction. When attempting to localize the site of mechanical obstruction, it is important to exclude colonic obstruction with a barium enema prior to administering contrast material orally. Barium retained proximal to a colonic obstruction can become inspissated and impacted. Barium should not be given orally if a perforated viscus is suspected, as it stimulates an intense inflammatory reaction upon exposure to the peritoneum. Use of a water-soluble contrast agent would be more appropriate in this circumstance.

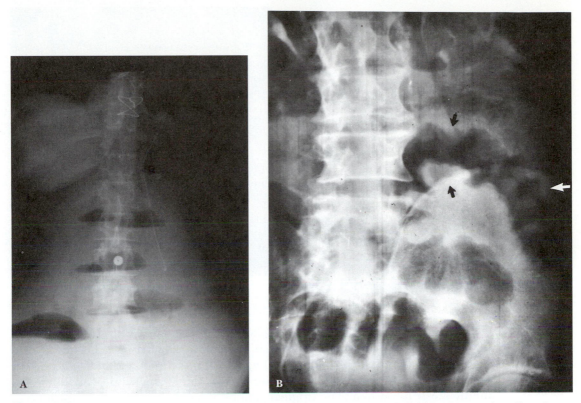

Figure 4-5. An abdominal radiograph in the upright position can demonstrate air-fluid levels suggestive of bowel obstruction (**A**). "Thumb-printing" on abdominal radiograph results from submucosal edema and is most often encountered in the setting of an ischemic process (**B**). (From Yamada T, Alpers DH, Owyang C, Powell DH, Silverstein FE, eds. Textbook of Gastroenterology, 2nd ed. Philadelphia: JB Lippincott, 1995:2514.)

ENDOSCOPY

Endoscopic examination is the most sensitive means of evaluating the mucosa of the upper gastrointestinal tract. Inflammation, ulceration, space-occupying lesions, and strictures can be fully evaluated both visually and histologically by way of biopsy (Fig. 4-6). In addition to diagnostic capabilities, endoscopy offers therapeutic options such as pneumatic dilatation in selected cases. Standard upper endoscopy, which allows examination of the esophagus, stomach, and proximal duodenum, has recently been joined by enteroscopy, which allows examination to the midjejunum. Disadvantages of endoscopy include the need for sedation, a small risk of aspiration or perforation, and relatively high cost.

STUDIES OF GASTRIC EMPTYING

The rate of emptying of liquids and solids can be quantified by a number of methods. The measurement of solid-phase gastric emptying is more sensitive than liquid-phase emptying in identifying those with gastroparesis. This is because solid-phase emptying requires vigorous antral contractions for grinding and propulsion, whereas liquid-phase emptying can occur simply by virtue of gravity or the pressure gradient generated by contraction of the gastric fundus.

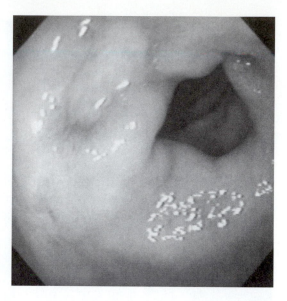

Figure 4-6. Endoscopic view of an ulcer in the antrum.

Gamma scintigraphy is the preferred method of measuring the emptying of both liquids and solids from the stomach. Liquids are labeled with chelates of technetium or indium, which prevent binding of the nuclides to either solid foods or gastric mucosa. Solids are labeled with technetium-99m sulfur colloid, which tightly binds to protein. The original studies of solid-phase gastric emptying utilized chicken livers injected with technetium-99m sulfur colloid. Most centers now use colloid intermixed with eggs or pancake batter prior to cooking. The rate of emptying is determined by performing sequential scans, typically over the course of 2 hours.

A number of other techniques to measure gastric emptying are being developed. These include real-time ultrasonography and magnetic resonance imaging. Regardless of the method used, a number of factors can influence the measure of gastric emptying, including contents and size of the test meal, time of day, body position (supine or erect), gender, age, and concomitant use of medications, alcohol, or tobacco. In addition, recall that gastric emptying in normal subjects can vary by up to 30% from one day to the next. These factors, coupled with the technical inadequacies of the tests themselves, explain why many patients with nausea and vomiting have normal studies of gastric emptying.

MANOMETRY

Manometry measures changes in gut intraluminal pressure either by water-perfused or solid-state catheters. In either case, changes in pressure are transferred from transducers to a chart recorder for interpretation. Manometry is best suited to record phasic motor activity rather than changes in luminal tone. Manometry loses sensitivity when performed in an organ of large diameter because small changes in intraluminal pressure are not accurately sensed. Manometry has traditionally been performed in a "stationary" manner, where the test subject stays in a prescribed location for a fixed amount of time. Newer technology allows the "ambulatory" recording of motor activity for more prolonged periods. This should eventually lead to a better understanding of both normal and abnormal motor activity under more physiologic conditions than the hospital or the physiology laboratory.

ELECTROGASTROGRAPHY

The gastric pacemaker is located in the body of the stomach and normally generates a gastric slow wave frequency of 3 to 4 cycles/minute. This electrical activity can be measured by electrodes surgically implanted into the serosa of the stomach, by peroral mucosal suction cup electrodes, or by cutaneously placed abdominal electrodes. The recording obtained is called an "electrogastrogram." Using this method, disturbances in gastric electrical rhythm, including tachygastria and bradygastria, can be identified. Electrogastrography remains investigational and as such is restricted to a limited number of medical centers. Wider acceptance of this technique may lead to the clear correlation of gastric slow wave disturbances with abnormalities in gastric emptying and the pathogenesis of nausea and vomiting.

CASE PRESENTATION

HISTORY AND PHYSICAL EXAMINATION

A 45-year-old male presents with a 5-month history of progressive nausea and emesis. The symptoms, which initially occurred only intermittently, have gradually progressed to a daily basis. Nausea reportedly began 1 to 2 hours after the completion of a meal. This was typically followed by emesis of "undigested food." Emesis led to relief of the nausea. Other features of the history included "feeling full after only a couple of bites of food," generalized weakness, and a 5-lb weight loss. The patient did not have fever, abdominal pain, gastrointestinal bleeding, hematuria, headache, visual disturbances, or dizziness. Pertinent medical history was remarkable for insulin-dependent diabetes mellitus complicated by retinopathy and peripheral neuropathy; congestive heart failure; and nephrolithiasis. The patient's current medications include daily NPH (neutral protamine Hajedorn) insulin, digoxin, and furosemide.

Physical examination revealed a thin white male with a pulse of 90 beats per minute and a blood pressure of 110/80 mmHg in the supine position. Pulse rose to 104 beats per minute and blood pressure fell to 80/50 mmHg when the patient assumed the standing position. Funduscopic examination revealed changes consistent with diabetic retinopathy. Pulmonary examination was unremarkable. Cardiovascular examination revealed no evidence of congestive heart failure. Abdominal examination was nontender with no hepatosplenomegaly. The abdomen was mildly to moderately distended, but normal bowel sounds were auscultated in all four quadrants. A succussion splash was present. Rectal examination revealed a normal prostate gland and decreased anal sphincter tone. Stool was negative for occult blood. Neurologic examination was remarkable for decreased joint position sense and decreased pinprick sensation in the distal lower extremities bilaterally.

Serum electrolyte examination revealed a blood urea nitrogen level of

25 mg/dl, creatinine of 1.6 mg/dl, and glucose of 235 mg/dl. A complete blood count, liver enzyme examination, and digoxin level were within normal limits. Upper endoscopic examination revealed normal mucosa throughout the esophagus, stomach, and proximal duodenum. The endoscope passed easily into the duodenum, excluding gastric outlet obstruction. A moderate amount of retained solid food was observed in the stomach. A solid phase scintigraphic study of gastric emptying revealed delayed emptying at 2 hours.

DISCUSSION

Although nausea and vomiting are relatively nonspecific complaints, a number of historical features can help to establish the underlying etiology. It is critical to determine whether the nausea and vomiting are acute or chronic in nature (>3 months), as the differential diagnoses vary accordingly. In the absence of pain, the acute onset of nausea and vomiting is most commonly due to infection, toxin exposure, or drug ingestion. Central processes such as head trauma, intracranial hypertension, or disturbances of the labyrinthine apparatus can manifest with the acute onset of nausea and vomiting. These cases are typically associated with symptoms such as changes in mental status, headache, visual disturbances, or vertigo. Projectile vomiting reportedly occurs more commonly in the setting of elevated intracranial pressure. The evaluation of acute nausea and vomiting associated with severe abdominal pain is usually dictated by the location, severity, and specific characteristics of the abdominal pain. Prescription and nonprescription medications are a common cause of acute and chronic nausea and vomiting. All medications taken by the patient should be carefully scrutinized by the evaluating physician.

Other clues, such as the timing of vomiting in relation to ingestion of meals, can prove helpful. Vomiting immediately or soon after eating is characteristic of psychogenic vomiting or eating disorders such as bulimia. Esophageal obstruction leads to postprandial regurgitation, not true vomiting. Vomiting more than an hour after eating is more typical of a mechanical gastric outlet obstruction or a motility disorder such as gastroparesis. Mechanical gastric outlet obstruction can result from malignancy, the edema and irritability of a pyloric channel ulcer, scarring related to chronic peptic ulcer disease, or stricture formation sometimes seen with Crohn's disease. The presence of bile in vomitus effectively excludes a mechanical gastric outlet obstruction. Significant anorexia and weight loss should raise the clinician's suspicion for a malignant etiology. Gastroparesis most commonly occurs as a consequence of surgical disruption of the vagus nerve, of longstanding diabetes mellitus, or of certain medications (e.g., narcotics, anticholinergics). Vomiting of undigested or partially digested food is characteristic of both mechanical and functional gastric outlet obstruction.

Feculent vomitus usually suggests a more obstruction. Unlike gastric outlet obstruction, mechanical small bowel obstruction typically presents primarily as pain. Pain is often transiently improved after vomiting. Other causes of feculent vomitus include ileus, gastrocolonic fistula, intestinal ischemia, small bowel bacterial overgrowth, and longstanding gastric outlet obstruction with bacterial overgrowth of the stomach.

A number of other diseases cause abdominal pain in addition to nausea and vomiting. As in mechanical small bowel obstruction, nausea and vomiting associated with uncomplicated peptic ulcer disease are often relieved by vomiting. However, the pain associated with pancreatitis or biliary tract disease is typically not relieved by vomiting. It is important to recall that severe pain from sources other than the gastrointestinal tract can also induce nausea and vomiting. Myocardial infarction and renal colic commonly cause nausea and vomiting.

On physical examination, the vital signs can assist in assessing the acuity of the patient's illness. Fever suggests an infectious etiology. Postural changes in pulse or blood pressure in addition to resting tachycardia or hypotension suggest intravascular volume depletion. Other physical findings consistent with volume depletion include dry mucous membranes and increased skin turgor. Purpura can be seen on the face and upper neck and can result from the sudden increases in intrathoracic pressure seen with vomiting. Calluses on the metacarpophalangeal joints can be seen in association with self-induced vomiting (bulimia). Oral examination can reveal dental erosions and caries in patients with chronic vomiting. Complaints referable to the central nervous system should prompt complete neurologic and funduscopic examinations. The neurologic examination is also useful in identifying peripheral neuropathy, which is often present in diabetics with gastroparesis. The presence of a succussion splash suggests a problem with gastric emptying. Exquisite tenderness on palpation suggests an intra-abdominal catastrophe. The presence of significant distention can suggest intestinal pseudo-obstruction. A hernia or abdominal scars should raise suspicion of incarcerated bowel or mechanical obstruction from adhesions, respectively. Clues can be obtained not only from the presence or absence of bowel sounds but also from their quality and pitch. High-pitched, tinkling bowel sounds occur in the setting of mechanical small bowel obstruction. Digital rectal examination establishes the presence of gross or occult fecal blood. Poor sphincter tone in the setting of chronic diabetes mellitus suggests significant autonomic neuropathy.

In the patient in our case presentation, progressive nausea and emesis of undigested food in the setting of insulin-dependent diabetes mellitus should raise suspicion for the diagnosis of gastroparesis. This diagnosis is confirmed by endoscopy, revealing only retained food in the stomach and an abnormal solid-phase scintigraphic study of gastric emptying. A more detailed discussion of diabetic gastroparesis is presented in the section on Disorders of Gastric Emptying.

SUMMARY

The elegant studies of Borison and Wang established the framework upon which our current understanding of nausea and vomiting is based. However, the concept of a discrete vomiting center is probably an oversimplification. New interactions between the brain, gastrointestinal tract, and extraintestinal locations continue to unfold. From our ever-expanding understanding of the pathophysiology of nausea and vomiting will arise new concepts regarding patient management and therapy.

SELECTED READING

Borison HL, Wang SC. Physiology and pharmacology of vomiting. Pharmacol Rev 5:193, 1953.

Feldman M. Nausea and vomiting. In: Sleisenger MH, Fordtran JS, eds. Gastrointestinal Disease, 4th ed. Philadelphia: WB Saunders, 1989 222–235.

Lumsden K, Holden SW. The act of vomiting in man. Gut 10:173, 1969.

Malagelada JR, Camilleri M. Unexplained vomiting: A diagnostic challenge. Ann Intern Med 101:211, 1984.

Ouyang A. Approach to the patient with nausea and vomiting. In: Yamada T, Alpers DH, Owyang C, Powell DW, Silverstein FE, eds. Textbook of Gastroenterology. Philadelphia: JB Lippincott, 1991: 647–659.

Lippincott's Pathophysiology Series: Gastrointestinal Pathophysiology, edited by Joseph M. Henderson. Lippincott–Raven Publishers. Philadelphia © 1996.

Pathophysiology of Diarrhea

W. Michael McDonnell and David C. Dawson

The gastrointestinal tract functions to absorb fluids, electrolytes, and nutrients. Diarrhea results when this process is disrupted and stool volume becomes excessive. Normal stool volume is about 100 g per day, but individuals with a high fiber intake can have stool volumes of 500 g per day. Clinically, the definition of diarrhea is daily stool volumes of more than 250 g. Notice that the definition of diarrhea does not depend on either the consistency of the stool or the number of bowel movements per day. Multiple loose stools a day with a volume less than 250 g are often called diarrhea but are better termed hyperdefecation or pseudodiarrhea. Hyperdefecation is often seen in individuals with irritable bowel syndrome or proctitis. Fecal incontinence is another condition often described as diarrhea. Patients who have any type of episode of fecal incontinence usually describe the experience as diarrhea, and this is complicated by the fact that incontinence usually involves unformed or liquid stool. Incontinence is a problem of neuromuscular control of the anus and rectum. In people who are prone to episodes of incontinence, these episodes usually occur when the stool is liquid or unformed because it takes a large degree of neuromuscular tone and coordination to retain a liquid stool in the rectum compared to a solid stool. One need only recall an experience with viral gastroenteritis as a child or adult to understand the difficulty in retaining a liquid stool. A careful history by the physician usually differentiates between incontinence and diarrhea. Water represents approximately 60 to 85% of stool weight and in diarrheal states the percentage is even higher. Of the remaining solid (dry weight), about half is bacteria.

Diarrhea is a problem of intestinal water and electrolyte balance. It results when excess water and electrolytes are actively transported into the lumen (secretory diarrhea) or when water is retained in the lumen by osmotically active agents (osmotic diarrhea). Osmotic diarrhea can be produced either by the ingestion of nonabsorbable substances that are osmotically active in the lumen of the intestine or by the malabsorption/maldigestion of nutrients that are normally absorbed. Ingestion of milk of magnesia is an example of a "pure" osmotic diarrhea, and cholera is an example of a "pure" secretory diarrhea. Diarrhea is often described as having either an osmotic or a secretory etiology, but most diarrheas are actually a combination of the two.

Another major contributor to diarrhea is gastrointestinal motility. Gastrointestinal motor activity can have a significant effect on the amount of water that reaches the rectum. The rate of transit through the gut determines the time available for intestinal absorption of water, and rapid transit can be the sole cause of diarrhea or can exacerbate pre-existing diarrheal states. The mechanism of action of most antidiarrheal drugs is to slow transit through the gut, resulting in increased absorption of water and decreased stool volume.

The purpose of this chapter is to discuss the physiology of fluid and electrolyte transport within the intestine and describe the pathophysiologic processes that lead to diarrhea. Intraluminal maldigestion and mucosal malabsorption (discussed in Chapter 6) are important causes of diarrhea that are only briefly touched upon here.

PATHOPHYSIOLOGY

FLUID AND ELECTROLYTE TRANSPORT

Average oral intake of water is about 2 L per day, but the amount of fluid passing through the duodenum is 8 to 10 L per day. The majority of water absorbed by the gut represents the recycling of salivary, gastric, pancreatic, biliary, and intestinal secretions needed for digestion. Most of this fluid is absorbed by the small intestine and about 1 to 1.5 L reach the colon (Fig. 5-1). The colon, where stool is formed and retained, continues to absorb water, reducing fecal water volume to about 100 ml per day. The maximum absorptive capacity of the colon is only about 4 L/day, so if volumes of fluid greater than this enter the small intestine, diarrhea will ensue despite normal colonic function. The capacity of the small intestine to absorb and secrete water is much greater than that of the colon. This is in part attributable to the tremendous surface area of the intestine provided by folds, villi, and microvilli (Fig. 5-2). Normal intestinal secretion is about 1 L per day but can be as much as 20 L per day. This striking difference of the absorptive and secretory capacity of the small intestine and colon dictates that large volume diarrhea is most often caused by small intestinal dysfunction.

Water movement into or out of the lumen of the gastrointestinal tract is passive. Water molecules follow the osmotic gradients created by electrolyte movement. Electrolytes are transported by active processes, and this ion transport controls water absorption and secretion. After an ingested meal enters the duodenum, fluids shift from plasma across the mucosa to make the luminal contents isotonic, and luminal contents remain isotonic throughout the gut. In the duodenum Na^+ and Cl^- concentrations are equivalent to those in serum. Sodium concentration decreases in the jejunum and is about 130 mEq/L in the ileum. In the colon Na^+ concentration continues to decline to about 30 mEq/L in stool owing to active Na^+ uptake and decreased mucosal permeability, preventing diffusion of Na^+ and water

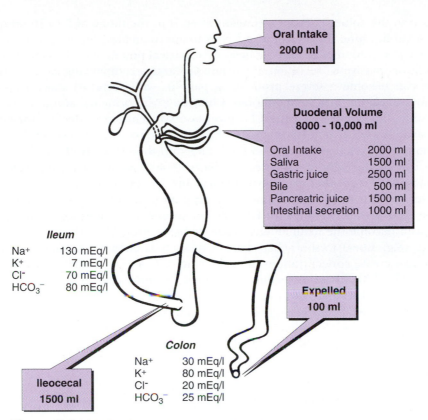

Figure 5-1. Fluid volumes through the digestive tract.

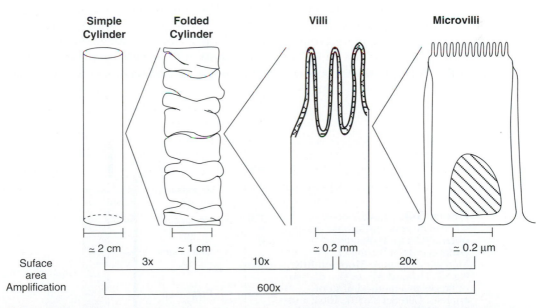

Figure 5-2. Amplification of the intestinal surface area by intestinal folds (plicae conniventes), villi, and microvilli. The numbers indicate the factor by which the surface area is amplified over a flat surface. Together the folds, villi, and microvilli amplify the surface area by approximately 600-fold. (Adapted from Yamada T, Alpers DH, Owyang C, Powell DW, Silverstein FE, eds. Textbook of Gastroenterology, 2nd ed. Philadelphia: JB Lippincott, 1995:327.)

back into the colon. Potassium concentration is in the range of 5 to 10 mEq/L in the small intestine. In the colon, K^+ rises to approximately 80 mEq/L because of the active secretion of K^+ and the negative electrical potential in the colonic lumen that favors passive K^+ secretion. Potassium loss and accompanying cardiac arrhythmias can become a severe problem in patients with secretory diarrhea so that serum potassium must be monitored. Chloride is the principal anion in the small intestine, but because of active Cl^- absorption concentrations decline throughout the small intestine to about 60 to 70 mEq/L before passing the ileocecal valve. Bicarbonate is exchanged for Cl^- in the lumen and therefore HCO_3^- concentration rises distally throughout the intestine. Bicarbonate loss and accompanying metabolic acidosis is another electrolyte abnormality that must be monitored when caring for patients with large volume secretory diarrhea. In the colon, Cl^- continues to be absorbed in exchange for HCO_3^-, but organic molecules from bacterial metabolism become the main anions. Bacterial breakdown of unabsorbable carbohydrates (e.g., fiber) to short-chain fatty acids such as butyrate, propionate, and acetate can create concentrations of organic anions as high as 180 mmol/L in the colon (Fig. 5-3). These molecules also serve as an important source of energy for colonic epithelial cells. Diverting the fecal stream away from a portion of the colon deprives epithelial cells of organic anions and can result in a condition known as diversion colitis with colonic inflammation, bleeding, purulent discharge, and tenesmus.

THE CELLULAR BASIS FOR INTESTINAL FLUID AND SOLUTE TRANSPORT

As suggested in Figure 5-4, the opposing absorptive and secretory transport processes that determine net fluid transport in the intestine are localized to specific regions of the intestinal epithelium. The cells of the villus tip are differentiated so as to promote fluid and solute absorption, whereas those in the crypt region promote fluid and solute secretion. A principle of fundamental importance in understanding the opposing fluid transport in these two regions of the intestine is that the opposing processes of fluid absorption and secretion are driven by op-

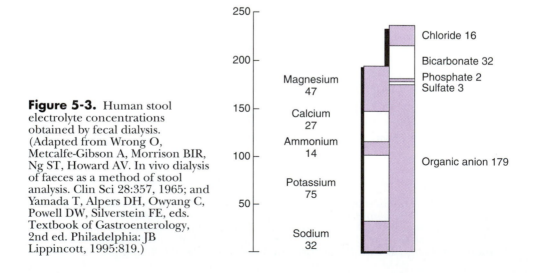

Figure 5-3. Human stool electrolyte concentrations obtained by fecal dialysis. (Adapted from Wrong O, Metcalfe-Gibson A, Morrison BIR, Ng ST, Howard AV. In vivo dialysis of faeces as a method of stool analysis. Clin Sci 28:357, 1965; and Yamada T, Alpers DH, Owyang C, Powell DW, Silverstein FE, eds. Textbook of Gastroenterology, 2nd ed. Philadelphia: JB Lippincott, 1995:819.)

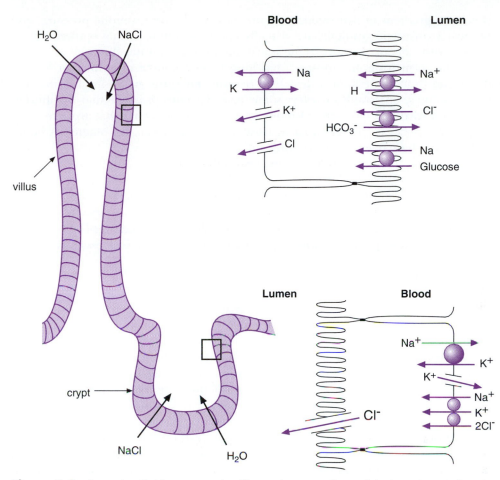

Figure 5-4. Opposing fluid transport in villus and crypt regions of the intestine. Cells of the villus tip are differentiated so as to promote fluid and solute absorption, whereas those in the crypt region promote fluid and solute secretion.

positely directed salt transport processes in these two cell types. As indicated above, the transport of water is entirely passive, that is, water will move only in response to osmotic gradients that are generated by solute transport, predominantly electrolytes. From this perspective, diarrhea can arise in two ways that are not mutually exclusive. Unabsorbed solute in the lumen can create an osmotic water secretion that is often referred to as "osmotic diarrhea" because it stems from the failure to absorb osmotically active solutes. In contrast, secretory diarrhea refers to the condition in which the normal transport of electrolytes is altered. Most often this is caused by stimulation of salt secretion, although attenuation of salt absorption also produces a net secretory effect.

WATER TRANSPORT IS PASSIVE

The implication of this phrase is that there are no molecular water pumps; no membrane proteins, analogous to the Na^+/K^+-ATPase, for example, that can couple free energy to the movement of water molecules. Thus, water only moves if there is a gradient of hydrostatic pressure or a gradient of osmotic pressure, and because hydrostatic gradients are virtually nil across the intestinal epithelium, we are left with osmotic pressure as the sole driving force for water flow.

The term "osmotic pressure" has long been a source of confusion for students and practitioners for at least two reasons. First, the name implies that dissolved solutes, or osmolytes, exert some sort of solute pressure that is different from the hydrostatic pressure. Osmotic pressure is a misnomer that arose because solute gradients can give rise to a hydrostatic pressure in an osmometer. A better name would have been "osmotic potential."

Osmotic pressure, π, is usually expressed as follows:

$$\pi = RTC_s$$

where C_s is the total concentration of dissolved solute in osmoles/Kg H_2O. The difference in osmotic pressure across the intestinal epithelium is expressed as $\Delta\pi$, i.e.:

$$\Delta\pi = RT\Delta C_s$$

Here we find the second point of confusion regarding osmotic pressure. $\Delta\pi$ is a measure of the passive driving force caused by a difference in the *concentration of water,* but it is expressed, for convenience, in terms of *solute* concentration. To keep this straight it is simply necessary to realize that the gradient of dissolved solute determines the gradient of water concentration; the two are oppositely directed so that the natural tendency for water to move down its concentration gradient means that it will move toward the compartment with the higher solute concentration.

Another important principle is that the overall osmotic effect of a dissolved solute is more profound if that solute is restricted to the compartment of interest. For example, in lactose intolerance, the unabsorbed glucose cannot leave the luminal compartment and exerts a significant osmotic effect, producing osmotic diarrhea. The term osmotic diarrhea focuses on the fact that the cause of water secretion is, in some cases, unabsorbed osmotic equivalents, but it should be remembered that all fluid movements must result from osmotic forces, although their origin (as in secretory diarrhea) is not always so obvious.

THE INTESTINE IS HIGHLY PERMEABLE TO WATER

The large movements of fluid across the small intestine imply that the layer of epithelial cells is highly permeable, or leaky, to water. Even enormous osmotic driving forces would produce little or no water flow if there were not pathways across the epithelium that permit water molecules to move down their concentration gradient. It is useful to think of water movement in terms of a relationship analogous to Ohm's law for electricity, in which water flow is proportional to the product of the osmotic driving force and the water permeability.

Water, like any other substance that traverses the intestinal epithelium, moves across cell plasma membranes or in between cells via the paracellular pathway composed of the tight junctions and lateral intercellular spaces between adjoining epithelial cells. The molecular basis for these water permeation pathways is not well worked out, but experience with artificial systems and other cell types, notably those in the kidney, provides some basis for speculation.

Measurements on planar lipid bilayers suggest that the lipid portion of the plasma membrane of many cells is probably highly permeable to water, and it was thought for some time that this might explain water permeation in most cells. Recently, however, definitive evidence has been obtained for the existence of a class of membrane proteins that function as water-conducting channels. This protein, or one like it, may be responsible for intestinal water permeation. Even less is known about paracellular paths, although it seems likely that some water flow traverses this route (Fig. 5-5).

ISOTONIC WATER TRANSPORT IS DRIVEN BY SALT TRANSPORT

It has been recognized since the earliest studies of intestinal transport that the normal absorption of salt and water occurs in such a way as to render the contents of the intestine virtually isotonic with plasma despite the prodigious movement of water and electrolytes from lumen to blood. This observation left early investigators to explain how water was transported in the absence of an osmotic gradient. It appeared that the intestine was capable of "active" water transport. Several decades later it is clear that water absorption is driven exclusively by osmotic

Fluid Absorption

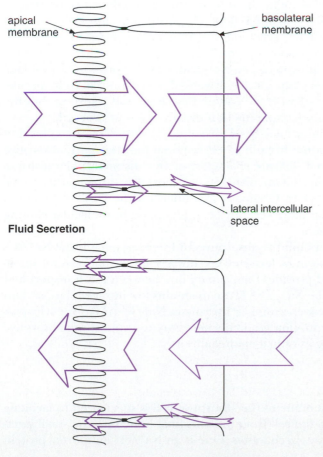

apical membrane

basolateral membrane

lateral intercellular space

Fluid Secretion

Figure 5-5. Cellular and paracellular paths for water transport.

forces that are generated by salt absorption, so that the two processes are tightly coupled. The absence of a readily discernible osmotic gradient across the intestine is probably a reflection of two factors. First, the high permeability of the intestine to water dictates that a very small transepithelial $\Delta\pi$ is required to support the observed rate of water absorption. This small $\Delta\pi$ might be difficult to detect in experimental situations. Second, there probably are *intra*epithelial compartments such as the lateral intercellular space in which salt accumulation can produce *local* gradients that contribute to the observed flow. The central principle is that intestinal fluid absorption is driven by salt transport, predominantly NaCl, so that the key to understanding derangements of this process is to be found in the molecular machinery for the transport of Na and Cl by the intestinal cells.

Intestinal fluid secretion is driven by the secretion of salt by the cells in the crypts of Lieberkühn. The term "secretory diarrhea" is a recognition of the fact that bacterial toxins and other agents that cause hyperstimulation of intestinal salt secretion result in the simultaneous secretion of an osmotically equivalent volume of water. The cause of these conditions is a derangement of the molecular control mechanisms that normally regulate intestinal secretion.

SURFACE CELLS AND CRYPT CELLS ARE SPECIALIZED FOR ABSORPTION AND SECRETION

The absorption and secretion of salt that underlie the movement of fluid across the small intestine are brought about by specialized epithelial cells. Absorption occurs in villous epithelial cells and is driven by the active transport of Na^+. Secretion occurs in crypt epithelial cells and is driven by active Cl^- transport. In order for either of these salt transport processes to take place, however, there must be a transepithelial pathway for the co-ion; Na^+-driven salt absorption cannot take place without a Cl^- absorptive path, and Cl^--driven salt secretion requires a permeation path for Na. Active transport is the engine that drives salt transport, but the co-ion permeation is an absolute requirement if the process is to proceed.

Figure 5-6 shows the molecular basis for solute transport by the villus and crypt cells of the small intestine. In both cases, vectorial ion transport, absorptive or secretory, is achieved by cells that are characterized by a distinctly polar distribution of the membrane proteins that mediate ion transport across the apical and basolateral membranes of the cells. Originally identified on the basis of function, each of these transporters has more recently been identified by molecular cloning as the product of a specific gene.

An essential element in both the absorptive and secretory cell is the Na^+/K^+-ATPase. This transport protein is localized exclusively in the basolateral membranes of intestinal cells and provides the primary link between ion transport and metabolic energy sources. The Na^+/K^+-ATPase maintains low intracellular Na^+ and high intracellular K^+ at the expense of ATP hydrolysis. Na^+/K^+-ATPase activity provides the Na^+ and K^+ concentration gradients necessary to support the absorptive and secretory activities of the intestinal epithelial cells.

ABSORPTIVE CELLS

The brush border membrane of the absorptive cell is specialized to facilitate the passive entry of Na^+ into the cell from the intestinal lumen. In the small intestine this occurs largely via two mechanisms. One is an Na^+/H^+ antiporter protein

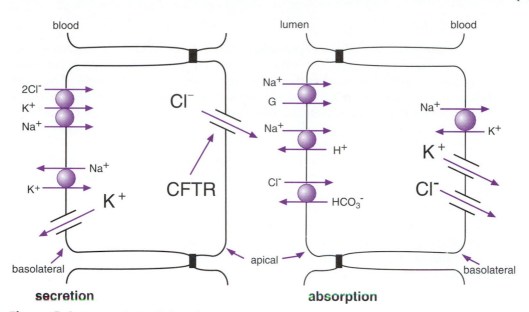

Figure 5-6. Molecular basis for solute transport by the villus and crypt cells of the small intestine. Shown are some of the membrane proteins that mediate salt transport across the apical and basolateral membranes. Note that the electrical potential difference (Vm) across the apical and basolateral membranes of the absorptive and secretory cells is oriented so that the cell is negative with respect to the extracellular fluid. The magnitude of the basolateral Vm, however, is greater than that of the apical Vm so that the transepithelial electrical potential, measured across the epithelial cell layer, is lumen negative.

specialized to catalyze the one-for-one exchange of sodium ions and protons, so that the entry of each Na^+ into the cell is coupled to the exit of one proton. The second is the Na^+-glucose cotransporter that mediates the coupled entry of Na^+ and glucose into the cell with a stoichiometry of either 1 Na^+:1 glucose or 2 Na^+:1 glucose, so that in the presence of glucose, Na^+ entry is coupled with glucose influx into the cell. The presence of this transporter permits the free energy in the Na^+ gradient to drive glucose absorption; but it is also important to note that the presence of glucose in the intestinal lumen actually enhances Na^+ absorption by increasing the rate of Na^+ entry into the cell. This effect is the basis for the use of glucose in oral rehydration solution therapy. The glucose in an oral rehydration solution is taken up by this cotransporter and enhances the absorption of Na^+ and therefore water in patients with diarrhea. A solution containing only much needed electrolytes is not as effective at rehydration because it does not activate glucose-coupled Na^+ entry into the cells.

The series arrangement of apical Na^+ entry mechanisms and basolateral Na^+/K^+-ATPase promotes the active transcellular transport of Na^+ from lumen to blood; active Na^+ transport is the engine that drives salt and water absorption. The required absorptive flow of Cl^- is provided in two ways. Some Cl^- is likely to be absorbed across the paracellular path owing to the small, lumen-negative transepithelial electrical potential. In addition, there is a cellular pathway for Cl^- absorption composed of an apical Cl-HCO_3^- antiporter and an as yet unidentified basolateral exit mechanism that could be a Cl-selective channel or a K^+/Cl^- cotransporter. The linkage between H^+ and HCO_3^- via carbonic acid and carbonic anhydrase provides a degree of coupling between the entry of Na^+ and Cl^-.

SECRETORY CELLS

In the secretory cell the expression of transport proteins is, as expected, very different from that seen in the villus cell (see Fig. 5-6). Apical Na^+ permeation mechanisms are lacking so that the Na^+ content of the cell is determined by basolateral transporters. Sodium enters the cell across the basolateral membrane via a cotransporter that, in each cycle, transports one Na^+, one K^+, and two Cl^- into the cell. Because the *net* charge transferred in one cycle is zero, the transport rate is not affected by membrane potential but depends only on the concentration gradients for the three ions. The net result of the inward gradients of Na^+ and Cl^- and the outward gradient of K^+ is that the inward movement of all three ions is favored. The Na^+ that enters via the cotransporter is "recycled" via the Na^+/K^+-ATPase so that the inward Na^+ gradient is maintained. This cotransport protein is similar to the one that is found on the *apical* membrane of cells in the kidney that are the sites of action of the loop diuretics (e.g., furosemide, bumetanide).

Chloride that enters the cell via the basolateral cotransporter exits via a Cl^- selective ion channel (CFTR, see below) in the apical membrane. Chloride exit from the cell is a passive process. The steady state intracellular Cl^- concentration is of the order of 30 mM, about one third of that in the luminal fluid, but the potential difference across the apical membrane is of the order of 50 to 60 mV, negative inside the cell, so there is a net outward driving force that promotes Cl^- exit when the channels are open (see Fig. 5-6). The net result is active Cl^- secretion, the engine of active salt secretion. The movement of the Na^+ required for NaCl secretion is thought to occur largely via paracellular pathways driven by the lumen-negative electrical potential. It is interesting to note that active Na absorption and active Cl^- secretion, although they promote salt transport in opposite directions, both produce a lumen-negative transepithelial potential (see the legend for Fig. 5-6). It is also noteworthy that the basic plan of this secretory machinery is widespread in the animal kingdom and is found in more primitive vertebrates such as sharks and birds in the form of so-called "salt glands" that are specialized for salt excretion.

CYTOSOLIC CYCLIC ADENOSINE MONOPHOSPHATE IS A KEY REGULATOR OF ABSORPTION AND SECRETION

Salt absorption and salt secretion are both regulated processes, and derangement of the regulatory mechanisms can cause diarrhea. Cytosolic cyclic adenosine monophosphate (cAMP) is a key factor in the regulation of both processes. Generally, events that bring about a rise in cytosolic cAMP increase salt secretion and decrease salt absorption, leading to a net secretory effect. To understand this regulation it is necessary to identify the transport elements (channels and transporters) that are modulated and the components of the cellular machinery that constitute the cAMP signaling system.

Figure 5-7 presents a schematic diagram of the cAMP second messenger signaling system as it is found in most cells. An agonist, stimulus, or drug can affect this system by influencing the synthesis of cAMP, the breakdown of cAMP, or both. Activating stimuli can interact with a regulatory G protein, either directly or via a receptor, to increase the activity of adenyl cyclase so as to increase the synthesis of cAMP from adenosine triphosphate. Cytosolic cAMP molecules bind to the regulatory subunits of another enzyme, protein kinase A, causing them to dissociate from the catalytic subunit so that the active catalytic subunit can catalyze the donation of a phosphate moiety to specific sites on cellular proteins.

Phosphorylation is a regulatory mechanism that is of major importance in many cell types, and the role of this process in intestinal fluid and electrolyte transport is particularly clear in the secretory cells of the intestinal crypt. As suggested in Figure 5-6, any change in the transcellular movement of Cl^- requires that both the entry of Cl^- into the cell across the basolateral membrane and the exit of Cl^- from the cell across the apical membrane be increased; both of these processes appear to be regulated by phosphorylation. Phosphorylation of the apical, Cl^- selective channel prolongs the opening of the channel, and phosphorylation of the Na:K:2Cl cotransporter increases the number of active transporters in the membrane, so that any stimulus that increases cAMP can potentially cause a massive increase in active Cl^- secretion.

The precise role of cAMP in the absorptive pathway is somewhat less clear, but there is convincing evidence that a rise in cytosolic cAMP inhibits salt absorption, probably by inhibiting the apical entry of Na^+ and Cl^-. Thus the net secretory effect of stimuli that lead to increases in cAMP is multiplied because secretion increases while absorption decreases. There is no evidence for any effect of cAMP on the apical entry of Na^+ and glucose via the Na^+-coupled glucose cotransporter; therefore this route for Na entry is not suppressed even in the face of stimuli that produce a potentially lethal increase in Cl^- secretion. This accounts for the efficacy of oral rehydration solution in the treatment of diarrhea.

Cyclic guanosine monophosphate also appears to be an important messenger in the control of active Cl^- secretion. This product of guanylate cyclase acts by activating a kinase known as protein kinase G. As with cAMP, increases in cyclic guanosine monophosphate have been shown to both promote salt secretion and attenuate salt absorption, although the molecular mechanisms are less well understood.

There is also evidence that another intracellular messenger, calcium, can play a role in modulating the rates of absorption and secretion, but the details of the mechanism are much less clear.

THE APICAL Cl CHANNEL IS THE CYSTIC FIBROSIS TRANSMEMBRANE CONDUCTANCE REGULATOR

Recently there has been intense interest in the protein that functions as the apical Cl^- channel in intestinal secretory cells because it is the product of the gene that is mutated in the inherited disease, cystic fibrosis. The gene encodes a 1480 amino acid protein named the cystic fibrosis transmembrane conductance regulator (CFTR), which functions as a cAMP-activated, Cl^- selective ion channel in cells of the airway, pancreas, intestine, liver, and reproductive organs, to name a few. Mutations in the gene cause alterations in Cl^- secretion that appear to be responsible for many symptoms of cystic fibrosis. Altered Cl^- transport can be directly traced to dysfunction of the CFTR Cl channel and can occur in at least three ways. Mutations can result in an incomplete protein that is degraded in the cell, in a protein that is complete but is not delivered to the apical membrane, or in a full-length protein that is delivered to the membrane but is functionally deficient. The most common mutation, the deletion of a phenylalanine at position 508 (ΔF508), results in nondelivery of a (nearly) full-length protein.

The molecular basis for the activation of CFTR was foreshadowed by the analysis of the amino acid sequence (see Fig. 5-8). A large cytosolic domain (R domain) was found to contain many consensus sites for phosphorylation by PKA (protein kinase A), and it has been shown that removal of these sites reduces the activation of the channel in response to elevation of cytosolic cAMP. The channel

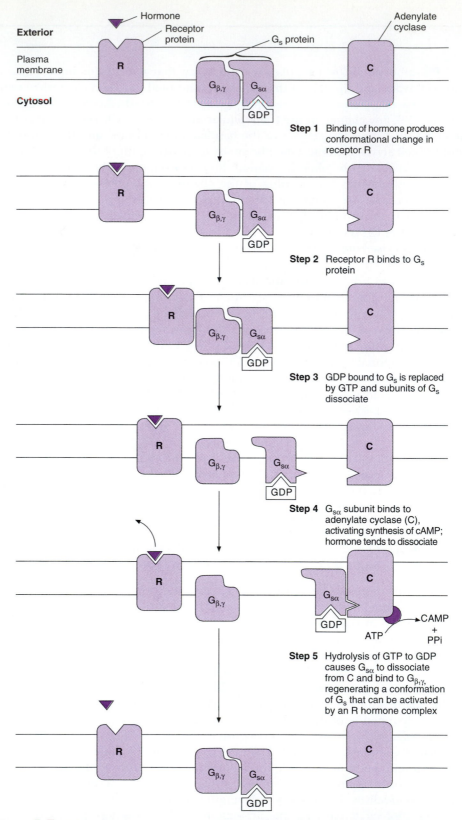

Figure 5-7. Schematic diagram of the cAMP second messenger signaling system as it is found in most cells. Binding of the hormone (or neurotransmitter) to its receptor forms an activated complex that interacts with a stimulatory G protein (G_s). *(continued)*

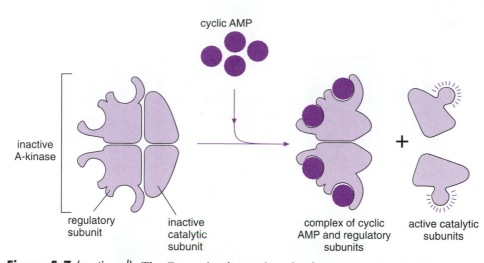

Figure 5-7 *(continued).* The G protein, thus activated, releases guanosine diphosphate (GDP) that is bound in the resting state, and binds guanosine triphosphate. This causes dissociation of the $G_{s\alpha}$ and $G_{\beta,\gamma}$ subunits, and the $G_{s\alpha}$ binds to adenylate cyclase, which catalyzes the synthesis of cAMP from adenosine triphosphate. The cAMP thus formed binds to the regulatory subunits of protein kinase A, causing them to dissociate from the catalytic subunits that can catalyze the deposition of a phosphate at an appropriate site on a protein. (Adapted from Darnell J, Lodish H, Baltimore D. Molecular Cell Biology, 2nd ed. New York: Scientific American Books, WH Freeman, 1990.)

has two other cytoplasmic regulatory domains that are called nucleotide binding folds because they share sequence homology with a family of proteins known to bind and hydrolyze ATP. A rise in cytosolic cAMP is thought to activate CFTR in the following way. cAMP binds to the catalytic subunit of protein kinase A and liberates an active catalytic subunit, which catalyzes the phosphorylation of one or more serines on the R domain of CFTR. The channel is then opened by the binding and hydrolysis of adenosine triphosphate at the nucleotide binding folds. The role of adenosine triphosphate is not to provide free energy to drive transport; the channel is a passive or permissive element. Rather, the free energy is presumably involved in changing the conformation of the channel so that the conduction pathway of the pore is open.

Unlike some other secretory tissues, notably the airway and sweat glands that also have a calcium-activated Cl channel in the apical membrane, in the intestinal secretory cells CFTR appears to be the only Cl channel that is expressed in the apical membrane. Accordingly, the intestine of cystic fibrosis patients is incapable of Cl secretion. Studies of mRNA distribution using in situ hybridization reveal that the message for CFTR is preferentially expressed in crypt cells in keeping with the localization of secretory processes in these cells.

BACTERIAL ENTEROTOXINS ACT BY ACTIVATING INTRACELLULAR SECOND MESSENGER SYSTEMS

Much of what is known about the cellular mechanisms that operate to regulate salt secretion and absorption is the result of studies aimed at understanding the mechanism of action of bacterial entertoxins that can produce severe, often life-threatening, diarrhea. The best studied of these is cholera toxin, the secretory product of *vibrio cholerae* and the cause of devastating epidemics in Asia and South America. The secretory effect of cholera toxin is the result of a persistent activation

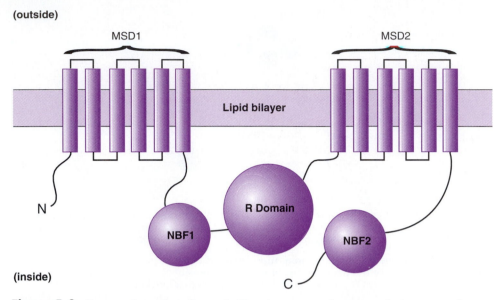

(outside)

Figure 5-8. Proposed topology for cystic fibrosis transmembrane conductance regulator (CFTR). The protein consists of 1480 amino acids that are organized into five more or less distinct domains: two membrane-spanning domains (MSD1, MSD2), each composed of six membrane spanning segments that are presumably organized so as to form a Cl-conductive pore; and three cytosolic domains (NBF1, NBF2, R) that serve to regulate channel activity.

of adenylate cyclase and resulting increases in cytosolic cAMP. The secreted toxin is an oligomeric 84 kilodalton (kd) protein composed of one A and five B subunits. Synthesized as a single polypeptide, the 29 kd A subunit is proteolytically reduced to two components, A1 (23 kd) and A2 (6 kd), linked by a disulfide bond. After the cholera toxin binds to the surface of the apical plasma membrane through its B subunits, the A subunit is internalized and the A1 component released. In the cytosol, it acts as an enzyme that catalyzes the covalent modification of the G protein, which activates adenylate cyclase. ADP ribose is added to an arginine residue in the α subunit of Gs, the G protein responsible for adenylate cyclase activation. The modified α subunit dissociates from the β and γ subunits and persistently activates adenylate cyclase. The resulting increase in cytosolic cAMP activates apical CFTR Cl channels in secretory cells and reduces the coupled entry of NaCl in absorptive cells, thus producing a robust secretory response and a potentially lethal loss of fluid. It has been suggested that the persistence in the human population of CFTR mutations that are associated with severe cystic fibrosis in homozygotic individuals is attributable to the fact that heterozygotic individuals, bearing only one functional CFTR gene, are less susceptible to some secretory diarrheas. Natural signals for cAMP-mediated secretion are thought to be secretory neurotransmitters, principally vasoactive intestinal polypeptide.

Another important tool for elucidating secretory control mechanisms is heat-stable *Escherichia coli* enterotoxin, STA, a family of 18-19 amino acid peptides that are activators of brush border guanylate cyclase. These secreted peptides act by binding to a receptor in the apical membrane that is apparently the normal target for the peptide hormone, guanylin. The receptor is apparently itself a guanylate cyclase, and ligand binding produces the secretory and antiabsorptive effects associated with cytosolic cyclic GMP.

ORAL REHYDRATION THERAPY

The dehydrating effect of diarrhea can be fatal, but the acute effects can be readily reversed by replacing fluids and electrolytes with intravenous solutions. An attractive alternative is the use of oral rehydration solutions that are composed of a mixture of salt and glucose designed to maximally stimulate salt and water absorptive processes in the villus cells. The oral rehydration strategy is based on the observation that secretory diarrhea induced, for example, by cholera toxin, reflects a net increase in salt and water secretion caused not only by stimulation of secretory processes but also by inhibition of absorption, probably on account of the inhibition of the coupled entry of Na^+ as Cl^- in the apical membrane of the villus cell. The Na^+-coupled glucose transporter, however, is unaffected so that if an intestine treated with cholera toxin is exposed to glucose in the luminal fluid, salt absorption is stimulated by increased apical Na^+ entry into the cell. The effect of luminal glucose is not to attenuate the secretory response but rather to induce a compensating absorptive Na^+ flux and to reduce or reverse net fluid loss despite the ongoing secretion in the intestinal crypts.

INHERITED DEFECTS IN ELECTROLYTE TRANSPORT

Specific, inherited defects in electrolyte transport that lead to diarrhea are rare but serve to highlight the role of specific membrane proteins in intestinal electrolyte transport. One example is glucose-galactose malabsorption, which produces a severe watery diarrhea in neonates that is ameliorated if glucose, galactose, and lactose are removed from the diet. Studies of mucosal biopsies showed that the villus cells of affected individuals fail to accumulate glucose or galactose and pointed toward a defect in the brush border Na^+-glucose cotransporter. Analysis of the DNA sequence of the sodium glucose cotransporter (SGLT-1) gene from an affected child revealed a single base change of guanine to adenine that resulted in an aspartic acid at position 28 in the protein being substituted for by arginine.

Two other apical transport proteins, the Cl^-/HCO_3^- antiporter and the Na^+/H^+ antiporter, have also been implicated in congenital defects of electrolyte absorption. Both conditions produce diarrhea caused by diminished salt absorption. In congenital chloridorrhea the ileum and colon are not capable of active Cl^- absorption, and the acidic pH of the stool implicates defective Cl^-/HCO_3^- exchange. Apical Na^+/H^+ exchange appears to be unaffected, and the absorption of Na^+ and HCO_3^- that occurs in affected individuals can be mimicked in normal subjects by perfusing the ileum with Cl-free salt solutions. Ion transport studies suggest that in congenital sodium secretory diarrhea Na^+/H^+ exchange is defective in the intestine, whereas Na^+ coupled glucose transport is unaffected. Affected individuals have elevated concentrations of Na^+ and HCO_3^- in the stool and metabolic acidosis. Perfusion of the intestine of one patient, in the absence of glucose, revealed net secretion of Na^+ and Cl^-.

APPLICATION TO DIARRHEA

This section applies the basic physiology just discussed to clinical conditions that result in diarrhea. Causes of diarrhea are many, and discussions of diarrhea are usually broken down into groupings such as acute versus chronic, osmotic versus secretory, infectious versus noninfectious, and inflammatory versus noninflammatory. Each of these categories serves a purpose for understanding the pathophysiology of diarrhea; yet in any particular disease state, diarrhea can be produced in many different ways. Diarrhea owing to malabsorption or maldigestion of intraluminal nutrients can result from a diseased intestine but can also occur in a completely normal intestine, as is the case in pancreatic insufficiency. These conditions are discussed in Chapter 6.

ACUTE DIARRHEA VERSUS CHRONIC DIARRHEA

Acute Diarrhea

Acute diarrhea is defined as being less than 2 to 3 weeks in duration, and chronic diarrhea is defined as lasting at least 4 to 6 weeks. This is an important distinction because, although numerous ill-defined conditions such as medications, transient change in bowel flora, and long-distance running can cause diarrhea, the vast majority of acute diarrhea in the United States is caused by infection. Acute diarrhea rarely warrants investigation unless the patient appears toxic or is immunosuppressed; such as those on steroids or other immunosuppressive therapy (organ transplant recipients) or those with acquired immunodeficiency syndrome. Most infectious diarrheas are self-limited and with some exceptions (e.g., that caused by parasites such as *Giardia* or *Entamoeba histolytica*) do not lead to chronic diarrhea (Table 5-1).

TABLE 5-1. *CAUSES OF ACUTE AND CHRONIC INTESTINAL INFECTIONS*

Acute	Parasites
Bacteria	*Strongyloides stercoralis*
	Others more rarely
Escherichia coli	
Salmonella	*Protozoa*
Shigella	
Vibrio species	*Giardia lamblia*
Campylobacter	*Cryptosporidium*
Yersinia	*Entamoeba histolytica*
Gonococcus	
Syphilis	**Chronic**
Clostridium difficile	
Clostridium perfringens	*Giardia lamblia*
Others	*Entamoeba histolytica*
	Strongyloides stercoralis
Viruses	Small intestinal bacterial overgrowth
	Tropical sprue
Rotavirus	*Yersinia enterocolitica*
Norwalk-like agents	*Aeromonas hydrophila*
Astroviruses	
Caliciviruses	
Herpes simplex	
Others	

From Kelley WN, ed. Textbook of Internal Medicine. Philadelphia: JB Lippincott, 1989:554.

Chronic Diarrhea

Chronic diarrhea usually merits a thorough investigation because of the possibility of more serious underlying disease and the desire on the part of the patient to resolve a life-disrupting situation. When interviewing a patient with chronic diarrhea, the physician attempts to quantitate the frequency and volume of bowel movements in part to decide if this is indeed diarrhea and next to assess the clinical features that will pinpoint the cause. For example, blood in the stool is a marker of inflammation or ischemia. It is also suggestive of colonic disease, since blood from the small intestine usually is not passed as red blood. Tenesmus along with diarrhea is suggestive of rectosigmoidal disease. Frequent small volume bowel movements suggest colonic disease, whereas less frequent large volume bowel movements suggest disease of the small intestine. Diarrhea that subsides with fasting is more suggestive of osmotic diarrhea. If other household members are also affected, infectious causes are suggested. Family history is important because about 10% of first-degree relatives of persons with inflammatory bowel disease are also afflicted. Most of the discussions that follow concern chronic diarrhea.

OSMOTIC VERSUS SECRETORY DIARRHEA

In diarrhea, water can be drawn into the lumen by either the osmotic effects of nonabsorbed particles (osmotic diarrhea) or by the active transport of ions into the lumen by mucosal epithelial cells (secretory diarrhea) (Tables 5-2 and 5-3). Osmotic diarrhea occurs with the ingestion of unabsorbable substances such as magnesium hydroxide or lactulose or when nutrients are malabsorbed, such as lactose in persons who are lactase-deficient. Any condition that causes malabsorption (e.g., pancreatic insufficiency, celiac sprue, Crohn's disease) can produce an osmotic load in the lumen and diarrhea. Unlike secretory diarrhea, osmotic diarrhea should stop with fasting (Table 5-4). Osmotic diarrhea is also characterized by an osmotic gap in the stool electrolyte composition. In osmotic diarrhea, stool electrolyte concentrations are significantly less than the actual stool osmolality because malabsorbed molecules rather than electrolytes are responsible for much of the stool osmotic activity (see below). In secretory diarrhea most of the stool osmotic activity can be accounted for by stool electrolytes. Understanding the mechanisms of osmotic and secretory diarrhea is important, but it is equally important to understand the limitations of these concepts. Few conditions are purely osmotic like lactulose ingestion or purely secretory like cholera. Most diarrhea involves both an osmotic and secretory component. For example, diarrhea involving mucosal damage is characterized by an osmotic component caused by malabsorption resulting from loss of brush border enzymes and absorptive cells, however, it also exhibits a secretory component because damage to villous epithelial cells, which are absorptive, leaves a relative excess of crypt secretory cells. In addition, cytokine release from inflammatory cells involved in mucosal damage can stimulate mucosal secretion.

Diminished diarrhea upon fasting is not necessarily diagnostic for osmotic diarrhea. Most secretory diarrheas have an osmotic component, and fasting usually results in decreased stool volumes. Also, eating stimulates large volumes of endogenous gastrointestinal secretion, which is prevented by fasting. Furthermore, the normal absorptive capacity of intestinal mucosa is diminished in many secretory diarrheas. Secretagogues inhibit absorptive cells in addition to stimulating secretory cells. Bile acid–induced diarrhea is secretory because bile acids induce net secre-

88

CHAPTER 5: PATHOPHYSIOLOGY OF DIARRHEA

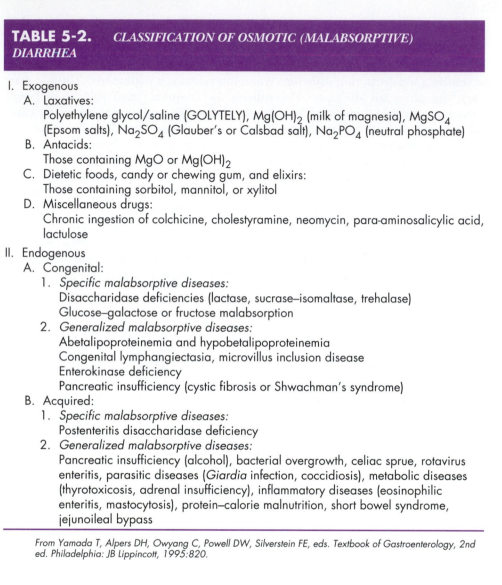

TABLE 5-2. *CLASSIFICATION OF OSMOTIC (MALABSORPTIVE) DIARRHEA*

I. Exogenous
  A. Laxatives:
    Polyethylene glycol/saline (GOLYTELY), $Mg(OH)_2$ (milk of magnesia), $MgSO_4$ (Epsom salts), Na_2SO_4 (Glauber's or Calsbad salt), Na_2PO_4 (neutral phosphate)
  B. Antacids:
    Those containing MgO or $Mg(OH)_2$
  C. Dietetic foods, candy or chewing gum, and elixirs:
    Those containing sorbitol, mannitol, or xylitol
  D. Miscellaneous drugs:
    Chronic ingestion of colchicine, cholestyramine, neomycin, para-aminosalicylic acid, lactulose

II. Endogenous
  A. Congenital:
    1. *Specific malabsorptive diseases:*
      Disaccharidase deficiencies (lactase, sucrase–isomaltase, trehalase)
      Glucose–galactose or fructose malabsorption
    2. *Generalized malabsorptive diseases:*
      Abetalipoproteinemia and hypobetalipoproteinemia
      Congenital lymphangiectasia, microvillus inclusion disease
      Enterokinase deficiency
      Pancreatic insufficiency (cystic fibrosis or Shwachman's syndrome)
  B. Acquired:
    1. *Specific malabsorptive diseases:*
      Postenteritis disaccharidase deficiency
    2. *Generalized malabsorptive diseases:*
      Pancreatic insufficiency (alcohol), bacterial overgrowth, celiac sprue, rotavirus enteritis, parasitic diseases (*Giardia* infection, coccidiosis), metabolic diseases (thyrotoxicosis, adrenal insufficiency), inflammatory diseases (eosinophilic enteritis, mastocytosis), protein–calorie malnutrition, short bowel syndrome, jejunoileal bypass

From Yamada T, Alpers DH, Owyang C, Powell DW, Silverstein FE, eds. Textbook of Gastroenterology, 2nd ed. Philadelphia: JB Lippincott, 1995:820.

tion in colonic crypt epithelial cells, but it resolves with fasting because bile acids are released by eating.

INFECTIOUS DIARRHEA

Acute infectious diarrhea is a leading cause of death worldwide, accounting for more than 4 million deaths of children under the age of 5. In the United States some groups are at greater risk than others (Table 5-5). Most acute diarrhea is caused by bacterial or viral agents but the exact cause is often unknown because most bacterial infections are self-limited and therefore not investigated. An estimate of the sources of diarrhea in the United States, in developing countries, and in travelers is shown in Table 5-6. Diarrhea from bacteria causes a wide spectrum of symptoms, but can generally be divided into two types, inflammatory and noninflammatory (Table 5-7). In *noninflammatory* diarrhea pathogens colonize the in-

TABLE 5-3. *CLASSIFICATION OF SECRETORY (DERANGED ELECTROLYTE TRANSPORT) DIARRHEA*

I. Exogenous
  A. Laxatives:
     Phenolphthalein, anthraquinones, bisacodyl, oxyphenisatin, senna, aloe, ricinoleic acid (castor oil), dioctyl sodium sulfosuccinate
  B. Medications:
     Diuretics (furosemide, thiazides); asthma medication (theophylline) Cholinergic drugs—glaucoma eye drops and bladder stimulants (acetylcholine analogues or mimetics); myasthenia gravis medication (cholinesterase inhibitors); cardiac drugs (quinidine and quinine); gout medication (colchicine)
     Prostaglandins (misoprostol); di-5-aminosalicylic acid (azodisalicylate); gold (may also cause colitis)
  C. Toxins:
     Metals (arsenic), plant (mushroom, e.g., *Amanita phalloides*), organophosphates (insecticides and nerve poisons), seafood toxins (ciguatera, scombroid poisoning, paralytic or neurotoxic shellfish poisoning), coffee, tea, or cola (caffeine and other methylxanthines), ethanol.
  D. Bacterial toxin:
     Staphylococcus aureus, Clostridium perfringens and *botulinum, Bacillus cereus*
  E. Gut allergy without histologic change
II. Endogenous
  A. Congenital:
     Microvillus inclusion disease
     Congenital chloridorrhea (absence of Cl:HCO_3 exchanger)
     Congenital Na diarrhea (absence of Na:H exchanger)
  B. Bacterial enterotoxins:
     Vibrio cholerae, toxigenic *E. coli, Campylobacter jejuni, Yersinia enterocolitica, Klebsiella pneumoniae, Clostridium difficile, S. aureus* (toxic shock syndrome)
  C. Endogenous laxatives:
     Dihydroxy bile acids and long-chain fatty acids, especially hydroxylated ones
  D. Hormone-producing tumors:
     Pancreatic cholera syndrome and ganglioneuromas (vasoactive intestinal peptide), medullary carcinoma of thyroid (calcitonin and prostaglandins), mastocytosis (histamine), villous adenoma (secretagogue unknown)

From Yamada T, Alpers DH, Owyang C, Powell DW, Silverstein FE, eds. Textbook of Gastroenterology, 2nd ed. Philadelphia: JB Lippincott, 1995:821.

testinal lumen and/or elaborate toxins that produce watery diarrhea without blood. These enterotoxins stimulate secretion but do not harm the mucosal cells. In *inflammatory* diarrhea pathogens invade the mucosa of the intestine and/or elaborate toxins, resulting in damage to mucosal cells and inflammation. This often presents as bloody diarrhea (dysentery), and patients usually have more pronounced systemic symptoms such as fever and abdominal pain.

SECRETAGOGUES

Secretagogues are molecules that induce secretion of electrolytes and water from the intestine, as described above. The molecules can be *endogenous,* such as cytokines, bile acids, hormones from neuroendocrine tumors, or enterotoxins

TABLE 5-4. *OSMOTIC VERSUS SECRETORY DIARRHEA*

DISTINGUISHING FEATURE	OSMOTIC	SECRETORY
Effect of fasting	Diarrhea stops	Diarrhea usually continues
Fecal pH	Frequently decreased	Normal
Fecal osmolality	330	290
Fecal electrolytes		
Na^+	30	100
K^+	30	40
$(Na^+ + K^+) \times 2$	160	280
Osmotic gap	210	10

From Kelly WN, ed. Textbook of Internal Medicine. Philadelphia: JB Lippincott, 1989:672.

TABLE 5-5. *HIGH-RISK GROUPS FOR INFECTIOUS DIARRHEA*

Recent Travel

Visitors to developing nations
Peace Corps workers
Campers (ground water)

Unusual Food

Seafood and shellfish, especially raw
Restaurants and fast-food houses
Banquets and picnics

Homosexuals, Prostitutes, and Intravenous Drug Users

"Gay bowel syndrome"
Acquired immunodeficiency syndrome

Day Care

Contact with children
Secondary contacts (family members)

Institutions

Mental institution patients
Nursing home inhabitants
Hospital patients

Modified from Yamada T, Alpers DH, Owyang C, Powell DW, Silverstein FE, eds. Textbook of Gastroenterology, 2nd ed. Philadelphia: JB Lippincott, 1995:825.

ORGANISM	UNITED STATES	TROPICS AND DEVELOPING COUNTRIES	TRAVELER'S DIARRHEA
TABLE 5-6. *EPIDEMIOLOGY OF ENTEROPATHOGENS (% OF TOTAL CASES)*			
Enterotoxigenic *Escherichia coli*	1–4%	7–50%	28–72%
Salmonella	2–4%	0–15%	3–15%
Shigella	1–25%	3–16%	3–25%
Campylobacter	3–15% (1–7% in children)	3–15%	3–17%
Parasites	True incidence unknown (4%—Giardia, 0.6%—Entamoeba histolytica, 2.8%—Cryptosporidium)	True incidence unknown (4–20%—Giardia, 2–15%—Entamoeba histolytica, 4–8%—Cryptosporidium)	0–9% (Giardia 1–4%)
Vibrio cholerae and other species	1–3%	1–6%	0–2% (cholera rare in travelers)
Viruses			
Rotavirus	8–50% (primarily in those younger than 2 years of age)*	5–45%*	0–36%
Norwalk	True incidence unknown (estimates in children: 10–17%)	1–2%	Unknown (15% of travelers develop seroconversion)
Unknown	40%	30–40%	10–15%

*Higher percentages seen during winter and in children with diarrhea requiring hospitalization. (In the general community: 12.5% incidence in United States, 5 to 19% in developing countries.)

From Yamada T, Alpers DH, Owyang C, Powell DW, Silverstein FE, eds. Textbook of Gastroenterology, 1st ed. Philadelphia: JB Lippincott, 1991:1448.

elaborated by bacterial pathogens in the intestine; or *exogenous,* such as castor oil or ingested bacterial toxins from a picnic potato salad.

Neuroendocrine. Pancreatic cholera or watery diarrhea-hypokalemia-achlorhydria is a syndrome of profound watery diarrhea caused by vasoactive intestinal polypeptide–secreting tumors (VIPomas), which are non–β-cell pancreatic islet cell tumors. Vasoactive intestinal polypeptide stimulates water and electrolyte secretion by binding to specific receptors on intestinal epithelial cell, activating adenylate cyclase, and increasing cAMP. This diarrhea behaves as a true secretory diarrhea, with most patients experiencing stool volumes of more than 3 L/day and in some as much 20 L/day. Hypochlorhydria results from the inhibitory effects of vasoactive intestinal polypeptide on gastric acid secretion, and hypokalemia is the result of the large amount of potassium lost in the diarrheal effluent. Hyper-

TABLE 5-7. *TWO MAJOR CLINICAL ACUTE DIARRHEA SYNDROMES*

WATERY, NONINFLAMMATORY	INFLAMMATORY*
Clinical Picture	
Watery stools	Mucoid and bloody stools
No blood, pus, tenesmus, or fever	May have tenesmus, fever, or severe abdominal pain
Abdominal pain not usually prominent	
Volume can be large and dehydration possible	Small volume, frequent bowel movements, dehydration unusual
No fecal leukocytes and rarely occult blood	Many fecal leukocytes and frequently occult blood
Causes	
Enterotoxin-producing bacteria, minimally destructive viruses, etc.	Invasive and cytotoxin-producing microorganisms
Vibrio cholerae	*Salmonella*
Enterotoxigenic *Escherichia coli*	*Shigella*
Staphylococcal and clostridial food poisoning	*Campylobacter*
Rotavirus	Invasive *Escherichia coli*
Norwalk agent, etc.	*Clostridium difficile*
Cryptosporidium	Ameba
Giardia	*Yersinia*

Some of the organisms may disseminate from the intestines to produce a systemic, enteric, fever-like syndrome (e.g., Salmonella typhi, other salmonellae, Yersinia).
From Kelley WN, ed. Textbook of Internal Medicine. Philadelphia: JB Lippincott, 1989:555.

glycemia, hypercalcemia, and flushing are also associated with this tumor. About 5% of VIPomas are associated with the multiple endocrine neoplasm tumors known as multiple endocrine neoplasia I (MEN-I).

Gastrinoma or Zollinger-Ellison syndrome is the most common and first described neuroendocrine tumor. This tumor causes aggressive, refractory peptic ulcer disease in 90% of patients but also causes a chronic secretory diarrhea in about 30% of patients. The mechanism of diarrhea is not completely understood but it does not appear to be caused by direct secretion of intestinal fluid, as is the case with vasoactive intestinal polypeptide. Diarrhea is induced by the high output of gastric secretion, inactivation of pancreatic enzymes, precipitation of bile salts, low intraluminal pH, and damage to the proximal intestinal mucosa by acid. In about 30% of patients the gastrinoma is associated with MEN-I. Gastrinomas are usually located in the pancreas but can also be located in the duodenum. Most gastrinomas are malignant at the time of diagnosis. In the past, the primary cause of death in patients with Zollinger-Ellison syndrome was complications of peptic ulcer disease, but with proper diagnosis and management this is no longer the case. Most patients now die of advanced metastatic disease.

Medullary carcinoma of the thyroid can occur alone or in association with MEN-II. Diarrhea is a common clinical presentation owing to the secretion of calcitonin and other peptides. Diarrhea is both secretory and associated with hypermotility of the intestine. Not all neuroendocrine tumors produce secretagogues that activate a true secretory diarrhea; some cause only mild diarrhea. Other endocrine causes of diarrhea are listed in Table 5-8.

Bacterial Toxins. Toxins elaborated by the bacteria that cause intestinal secretion are called enterotoxins. Cholera toxin is the classic bacterial secretagogue. It binds to the Gs protein of the adenylate cyclase complex, resulting in increased cytosolic cAMP levels and sustained secretion of chloride. A severe case of cholera can induce a secretory diarrhea of more than 10 L/day and rapidly progress to death if untreated. Cholera exemplifies the type of infection in which pathogenicity is primarily caused by bacterial colonization of the intestine and production of toxin. In contrast, other pathogenic bacteria such as *Shigella,* not only secrete an enterotoxin but also invade the mucosa of the intestine and cause cell damage. Other bacteria are pathogenic primarily through their invasiveness (Table 5-9). *Escherichia coli* is usually not a pathogenic bacteria in the intestine, but several pathogenic strains are well known. Enterotoxigenic *E. coli* is a noninvasive but toxin-producing strain of *E. coli* responsible for most of the diarrhea in developing countries and the associated morbidity and mortality of childhood diarrhea. It is also responsible for a large percentage of traveler's diarrhea or "Montezuma's revenge" experienced by travelers from the United States in developing countries. Other bacterial infections that express enterotoxins include those caused by *Clostridium difficile, Staphylococcus aureus, Campylobacter jejuni, Yersinia enterocolitica,* and the enterohemorrhagic *E. coli* strain O157:H7, which in 1993 killed several children in Oregon and Washington. Many of these bacterial toxins (e.g., *Clostridium difficile, E. coli* O157:H7) are cytotoxic and should also be listed in the section on mucosal damage as the mechanism of diarrhea (see page 95).

Food poisoning refers to the ingestion of contaminated food followed within

TABLE 5-8. *NEUROHUMORAL AGENTS THAT STIMULATE SECRETION*

AGONIST	MEDIATOR	DISEASE
Vasoactive intestinal polypeptide	cAMP	Pancreatic cholera
Serotonin	Calcium	Neural tumors
Calcitonin	Unknown	Carcinoid syndrome
Gastrin	? Calcium	Medullary thyroid carcinoma
Histamine	Unknown	Zollinger-Ellison syndrome
Adenosine	cAMP	Systemic mastocytosis
Cholinergic muscarinic agonists	Calcium	? Mesenteric ischemia
Secretin	cAMP	? Diabetic diarrhea
Substance P	Calcium	
Neurotensin	Calcium	
Cholecystokinin	Unknown	
Glucagon	Unknown	

From Kelley WN, ed. Textbook of Internal Medicine. Philadelphia: JB Lippincott, 1989:673.

TABLE 5-9. *CORRELATIONS BETWEEN PATHOPHYSIOLOGY AND SYMPTOMS OF INFECTIOUS DIARRHEA*

PATHOPHYSIOLOGY	MICROORGANISMS	SYMPTOMS
I. Preformed toxins (food poisonings)	*Bacillus cereus, Staphylococcus aureus, Clostridium perfringens, C. botulinum*	Nausea, vomiting, watery diarrhea, low-grade fever, mild–moderate pain
II. Enterotoxin production		
Adherent organisms:	*Vibrio cholerae*, enterotoxigenic *Escherichea coli*, *Klebsiella pneumoniae*	Watery diarrhea; may contain mucus (i.e., "rice water" stool), low-grade fever, mild–moderate pain
Invading organisms:	*Campylobacter, Aeromonas, Shigella*, noncholera *Vibrio*	Initially watery diarrhea, then bloody; high fever, severe pain
III. Invasive organisms		
Enterocyte invasion and destruction		
Minimal inflammation:	Rotavirus, Norwalk agent	Watery diarrhea and malabsorption, high fever, moderate pain
Severe inflammation:	*Shigella*, enteroinvasive *E. coli, Entamoeba histolytica Campylobacter, Salmonella, Aeromonas, ? Plesiomonas,*	Bloody diarrhea, high fever, severe pain
Mucosal penetration with multiplication in lamina propria and inflammation:	*Yersinia, V. parahaemolyticus* and *fulnificus, Mycobacterium avium- intracellulare* and *tuberculosis, Histoplasma*	Either watery or bloody diarrhea depending on degree of mucosal destruction, high fever, severe pain
IV. Attachment or colonization		
Local cytotoxin and inflammation:		
Adherent:	Enteropathogenic (enteroadherent) *E. coli, Giardia*, cryptosporidiosis, helminths, *Clostridium difficile*	Watery diarrhea, low–moderate fever, moderate–severe pain Usually watery diarrhea, occasionally bloody diarrhea, low–moderate fever, severe pain
Cytotoxic:	Enterohemorrhagic *E. coli*	Watery diarrhea for short time, then bloody diarrhea; low–moderate fever, severe pain
V. Systemic infection:	Hepatitis, listeriosis, legionellosis, Rocky Mountain spotted fever, psittacosis, otitis media in infants, toxic shock syndrome (*S. aureus*), measles	Watery diarrhea may be initially a part of disease or it may accompany disease; clinical manifestations are overwhelmingly those of the organs and tissues primarily involved by the organisms

From Yamada T, Alpers DH, Owyang C, Powell DW, Silverstein FE, eds. Textbook of Gastroenterology, 1st ed. Philadelphia: JB Lippincott, 1991:745.

hours by diarrhea and/or nausea and vomiting. Bacterial toxins can be ingested with food as preformed toxins (e.g., *Bacillus cereus*, *Staphylococcus aureus*) or the toxin can be made in vivo (e.g., *Clostridium perfringens*, *C. botulinum*, *E. coli* O157:H7) (Table 5-10).

Other. Amphipathic molecules such as bile acids and long-chain free fatty acids that escape absorption in the small bowel can cause secretion of fluid in the colon and result in diarrhea. The mechanism for this form of secretion is not completely clear but probably involves inflammatory mediators. Disease or surgical resection of the terminal ileum (as in Crohn's disease) can produce diarrhea as a result of malabsorbed bile acids and free fatty acid stimulation of the colon. In mild forms of disease or resection, bile acids are malabsorbed and enter the colon causing colonic secretion and ensuing diarrhea. With more extensive disease, such as the surgical removal of 100 cm of the terminal ileum, not only are bile acids malabsorbed but the bile salt pool is also diminished sufficiently to produce maldigestion of fat so that free fatty acids reach the colon and induce diarrhea. This is generally known as the "100-cm rule," i.e., if less than 100 cm of terminal ileum has been removed, the diarrhea is likely to be caused by bile acid malabsorption, and if more than 100 cm has been removed diarrhea will be exacerbated by long-chain fatty acid maldigestion. In other forms of steatorrhea, such as pancreatic insufficiency in which malabsorbed triglycerides reach the colon, bacteria in the colon hydrolyze the molecule to free fatty acids with ensuing diarrhea. Castor oil contains ricinoleic acid, a hydroxy fatty acid, which is the active agent and responsible for the catharsis induced by this product.

Some patients exhibiting secretory diarrhea of no apparent cause are surreptitious laxative abusers. These people can be quite ill, with weight loss, 10 to 20 bowel movements per day, and high stool volumes. Laxatives commonly used for this purpose are those that induce a secretory diarrhea such as phenolphthalein (Fenn-A-Mint), and anthraquinones such as senna, cascara, aloe, and rhubarb. Patients who, after extensive evaluation, have no identifiable cause for their secretory diarrhea are given a diagnosis of chronic idiopathic diarrhea if their stool volumes are less than 700 ml per day and pseudopancreatic cholera syndrome if their diarrhea is more than 700 ml per day.

MUCOSAL DAMAGE (LOSS OF VILLUS CELLS AND INFLAMMATION)

The architecture of the mucosa of the small intestine consists of villi and crypts (Fig. 5-9). Stem cells in the crypts produce enterocytes and other specialized epithelial cells that migrate up the cypt-villous axis as they become differentiated. As they continue to move up the villi, they become senescent and eventually slough off into the lumen. In humans migration of enterocytes takes about 3 to 5 days. Enterocytes in the villi are primarily absorptive and those in the crypts are primarily secretory so that, in conditions in which the villi are lost or damaged, the remaining intestinal mucosa is composed largely of crypts, and secretory diarrhea results. Because the damaged mucosa cannot absorb nutrients, eating produces an additional component of osmotic diarrhea. In conditions that are primarily inflammatory (e.g., certain infections, ulcerative colitis, or Crohn's disease), inflammatory cells act in two ways—by damaging enterocytes and by producing a large array of inflammatory mediators that induce secretion. The cytokines prostaglandin E_1, prostaglandin E_2, hydroxyeicosatetraenoic acid, and hydroxyperoxyeicosatetra-

TABLE 5-10. *PARTIAL LIST OF ETIOLOGIES OF CONFIRMED FOOD-BORNE OUTBREAKS OF GASTROENTERITIS REPORTED TO THE CENTERS FOR DISEASE CONTROL—1982*

ETIOLOGIC AGENT	% OUTBREAKS	% CASES
Bacterial		
Salmonella	25.0	18.6
S. aureus	12.7	6.0
Clostridium perfringens	10.0	10.8
Clostridium botulinum	9.5	0.3
Bacillus cereus	3.6	1.8
Shigella	1.8	1.1
Vibrio parahaemolyticus	1.4	0.4
Escherichia coli	0.9	0.4
Yersinia entercolitica	0.9	1.7
Vibrio cholerae	0.5	8.0
Campylobacter	0.9	0.3
Total for all bacterial pathogens	68.7	49.9
Viral		
Norwalk	0.9	45.2
(hepatitis A)	(8.5)	(2.9)
Chemical		
Ciguatoxin	3.6	0.3
Scombrotoxin	8.2	0.5
Shellfish	0.5	<0.1
Other	3.6	0.7

Etiology of Confirmed Water-Related (Intended for Drinking) Outbreaks of Gastroenteritis Reported to the Centers for Disease Control 1985

Giardia	20.0	48.3
Campylobacter	13.3	11.2
Staphylococcus typhi	6.7	1.8
Shigella	6.7	3.9
Virus	0.0	0.0
Unknown	53.3	34.8

Adapted from Centers for Disease Control. Food-borne disease outbreaks, annual summary, 1982. Atlanta: Centers for Disease Control, 1986; from St. Louis, ME. Water-related disease outbreaks, 1985 MMWR CDC Surveillance Summary 1988;37(55–2):15; and from Yamada T, Alpers DH, Owyang C, Powell DW, Silverstein FE, eds. Textbook of Gastroenterology, 2nd ed. Philadelphia: JB Lippincott, 1995:1609.

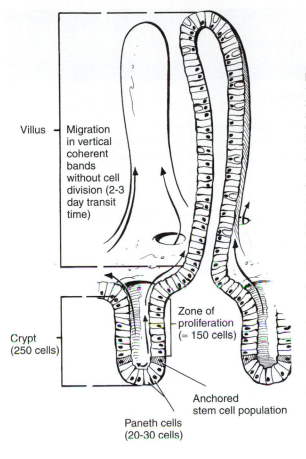

Villus

Migration
in vertical
coherent
bands
without cell
division (2-3
day transit
time)

Crypt
(250 cells)

Zone of
proliferation
(≈ 150 cells)

Paneth cells
(20-30 cells)

Anchored
stem cell population

Figure 5-9. Schematic representation of the crypt-villus relationship in the adult mouse small intestine. Six to fourteen crypts surround each villus base, less proximally and more distally in the ileum (horizontal gradient). The lower five cell positions contain a total of 40 to 50 cells with an average cycle time of 26 hours and with 20 to 30 nonproliferative Paneth's cells. Anchored stem cells exist at the fifth position with maximal rates of proliferation. Cells migrate from this position toward both the villus tip and the crypt base (the Paneth cells). The upper portion of the crypt contains proliferating cells that undergo upward migration; 275 cells are delivered to the villus base from each crypt. This migration occurs in strict vertical coherent bands toward the villus tip, where the cells are extruded. (Adapted from Yamada T, Alpers DH, Owyang C, Powell DW, Silverstein FE, eds. Textbook of Gastroenterology, 2nd ed. Philadelphia: JB Lippincott, 1995:562.)

enoic acid all have secretory effects on intestinal mucosa. Ischemia of the small bowel or colon results in epithelial death and damage. Bloody diarrhea is a common presentation of both ischemic colitis and radiation colitis. The term "colitis" in these two conditions is somewhat of a misnomer because the mechanism of injury is vascular rather than inflammatory. Conditions that result in mucosal damage are outlined in Table 5-11.

NONABSORBABLE INGESTION

Ingestion of nonabsorbable compounds and the resulting osmotic diarrhea constitute another broad category in the etiology of diarrheas. Agents such as milk of magnesia are easily identified as a cause of osmotic diarrhea. Other products such as magnesium-based antacids (e.g., Maalox or Mylanta) are not as obvious to the patient. Sorbitol in chewing gum and other dietetic foods is yet another possible cause of diarrhea. Most adults in the world are lactase-deficient. In humans, as in other mammals, lactase levels decline after weaning, and lactose becomes a relatively nonabsorbable compound. Lactose intolerance is a common cause of bloating, abdominal pain, and osmotic diarrhea.

TABLE 5-11. *CLASSIFICATION OF DIARRHEAS DUE TO BRUSH BORDER OR ENTEROCYTE DAMAGE/DEATH WITH INFLAMMATION*

I. With minimal to moderate inflammation
   A. Infections:
      Bacteria (enteroadherent or enteropathogenic *Escherichia coli*)
      Viruses (rotavirus and Norwalk agent, human immunodeficiency virus)
      Parasites (*Giardia, Cryptosporidium, Isospora, Ascaris, Trichinella*)
      Mixed organisms (tropical sprue, bacterial overgrowth)
   B. Cytostatic (anticancer) agents:
      Chemotherapy (mucositis)
      Radiation therapy (acute or chronic radiation enteritis, radiation sickness)
   C. Hypersensitivity:
      Nematode infestation, ? food allergy
   D. Idiopathic or autoimmune:
      Microscopic (lymphocytic) and collagenous colitis, Canada–Cronkhite syndrome,
      graft-versus-host disease
II. With moderate–severe inflammation ± ulceration
   A. Infections:
      Destruction of enterocytes (*Shigella,* enteroinvasive *E. coli, Entamoeba histolytica,*
      hookworm)
      Penetration of mucosa (*Salmonella, Campylobacter jejuni, Yersinia enterocolitica,
      Mycobacterium avium-intracellulare,* Whipple's disease)
   B. Hypersensitivity:
      Celiac sprue, milk or soybean protein hypersensitivity, eosinophilic gastroenteritis,
      nematode infestation (reinfection)
      Drug-induced colitis (gold, methyldopa)
   C. Idiopathic or autoimmune:
      Ulcerative colitis/proctitis, Crohn's disease, lymphoma

From Yamada T, Alpers DH, Owyang C, Powell DW, Silverstein FE, eds. Textbook of Gastroenterology, 1st
ed. Philadelphia: JB Lippincott, 1991:743.

MOTILITY

The human gastrointestinal tract is one of the largest muscle masses in the body. It is controlled by its own nervous system, the enteric nervous system, in conjunction with parasympathetic and sympathetic input. Gut motility is constant and finely regulated, although most people are completely unaware of the movements of their gastrointestinal tract. Altered motility, increased or decreased, can result in accompanying diarrhea or constipation. Many people suffer from frequent episodes of abdominal pain, bloating, alternating diarrhea and constipation, or any combination of symptoms. This condition is commonly known as *irritable bowel syndrome* (IBS) or functional bowel. The cause is unknown and the lack of any physical abnormalities or abnormal tests is characteristic. (Before lactase deficiency was understood as a cause of bloating and diarrhea, patients with lactose intolerance were given a diagnosis of functional bowel.) IBS is a functional disorder, but most investigators believe that these symptoms are caused by dysmotility of the gut. Functional bowel is important because these people represent a large percentage of the patients seen in any primary care practice despite the fact that most people with functional bowel symptoms do not seek medical attention. Approximately 10 to 30% of the population have symptoms of functional bowel. The "diarrhea" experienced by patients with IBS may not meet the criteria for diarrhea in that stool volumes are less than 250 ml, but it is nevertheless often their chief complaint.

Postsurgical Diarrhea. Patients who have had surgical procedures that disrupt the normal function of the pylorus and antrum such as pyloroplasty, vagotomy, gastrectomy, and antrectomy can develop diarrhea as a consequence of rapid gastric emptying known as dumping. Diarrhea is caused by the large volumes dumped into the duodenum with associated fluid shifts into the small bowel from plasma, dilution, and poor mixing of bile and pancreatic juices, stimulation of intestinal motility, and decreased transit time. Patients may have a more specific constellation of symptoms known as *dumping syndrome.* Early dumping syndrome occurs within an hour of eating, with symptoms of early satiety, nausea, diarrhea, bloating, and abdominal pain and possibly vasomotor symptoms of sweating, tachycardia, and flushing. These symptoms arise from dumping of large quantities of hypertonic chyme from the stomach or gastric remnant to the upper small intestine after meals. This results in distention of the upper intestine with reflex stimulation of motility; fluid shifts into the small bowel due to the osmotic load that may result in hypovolemia; and release of vasoactive substances including bradykinin, serotonin, and vasoactive intestinal peptide. Late dumping syndrome can occur in the next hour or two and consists of more symptoms of sweating, palpitations, weakness, confusion, and, rarely, loss of consciousness. The late dumping symptoms are caused by reactive hypoglycemia. During the initial dumping rapid absorption of carbohydrates results in an exaggerated release of insulin. This excess release of insulin outlasts the transient bolus of glucose, resulting in hypoglycemia. Postsurgical diarrhea has occasionally been reported after cholecystectomy, although the mechanism is unclear. Total colectomy results in diarrhea because the small bowel is not as efficient as the colon in removing water. The average ileostomy output after colectomy is 500 ml per day.

Fecal Impaction. Fecal impaction in elderly or demented patients may manifest as paradoxical diarrhea when unformed stool escapes around the area of impaction. Impaction can cause distention and a secretory diarrhea proximal to the site. Therefore in elderly hospitalized patients with diarrhea a good rectal, abdominal examination and, if necessary, abdominal x-ray films are particularly important.

DRUGS

Diarrhea is a side effect of numerous medications. The mechanism is obvious in some cases, such as magnesium-based antacids or oral phosphorus compounds such as Neutra-Phos but less obvious or unknown in other cases. Drugs that produce an osmotic diarrhea directly also include elixirs containing sorbitol, mannitol, or xylitol, lactulose, and Epsom salt. Drugs that cause a mild malabsorptive state from enterocyte damage and therefore osmotic and secretory activity include colchicine, quinidine, quinine, gold, and para-aminosalicylic acid. Other drugs that produce a secretory diarrhea include furosemide, thiazides, misoprostol (prostaglandin E_1), olsalazine (Dipentum), and ethanol. Drugs that have a secretory and/or motility component include cholinergic drugs, both acetylcholine analogues (pilocarpine, muscarine, metoclopramide) and cholinesterase inhibitors (neostigmine, edrophonium, physostigmine), erythromycin and arsenic, and methylxanthines such as theophylline and caffeine-containing compounds including chocolate. Cholestyramine is normally constipating, but with chronic use binding enough bile salts can lead to bile acid insufficiency and steatorrhea.

The rapid turnover of epithelial cells along the crypt-villous axis makes them particularly sensitive to the antimetabolic activity of cancer drugs. Mucosal damage can be minor with loss of brush border enzymes or extensive with sloughing and ulceration of much of the mucosal epithelium, depending on the drug and dose. Chemotherapeutic agents that cause severe diarrhea include cytosine arabinoside, amsacrine, mithramycin, doxorubicin, daunorubicin, actinomycin D, 6-mercaptopurine, and methotrexate.

Antibiotic-Associated Diarrhea and Antibiotic-Associated Colitis

Antibiotics commonly cause a mild form of diarrhea known as antibiotic-associated diarrhea. This type of diarrhea is not associated with inflammation of the colon, (as in colitis). Symptoms of antibiotic-associated diarrhea are milder than symptoms of colitis and usually develop several days after beginning antibiotic therapy and resolve 5 to 10 days after stopping. The cause is not clear but is probably related to changes in colonic flora. Antibiotic use can also lead to diarrhea and inflammation of the colon known as antibiotic-associated colitis. Antibiotic-associated colitis is most often caused by *Clostridium difficile*, which typically presents with mucosal destruction and pseudomembrane formation. *C. difficile* colitis is a severe, often life-threatening infection that can lead to toxic megacolon and death. Antibiotic-associated colitis is most commonly seen in patients who are taking antibiotics and/or are hospitalized and can arise after the first dose of antibiotics or months after a course of antibiotics is completed. Diagnosis of *C. difficile* colitis can be made presumptively based on the clinical presentation of diarrhea, abdominal pain, fever, and especially with the presence of pseudomembranes on sigmoidoscopic examination (Fig. 5-10), but a firm diagnosis requires the identifi-

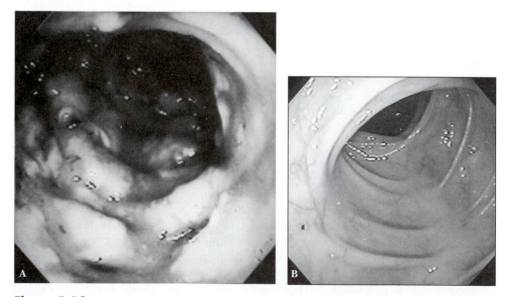

Figure 5-10. Pseudomembranous colitis. (**A**) Endoscopic view of the colon in a patient with pseudomembranous colitis. Note the patches of pseudomembranes throughout the lumen in addition to the edematous mucosa and loss of normal vascular pattern. (**B**) This figure shows the normal, smooth, mucosal pattern of the colon.

cation of *C. difficile* toxin in the stool. This is because *C. difficile* is commonly found in hospitalized patients or small children in the absence of toxin. Conversely, although colitis is not present in antibiotic-associated diarrhea, *C. difficile* toxin can be found in about 20% of cases, and in about 40% of cases stool cultures are positive for *C. difficile*.

Bacterial Overgrowth. Although the lumen of the stomach and small intestine is not sterile, the bacterial counts in the upper gut are low, in the range of 0 to 10^3 colony-forming units/ml. Conditions in which the normal flow of luminal contents is upset can lead to bacterial overgrowth and diarrhea. Bacteria in the gut can deconjugate bile acids and directly damage intestinal mucosa, and both effects can result in diarrhea owing to malabsorption and steatorrhea. Bacteria also compete for luminal vitamin B_{12}, which can result in vitamin B_{12} deficiency and macrocytic anemia. Overgrowth can occur, with impaired motility seen in scleroderma, diabetes mellitus, and idiopathic pseudo-obstruction. Surgical conditions are a common cause, especially when a "blind loop" is created, such as in the Billroth II procedure. Crohn's disease patients are susceptible to bacterial overgrowth because of the formation of enteroenteric fistulas, stricture formation, and partial obstruction or loss of the ileocolic valve after ileal resection. A more complete list of conditions that can lead to bacterial overgrowth is provided in Table 5-12.

CLINICAL TESTING

Stool Electrolytes

The osmolality of diarrheal stool is generally found to be the same as that of serum, i.e., 290 mOsm/kg H_2O. In secretory diarrhea the osmotic activity of stool is the result of stool electrolytes, whereas in osmotic diarrhea the osmotic activity of the stool derives in large part from malabsorbed food or some other osmotically active substance. Therefore measurement of stool electrolytes can help to distinguish between secretory and osmotic diarrheas. A liquid stool sample is spun down to remove solid material and sent to the laboratory to determine stool osmolality, Na^+, and K^+ concentrations. The major solutes in luminal secretions are Na^+, K^+, Cl^-, and HCO_3^-; therefore, the osmotic activity of secretory diarrhea should equal approximately $2 \times ([Na^+] + [K^+])$. This formula is derived from the fact that Na^+ and K^+ represent most of the cationic activity in stool, and since anionic activity must equal the cationic activity, doubling the sum should equal total ion activity (see Fig. 5-3). In an osmotic diarrhea a portion of the osmotic activity of the stool is contributed by some other unmeasured molecule and therefore the electrolyte osmotic activity should be significantly less than the actual osmotic activity (Table 5-13).

Stool osmolality is often not measured because it can usually be assumed that it approximates 290 mOsm/kg H_2O. Measuring stool osmolality, however, can be informative with regard to the reliability of the stool sample and can reveal possible tampering. Stool osmolality significantly less than 290 mOsm/kg H_2O indicates that the stool specimen has been diluted, either with water or unconcentrated urine. A stool osmolality significantly greater than 290 mOsm/kg H_2O may be the result of contamination with concentrated urine. In old specimens bacteria can increase the osmolality through normal metabolism. Such findings may indicate that the specimen has been altered to give the appearance of diarrhea, as can be seen in patients with factitious diarrhea. About 15% of patients referred to tertiary med-

TABLE 5-12.	*CONDITIONS ASSOCIATED WITH BACTERIAL OVERGROWTH*

Postsurgical Conditions

Billroth II anastomses (afferent limb overgrowth)
Jejunoileal bypass
Gastrectomy
Vagotomy and pyloroplasty
Adhesions (strictures leading to partial obstruction)
Resection of ileocecal valve

Motor Dysfunction

Diabetic autonomic neuropathy
Scleroderma
Intestinal pseudo-obstruction
Medications (opiates, antimotility agents)

Structural Abnormalities

Strictures
    Postsurgical (anastomotic)
    Crohn's disease
    Radiation enteritis
    Small bowel stenosis
    Nonsteroidal antiinflammatory drug induced stricture
Fistulas
    Postsurgical
    Crohn's disease
    Gallstone induced
    Foreign-body induced (e.g., PEG tube)
Small bowel diverticula
Malrotation

Hypochlorhydria

Atrophic gastritis
Medications (e.g., omeprazole)
Vagotomy
Partial gastrectomy

Malabsorptive conditions

Celiac sprue
Crohn's disease
Protein-calorie malnutrition

Primary immunodeficiencies

TABLE 5-13. *STOOL OSMOTIC GAP AS A GUIDE TO THE PATHOPHYSIOLOGY OF DIARRHEA*

Stool osmolality or 290 mOsm/kg H_2O – 2 [Na + K] mmol/L	=	Stool osmotic gap
Stool [Na] > 90 mmol/L and Osmotic gap < 50 mOsm/kg H_2O	=	Secretory diarrhea; rarely, osmotic diarrhea due to Na_2SO_4 or Na_2PO_4 ingestion*
Stool [Na] < 60 mmol/L and Osmotic gap > 100 mOsm/kg H_2O	=	Osmotic diarrhea; if stool volume does not return to normal on fast, suspect surreptitious Mg ingestion†
Stool [Na] > 150 mmol/L and Stool osmolality > 375–400 mOsm/Kg H_2O	=	Suspect contamination of specimen with concentrated urine
Stool osmolality < 200–250 mOsm/ Kg H_2O	=	Suspect contamination of specimen with dilute urine or water

*Normal stool SO_4 and PO_4 levels are usually < 5 mmol; exact values not established.
†Normal stool Mg on regular diet is 20–50 mmol/L; on fast, the concentration should be less than 10 mmol/L. Exact values not well established.
From Yamada T, Alpers DH, Owyang C, Powell DW, Silverstein FE, eds. Textbook of Gastroenterology, 2nd ed. Philadelphia: JB Lippincott, 1995:820.

ical centers for diarrhea are found to have factitious diarrhea, usually induced by surreptitious laxative abuse.

Small Bowel Perfusion Study

A definitive test to identify whether the small bowel is in a net absorptive state as it should be or a net secretory state is done in specialized medical centers. This is accomplished by placing a tube in the small intestine and instilling a known amount of Na^+, Cl^-, HCO_3^{2-} solution in a proximal port and then collecting luminal aspirates from two distal ports. Polyethylene glycol (PEG), which is not absorbed, is also infused and collected in the distal aspirates as a marker of fluid absorption. Because PEG is neither secreted nor absorbed, changes in the luminal concentration reflect the movements of fluid into or out of the lumen. By knowing the amount of PEG placed in the proximal port and collected in the distal ports, it can be calculated whether the amount of electrolytes collected in the distal ports represents net secretion or net absorption of electrolytes by that portion of the small bowel.

For each electrolyte the net secretion can be calculated from the following formula, with positive values representing net secretion and negative values representing net absorption:

$$\text{Secretion rate of } Na^+ (\text{mmol/hr}) = ([Na^+]_{OUT} - [Na^+]_{IN}) \times [PEG]_{IN} / [PEG]_{OUT} \times \text{perfusion rate (ml/hr)}$$

An advantage of this method is that patients with chronic secretory diarrhea can be tested for response to drugs to see what medication is most likely to help them. For example, somatostatin can be given after determining that a secretory state exists in the small bowel, and repeating the study may show that bowel is now in a net absorptive state.

Fecal Fat

Fecal fat is a measure of luminal digestion and mucosal absorption. Stool fat is measured either qualitatively as a stool spot check (Sudan stain) or quantitatively as a 72° fecal fat collection. The 72° fecal fat collection is the most definitive test for the diagnosis of maldigestion. This is performed by placing the patient on a 100 g fat/day diet to ensure an adequate fat load for the intestine to absorb and then collecting all stools for 72 hours in a paint can. The stool is collected over 3 days to overcome the normal variation that can be seen in bowel habits. Total fat concentration is determined and reported as grams/100 g wet weight/24 hours. Normal stool fat is less than 7 g. Most of this fat is endogenous phospholipids from bile, sloughed enterocytes, bacteria, and other sources rather than dietary triglycerides. Steatorrhea can be seen in either mucosal disease or pancreatic disease, but stool concentration of fat greater than 10 g is more common in pancreatic disease.

β-Carotene/D-Xylose

Compounds that are absorbed directly by intestinal mucosa without undergoing luminal digestion are used to determine if mucosal absorption is intact. Measuring serum β-carotene is a useful test of mucosal integrity. Normal levels suggest normal mucosal absorption. Low levels suggest mucosal disease but can also be seen in pancreatic disease and malnutrition. The D-xylose test is a more specific test of mucosal absorption. This five-carbon sugar is absorbed in the duodenum and jejunum. It is poorly metabolized and therefore much of it is secreted into the urine. After an overnight fast, patients are given 25 g of D-xylose orally. A serum sample is taken at 2 hours and urine is collected for 5 hours to determine D-xylose levels. Normal serum levels should be 30 mg/dl or higher and more than 4.5 g should be excreted in the urine. Abnormal levels suggest mucosal malabsorption.

Hydrogen Breath Test

A wide array of breath tests are available for the diagnosis of diarrhea, but the most widely used is the hydrogen breath test. Here oral glucose is given to the patient, and breath hydrogen is measured before and after ingestion. A high baseline (before glucose) breath hydrogen is suggestive of bacterial overgrowth. In the normal individual oral glucose is completely absorbed in the small intestine and no increase in breath hydrogen is seen. If significant numbers of bacteria are in the small intestine, however, some of the glucose will be metabolized, hydrogen liberated, absorbed into the circulation, and ultimately exhaled. Breath samples are taken every 30 minutes for 3 hours and hydrogen is reported as parts per million.

Sigmoidoscopic Examination

In patients who appear ill and have any risk factors for *Clostridium difficile* colitis, flexible sigmoidoscopic examination can provide a rapid diagnosis of pseudomembranous colitis. However, a negative examination would not exclude the diagnosis, since pseudomembranes may not be evident or may be located beyond the reach of the sigmoidoscope. Sigmoidoscopy can also be helpful in examining the distal colon for evidence of ulcerative colitis, *Entamoeba histolytica* infection, ischemic colitis, lymphocytic colitis, or collagenous colitis. However, in most of these cases a more complete examination of the colon may be needed to completely exclude these diseases.

Neuroendocrine Screen

If neuroendocrine tumor is a diagnosis being considered in a patient with diarrhea, serum neuroendocrine hormone levels can be obtained either individually or as part of a screening profile. In patients with peptic ulcer disease, especially if the ulcers are present in the second part of the duodenum (beyond the bulb), obtaining a serum gastrin level is mandatory. For other high-volume secretory diarrheas of unclear etiology, a neuroendocrine panel consisting of vasoactive intestinal peptide, gastrin, somatostatin, pancreatic polypeptide, motilin, and substance P can be obtained from a reference laboratory. These hormone levels are measured by radioimmunoassay.

Stool Culture/Ova and Parasites

Fresh stool specimens are cultured to look for important stool bacterial pathogens and are often obtained in the evaluation of diarrhea, but the return of useful information is usually minimal. Stool culture is most helpful in those with evidence of inflammatory diarrhea (bloody stool or fecal leukocytes present) of an acute nature. Bacterial infection is rarely a cause of chronic diarrhea, and therefore stool cultures usually do not provide helpful information in the evaluation of chronic diarrhea. However, in patients who have had a more prolonged course of symptoms or more severe symptoms, identification of bacterial pathogens is important in deciding appropriate treatment. The pathogens routinely checked for on stool cultures include *Salmonella, Shigella, Campylobacter,* and possibly *Yersinia,* depending on the patient's location. Pathogenic strains of *Escherichia coli* are not routinely sought but can be obtained on request. *C. difficile,* the causative agent in most cases of pseudomembranous colitis (antibiotic-associated colitis), is cultured separately. This pathogen should always be checked for in any patient recently on antibiotics or discharged from the hospital, and especially in patients who develop diarrhea while in the hospital. Patients are routinely tested for the presence of *C. difficile* by culture and the presence of *C. difficile* toxin by enzyme-linked immunosorbent assay or a cytotoxic assay. *C. difficile* toxin is required to make the diagnosis of *C. difficile* colitis because culturing *C. difficile* is a relatively nonspecific finding; it is found in many hospitalized patients and many patients taking antibiotics. Microscopic stool examination for ova and parasites is done on either fresh stool specimens or preserved specimens and is usually done in triplicate. The pathogens most commonly seen in the United States are the protozoa *Giardia lamblia, Entamoeba histolytica,* and *Cryptosporidium. Strongyloides sterocoralis* is also seen, especially in the Southern states. The yield of stool parasite examination usually correlates with the patient's travel history.

CASE PRESENTATION

A.T. is a 55-year-old male who was well until 4 months prior to hospital admission, when he began having two to three loose stools per day. There was no blood in his stool and other people in his neighborhood were experiencing diarrhea, so he refrained from seeking medical attention. However, family

members were not having diarrhea. The diarrhea progressed over the next few months to four to six watery loose stools per day. He treated himself by taking in less fluids and started taking psyllium to decrease his diarrhea, but these measures were not helpful. His diarrhea progressed to 10 bowel movements per day, which were of large volume and frequently got him up at night. He began experiencing fevers to 101.0°F and chills. His family physician admitted him to the hospital for further evaluation. His major complaint on admission was extreme fatigue and a 40-lb weight loss. The patient did not have any complaints of nausea, vomiting, hematochezia, or melena. He did not have complaints of back pain, joint pain, rashes, or eye problems. He had never had colitis or diarrhea before. He had traveled to northern Michigan on camping vacations and used well water at home. Over the summer he was treated for a presumed sinus infection with ampicillin, but he had not been taking any medications recently.

On admission the patient was found to be markedly hypotensive and hypovolemic. His temperature was 98.0°F, pulse 110 beats/minute, respiration 20 breaths/minute, and blood pressure 82/40 mmHg. On physical examination his oral mucosa was dry and his liver was palpable 5 cm below the costal margin in the midclavicular line. His admitting laboratory evaluation revealed a hemoglobin 19, hematocrit 55%, white blood cells 11,000 cells/cu mm with a normal differential count, sodium 135, potassium 2.5, HCO_3 8, blood urea nitrogen 44, creatine 1.7, glucose 148, calcium 14.2, phosphorus 4.3, protein 8.4, albumin 4.7, alanine transaminase 62, aspartate transaminase 54, alkaline phosphatase 113, total bilirubin 0.7. He was transferred to the intensive care unit for aggressive fluid and electrolyte resuscitation. He went on to have an extensive evaluation, including:

Stool volume: 6 L/24 h
Stool electrolytes: Na^+ 56 mEq/L, K^+ 80 mEq/L, Cl^- 99 mEq/L

Stool Gram's stain: no fecal leukocytes
Stool culture: negative; stool for ova and parasites: negative.

Barium swallow and small bowel follow-through: normal
Barium enema: normal

Esophagogastroduodenoscopy: erythema of the antrum but no evidence of ulcers; normal duodenum and esophagus

Colonoscopy: normal

Gastrin: 124 pg/ml

This patient developed watery diarrhea in the summer; it was not bloody or causing other systemic problems. He knew that other members of his community were having diarrhea, and he was not concerned. At this point in his illness he was having *acute* nonbloody diarrhea without fever, and therefore from a medical point of view there was not much concern or the need to begin a diagnostic evaluation. The most likely diagnosis at this time was viral infection. As the patient's illness progressed, it became clear to him that he had a problem. He still had no systemic complaints except that the diarrhea was interfering with his sleep. Later on his diarrhea became even more severe, with 10 large volume bowel movements a day, and he developed severe fatigue and fever. He saw his personal physician, who found him to be extremely dehydrated and immediately hospitalized him. The patient now has chronic diarrhea, and from the history it is clear that it is a noninflammatory diarrhea. His diarrhea has never been bloody; he had not had fever or much abdominal discomfort throughout his illness except at the very end, when he was extremely ill, hypotensive, and hypovolemic. Therefore, causes of diarrhea that are primarily inflammatory, such as infection with *Shigella* or *Campylobacter* or Crohn's disease or ulcerative colitis, are unlikely. The patient was recently on antibiotics; therefore pseudomembranous colitis should be considered despite the lack of systemic symptoms. The patient began by having a few large volume stools per day, progressing to more frequent large volume. This would suggest that the small bowel is involved more than the colon. Generally, stool volumes greater than a liter are of small bowel origin and volumes less than a liter are of colonic origin. Remember that large fluid volumes pass through the small bowel. If normal absorption through the small bowel is decreased by 50%, about 5 L of fluid would be delivered to the colon rather than the usual 1.5 L, and this would overwhelm the normal absorptive capacity of the colon. In secretory small bowel diarrhea the volume reaching the colon can be extremely high (up to 20 L/day). Small bowel diarrheal bowel movements are often reported as being large volume but smaller in number. Diarrheas involving primarily the large intestine often involve inflammation or colitis. People with colitis, especially of the sigmoid colon and rectum, frequently complain of having numerous bowel movements per day of small volume. These patients often have a sense of incomplete defecation, that is, after a bowel movement they still feel like they have to go. They may also complain of tenesmus and urgency, feeling like they have to run to the bathroom to avoid an accident.

On admission the patient's physical examination and serum chemistry results were consistent with dehydration and hypovolemia. He was tachycardic at rest and orthostatic, suggesting at least a 20% loss of intravascular volume. He had an elevated blood urea nitrogen level and creatinine with a ratio >20:1. Patients suffering from dehydration and hypovolemia from lack of oral intake (rather than diarrhea) are more likely to develop a contraction alkalosis, but this patient was acidotic with a low serum bicarbonate concentration, suggesting HCO_3 loss in the stool. His low serum K^+ was also most likely from stool loss. The elevated calcium level was most likely caused by dehydration, but it raised the possibility of medullary carcinoma of the thyroid or another MEN tumor. The microscopic stool examination did not show fecal leukocytes or blood. Although this does not exclude an inflammatory cause of the diarrhea, it is consistent with the other features pointing away from an inflammatory process. Fecal leukocytes are helpful when present but can be misleading when results are negative. About half of patients with pseudomembranous colitis do not have fecal leukocytes on stool examination. The patient's stool electrolyte levels were quite helpful: $2 \times (Na^+\ 56\ mEq/L + K^+\ 80\ mEq/L) = 272\ mOsmol/L$. Therefore, all the osmotic activity could be accounted for by the stool electrolytes, confirming that this is a pure secretory diarrhea; and since the patient is putting out about 6 L of stool per day, this is a small bowel secretory diarrhea.

Looking over the patient history, it was noted that he had been camping in Michigan and drinking well water. *Giardia* is a common parasite in many places in the United States and is often found in hikers and campers. *Giardia* is a small bowel parasite that produces watery diarrhea and abdominal bloating. Since *Giardia* colonizes the small intestine, stool examination for the trophozoites or cysts is often negative, being found in only about half of cases. However, *Giardia* does not cause this profound a diarrhea. Toxin-forming bacteria like those causing cholera can be a cause of profound secretory diarrhea, but most bacterial infections are self-limited and do not drag on over such a prolonged period with worsening diarrhea. The patient's low serum potassium concentration coupled with the prolonged and worsening high volume nature of his illness is a clue, suggesting the possibility of a VIPoma. The patient's elevated serum calcium level suggests that this may not only be a neuroendocrine tumor but may be part of a MEN syndrome. The patient had mildly elevated transaminase levels on admission, which at that low level are nonspecific findings; however, he also had an enlarged palpable liver on admission. This would suggest the possibility of liver metastasis from a primary VIP-secreting neuroendocrine tumor.

A computed tomographic scan of the abdomen was obtained, which showed several low attenuation masses (1 to 2 cm) in the body and tail of the pancreas and multiple low attenuation masses throughout the liver. Fine-needle aspiration of the liver showed positive findings for neoplastic cells consistent with neuroendocrine tumor. Serum vasoactive intestinal polypeptide levels were 3337 pg/ml (normal is 0 to 50 pg/ml).

This patient was started on a long-acting somatostatin analogue resulting in marked improvement of his diarrhea. He then underwent a noncurative debulking operation for removal of most of the body and tail of his pancreas. His serum vasoactive intestinal polypeptide level returned to normal after this operation, but because of the metastatic nature of his disease he was expected to have a relapse in the future. Evaluation of his thyroid gland was unremarkable, and his serum calcium level returned to normal after rehydration.

SUMMARY

In any given patient presenting with diarrhea, the diagnostic possibilities are vast. To identify the cause requires an understanding of the pathophysiology of diarrhea, or the physician will be lost in a forest of possibilities with no idea as to which direction to proceed in. Applying basic concepts of gastrointestinal physiology should allow many possible diagnoses to be eliminated and several diagnoses to be considered more likely. It should also allow for an intelligent approach to evaluating and treating the patient with diarrhea.

SELECTED READING

Dobbins J. Approach to the patient with diarrhea. In: Kelley WN, ed. Textbook of Internal Medicine. Philadelphia: JB Lippincott, 1989:669–680.

Gianella RA. Gastrointestinal infections. In: Kelley WN, ed. Textbook of Internal Medicine. Philadelphia: JB Lippincott, 1989:554–562.

Powell DW. Approach to the patient with diarrhea. In: Yamada T, Alpers DH, Owyang C, Powell DW, Silverstein FE, eds. Textbook of Gastroenterology, 2nd ed. Philadelphia: JB Lippincott, 1995:813–863.

Lippincott's Pathophysiology Series: Gastrointestinal Pathophysiology, edited by Joseph M. Henderson. Lippincott–Raven Publishers. Philadelphia © 1996.

CHAPTER

6

Malabsorption

John M. Carethers

Digestion and absorption are often taken for granted until a problem arises with the process of breaking down and assimilating food. An understanding of the normal mechanisms of digestion and absorption is necessary in order to understand the disease processes that lead to malabsorption.

Malabsorption is a syndrome characterized by disordered or inadequate absorption of nutrients from the intestinal tract. Malabsorption can be caused by diseases affecting the stomach, small intestine, liver, or pancreas. Examples include postsurgical states such as gastric resection and intestinal bypass or resection, intestinal mucosal lesions such as tropical sprue or gluten-sensitive enteropathy (celiac or nontropical sprue), and pancreatic insufficiency. The patient afflicted with malabsorption often experiences weight loss and foul-smelling stools as well as vitamin deficiencies. Malabsorption can lead to death if the disease process is not reversed or compensated for by nutritional supplementation.

This chapter focuses on the normal processes of absorption and nutrient assimilation. Symptoms of malabsorption are discussed, and common clinical entities of malabsorption are highlighted.

PATHOPHYSIOLOGY

DIGESTION

Mastication and Salivary Secretion

Mastication (chewing) is the process by which large food particles are physically ground to smaller particles in the oral cavity, thus increasing the total surface area for the subsequent action by digestive juices. The temporomandibular joint (TMJ) is important for this action, as are the grinding surfaces provided for by the teeth. Diseases affecting the TMJ, such as rheumatoid arthritis, can interfere with this process. Patients who have severe TMJ disease or are edentulous often must restrict their diet to soft foods. Unless their diet is well balanced, nutritional deficiencies can occur.

Salivary secretion is necessary for lubrication, which is extremely important for swallowing. This is accomplished by mucins, glycoproteins present in the saliva that coat the food. Saliva also contains salivary amylase (ptyalin), which plays a very minor role in carbohydrate digestion. These secretions also facilitate speech, act as a solvent for molecules that stimulate taste buds, keep the mouth and teeth clean by preventing bacterial accumulation, and act as a bicarbonate buffer that keeps oral pH at about 7.0. Control of salivary secretion is primarily neural (autonomic nervous system), although hormones such as estrogens, androgens, glucocorticoids, and peptide hormones exert some control over secretion. The most potent stimulation for salivary secretion is taste. Salivation is inhibited during sleep. Salivary secretions total approximately 1500 ml/day, and 90% of saliva comes from the parotid and submandibular glands (Figs. 6-1A and B). Parotid secretions tend to be serous (low in organic elements), whereas the submandibular gland tends to secrete mixed serous and mucus saliva.

Saliva is secreted by acinar cells and modified by ductal cells in the salivary gland (Fig. 6-2). The acini, with Na^+/K^+ adenosine triphosphatase (ATPase) on the basolateral aspect of each cell, actively secrete potassium and bicarbonate and passively secrete chloride into the lumen. The ductal cells modify the saliva by reabsorbing chloride and sodium with the aid of basolateral Na^+/K^+ ATPase, while secreting bicarbonate and potassium. The final saliva contains bicarbonate and water and is hypotonic. Rates of secretion and hormonal influences can modify the final composition of saliva.

Xerostomia is a symptom caused by lack of salivary secretion. Medications such as antidepressants, through their anticholinergic effect, are the most common cause of xerostomia. Diseases that affect the salivary glands, such as Sjögren's disease or radiation damage during therapy for head and neck tumors, can also

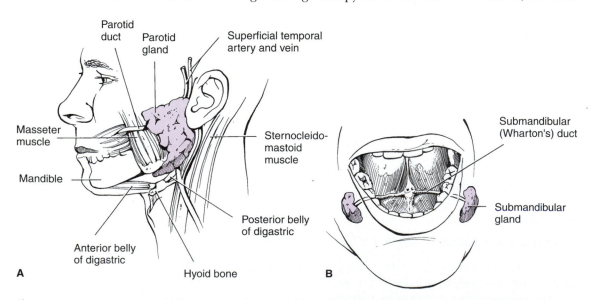

Figure 6-1. Location of parotid (**A**) and submandibular salivary glands (**B**). (Adapted from Akesson EJ, Loeb JA, Wilson-Pauwels L, eds. Thompson's Core Textbook of Anatomy, 2nd ed. Philadelphia: JB Lippincott, 1990:335, 370.)

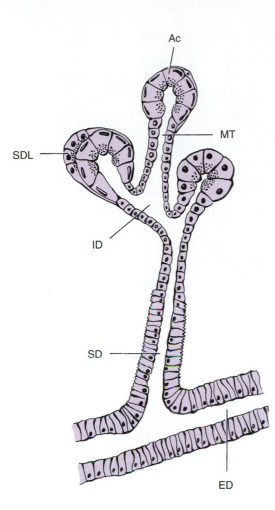

Figure 6-2. Diagrammatic representation of the secretory endpieces and duct system of the human submandibular gland. In this gland the end pieces may be seromucous acini (Ac) or mucous tubules (MT) with seromucous demilunes (SDL). Both types of end pieces are drained by relatively large intercalated ducts (ID), striated ducts (SD), and excretory ducts (ED). (Adapted from Johnson LR, ed. Physiology of the Gastrointestinal Tract, 2nd ed. New York: Raven Press, 1987:774.)

cause xerostomia. Xerostomia leads to dysfunction of speech, taste, and swallowing as a result of loss of the saliva's lubricating function.

Gastric Acid and Pepsin: Grinding and Sieving

The stomach receives masticated food via the esophagus, and then chemically and physically breaks down the food particles into a liquid mixture (chyme) in preparation for processing and absorption by the small intestine. These steps are accomplished by two remarkable processes that coordinate stomach digestion: secretion of acid and pepsinogen to begin the chemical process of digestion, and grinding and sieving by the stomach driven by specialized muscle layers to physically break down particles. The stomach also secretes intrinsic factor, which is a necessary cofactor for vitamin B_{12} absorption. Gastrin, a peptide hormone released by G cells in the gastric antrum, aids in stimulating acid secretion.

Hydrochloric acid secretion is achieved by the parietal cell located primarily in the fundus and body of the stomach. Parietal cells are microscopically located in the neck of oxyntic glands (Fig. 6-3) along with mucus-secreting cells. Oxyntic glands extend into the lamina propria from a microscopic gastric pit and secrete their contents into the lumen of the stomach. The parietal cell secretes acid via an active transport mechanism, the H^+/K^+ ATPase on its apical membrane (Fig. 6-4),

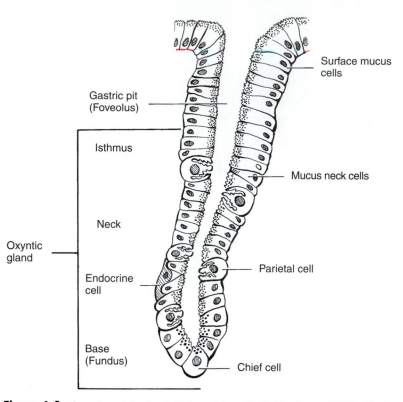

Figure 6-3. Oxyntic gastric gland. (Adapted from Ito S, Winchester RJ. The final structure of the gastric mucosa in the bat. J Cell Biol, 16:541, 1963, from Yamada T, Alpers DH, Owyang C, Powell DW, Silverstein FE, eds. Textbook of Gastroenterology, 2nd ed. Philadelphia: JB Lippincott, 1995;1:297.)

and pumps hydrogen ion out of and potassium ion into the cell. Hydrochloric acid is secreted at a pH of 0.8 from the parietal cell, which has an intracellular pH of 7.2. For each hydrogen ion secreted, a hydroxyl ion (OH^-) is generated that reacts with CO_2 (catalyzed by carbonic anhydrase) to form bicarbonate (and water). Intracellular bicarbonate is exchanged for extracellular chloride at the basolateral membrane, which provides a pool of chloride for transport out of the apical membrane; this, along with hydrogen ion, produces isotonic HCl. The stomach secretes approximately 2 L of fluid per day. Although acid is not absolutely necessary for digestion, it provides a low pH for initiation of protein digestion and iron absorption and acts as a protective barrier against ingested microorganisms.

Stimulation of acid is under both neural and humoral control (Fig. 6-5) and is traditionally divided into three phases initiated by the physiologic stimulus of food. These phases refer to the site of origin, not mechanisms by which acid is stimulated or inhibited. The cephalic phase is caused by the sight, smell, and taste of food and produces stomach acid by virtue of the action of the vagus nerve on parietal cells. The gastric phase leads to acid production by physiologic distention of the stomach by the food bolus as sensed by stretch receptors present in the stomach wall and a reflex arc involving the vagus nerve. The gastric phase is also influenced by specific components of food (peptides/amino acids, caffeine, ethanol,

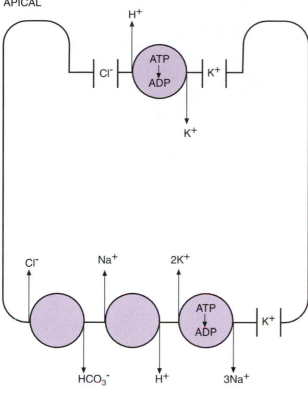

APICAL

BASOLATERAL

Figure 6-4. Ion transport pathways in parietal cells. The apical membrane contains the H$^+$, K$^+$-ATPase pump as well as K$^+$ and Cl$^-$ conductances. The basolateral membrane also has a K$^+$ conductance as well as Cl$^-$/HCO$_3$$^-$ exchanges, Na$^+$/H$^+$ exchanges, and Na$^+$, K$^+$-ATPases to maintain cellular homeostasis during secretory and resting states. (Adapted from Yamada T, Alpers DH, Owyang C, Powell DW, Silverstein FE, eds. Textbook of Gastroenterology, 2nd ed. Philadelphia: JB Lippincott, 1995;1:312.)

and calcium), which stimulate release of the peptide hormone gastrin, the principal mediator of postprandial gastric acid secretion. The intestinal phase of acid secretion may be caused by circulating absorbed amino acids and wall distention when chyme enters the small intestine.

Pepsinogen is produced by chief cells, located in the base of oxyntic glands in the fundus and body of the stomach. Pepsinogen is stored in zymogen granules and is released into the lumen when stimulated by vagal (acetylcholine) input and possibly by peptide hormones such as gastrin and cholecystokinin (CCK). Pepsinogen is autocatalytically cleaved in the acid environment of the stomach to pepsin, a protease with optimal activity at acid pH, and initiates protein digestion, especially the breakdown of collagen. Peptides produced by pepsin cleavage of proteins stimulate gastrin and CCK production, thus initiating the coordinated digestive response necessary for nutrient absorption. In addition, the acid chyme released into the small intestine stimulates not only CCK but also secretin, a hormone important in stimulating secretion of bicarbonate-rich biliary and pancreatic juices. Gastric lipase secreted in the fundus of the stomach may also have a limited catabolic action on ingested lipids.

The stomach also functions in the storage and mixing of food. The stomach wall contains smooth muscle organized in outer longitudinal, median circular, and inner oblique layers. The circular layer predominates throughout, and the distal body and antrum of the stomach have thicker muscle compared with the proximal

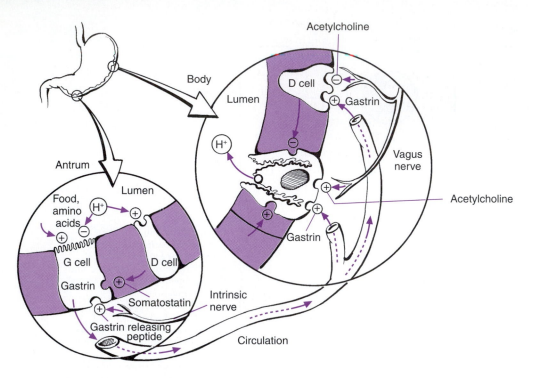

Figure 6-5. Regulation of gastric acid secretion. Major gastric mucosal ligand–receptor interactions regulating parietal cell HCl secretion are shown. *D cell*, somatostatin cell; *G cell*, gastrin cell. (Adapted from Feldman M. Acid and gastrin secretion in duodenal ulcer disease. Regul Pept Lett 1:1, 1989 and Yamada T, Alpers DH, Owyang C, Powell DW, Silverstein FE, eds. Textbook of Gastroenterology, 2nd ed. Philadelphia: JB Lippincott, 1995;1:308.)

stomach. This is important for the way the stomach physically handles food. When food distends the esophagus or there is mechanical stimulation of the throat, the proximal stomach (fundus and body) relaxes in order to receive the masticated food (receptive relaxation). This is a vagally-mediated event. Distention of the stomach beyond a threshold volume initiates antral peristaltic contractions, which propel the food toward the pylorus and duodenum. Digestible solids are reduced to particles smaller than 1 mm for further efficient digestion in the small intestine. The increased surface area-to-mass ratio generated by stomach grinding facilitates enzymatic attack on the minute particles once inside the small intestine. Selective retention of larger particles (gastric sieving) until they are smaller prevents poor overall absorption of nutrients. Gastric sieving and grinding are achieved when muscular antral contractions forcefully propel chyme toward the pylorus but also move chyme forcefully backward with the closure of the pylorus at the end of an antral contraction. This turbulence is sufficient to break down the larger particles as they are retropelled but allows smaller (≤1 mm) particles through into the duodenum. Meals that are more nutrient-rich are delayed from exiting the stomach by an enterogastric reflex arc, presumably to allow thorough breakdown for proper small intestinal absorption. Carbohydrate-rich meals exit the stomach the fastest, followed by protein and then fat meals. Hyperosmolar meals are delayed from emptying from the stomach via intestinal feedback inhibition. Liquid meals emptied from the stomach are proportional to the volume of the meal, called "first-order" kinetics. Liquid emptying in general precedes solid emptying from the stomach. The emptying of solids follows a sigmoidal time course. There is often an initial lag period, followed by a prolonged linear phase, and then a much slower phase. Since the linear phase is independent of the meal volume, solid emptying follows "zero-order" kinetics. The antrum, pylorus, and duodenum function as a unit rather than individually to empty the stomach. Contraction is sequential from the antrum to the pylorus to the duodenum (aboral). Even if the pylorus is surgically resected (pyloroplasty), gastric emptying is often normal. Denervation of the proximal stomach may accelerate liquid emptying without much effect on solids; however, denervating the antrum as well as the proximal stomach accelerates liquid emptying while slowing solid emptying.

Biliary Secretions

Bile is made by hepatocytes and accounts for 500 ml/day of total intestinal secretions. Bile contains bile salts, bile pigments, cholesterol and other lipids, and alkaline phosphatase. Important for fat absorption are the bile salts, the sodium and potassium salts of bile acids. These salts are conjugated to taurine or glycine, enhancing their hydrophilicity and stability in the small intestine, and have structures similar to that of cholesterol. Hepatocytes make cholic acid and chenodeoxycholic acid, the primary bile acids, but intestinal bacteria can modify these to make the secondary bile acids deoxycholic, lithocholic, and ursodeoxycholic acids. When secreted out of the bile duct and sphincter of Oddi all bile acids combine spontaneously with ingested lipids and fat-soluble vitamins to form micelles, water-soluble complexes from which lipids can be more easily absorbed. The formation of micelles is stabilized by the presence of phospholipids and monoglycerides in the intestinal lumen. These lipids reduce the surface tension of the micelle. Micelles emulsify ingested lipids and increase the surface area for enzyme hydrolysis in preparation for absorption in the small intestine. Bile salts themselves are the primary regulators of bile production by the liver. Bile salts are reabsorbed 4 to 15 times/day in the ileum by secondary active transport processes in enterocytes; bile acids subsequently enter the portal circulation and return to the liver for re-excretion. As bile is returned to the liver, negative feedback inhibition occurs on new bile acid synthesis. This is the process of enterohepatic circulation (Fig. 6-6). Without the enterohepatic circulation, fat malabsorption would occur, since the liver could not keep up with intestinal losses and make an adequate amount of new bile acids to handle dietary lipids. A balance is achieved between small daily fecal losses and synthesis of bile salts by hepatocytes.

Bile duct cells, like salivary ductal cells, modify secretions by adding bicarbonate and water, with the final bile product being alkaline and iso-osmotic with plasma. This aids in the neutralization of acid chyme from the stomach. The gallbladder, if not removed by cholecystectomy, concentrates bile made by the liver and releases it into the bile duct and into the duodenum in response to CCK. Bile duct cells increase water and bicarbonate secretion in response to secretin. Both secretin and CCK are made by cells found deep in the mucosa of the proximal small intestine. These hormones complement each other by augmenting each other's effects on biliary and pancreatic secretions.

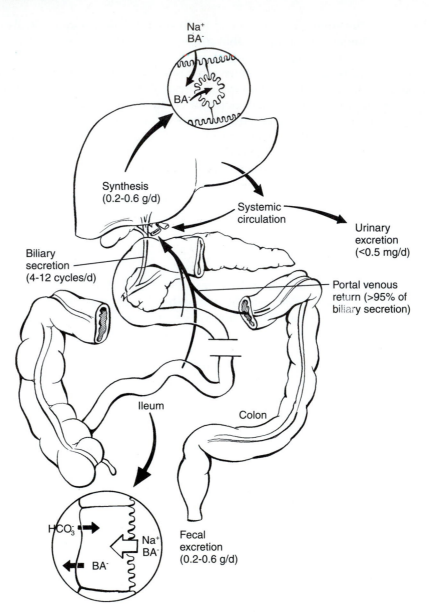

Figure 6-6. Enterohepatic circulation of bile salts showing typical kinetic values for healthy humans. (Adapted from Carey MC, Cahalane MJ. Enterohepatic circulation. In: Arias IM, Jakoby WB, Popper H, Schachter D, Shafritz DA, eds. The Liver: Biology and Pathology, 2nd ed. New York: Raven, 1988:576; and Yamada T, Alpers DH, Owyang C, Powell DW, Silverstein FE, eds. Textbook of Gastroenterology, 2nd ed. Philadelphia: JB Lippincott, 1995;1:395.)

Pancreatic Secretions

The exocrine portion of the pancreas contributes 1500 ml/day of fluid to the small intestine and produces enzymes important in protein, lipid, and starch hydrolysis. Primary control of secretion is hormonal. CCK is primarily important for enzyme secretion, and secretin is primarily responsible for bicarbonate secretion. There is also some evidence for vagal stimulation of secretion. Regulation of pancreatic secretions is balanced between stimulatory and inhibitory factors. The peptide hormones human pancreatic polypeptide, glucagon, and somatostatin have been shown to inhibit pancreatic secretion. Human pancreatic polypeptide is released from pancreatic islets via a vagal response to inhibit pancreatic and biliary secretions postprandially. Glucagon inhibits pancreatic secretion in the hyperglycemic state. Pancreatic secretion can be conveniently characterized by three phases, similar to those of gastric acid secretion. The cephalic phase commences secretion in response to the taste and smell of food and is vagally-mediated. The gastric phase stimulates pancreatic secretion upon gastric distention and is also vagally-mediated. The most potent is the intestinal phase, predominantly mediated by CCK and secretin; it is initiated by luminal amino acids and fatty acids as well as intestinal distention. The pancreatic ductal cells modify pancreatic juice by adding bicarbonate and water to the final secretion.

Important for nutrient absorption are the enzymes released by the pancreas into the intestinal lumen via the pancreatic duct and sphincter of Oddi. The proteases, including trypsinogen, chymotrypsinogen, procarboxypeptidase A and B, and proelastase are released from the pancreas as inactive precursors. Trypsinogen is converted in the duodenum to trypsin by enterokinase, an enzyme secreted by the duodenal mucosa (Fig. 6-7). Trypsin subsequently can convert the other proteases to their active forms of chymotrypsin, carboxypeptidase A and B, and elastase. Trypsin can also convert more trypsinogen to trypsin and therefore enhance activation of the remaining pancreatic proteases. Secretion of inactive enzymes is thought to protect the pancreas from autodigestion; if trypsin is formed within the pancreas, proteolysis of the pancreas can take place, causing severe inflammation. A trypsin inhibitor is secreted by the pancreas and is active at a pH of 3 to 7, but it is only made in minute quantities as compared to the full proteolytic capacity of the pancreas. Proteases break down the ingested protein present in the intestinal lumen. Pancreatic amylase cleaves polysaccharides to oligosaccharides, lipase breaks down emulsified triglycerides, and esterase hydrolyzes cholesterol esters. These last three enzymes are secreted in their active forms, in contrast to proteases, which are secreted as inactive precursors. Colipase, also made by the exocrine pancreas, is a required cofactor for lipase action on triglycerides. Colipase displaces the bile salt–triglyceride interaction in micelles to facilitate lipase hydrolysis of the triglyceride.

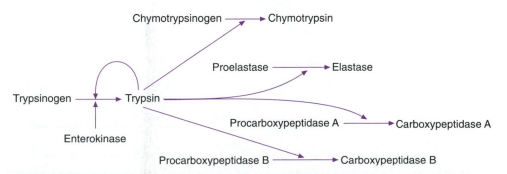

Figure 6-7. Activation of pancreatic proteolytic enzymes. Enterokinase (enteropeptidase) plays a critical role in activating trypsinogen to form trypsin. Trypsin, in turn, activates not only more trypsinogen but also the other proteolytic enzyme precursors. (Adapted from Sleisenger MH, Fordtran JS, eds. Gastrointestinal Disease, 5th ed. Philadelphia: WB Saunders, 1993;1:994.)

INTESTINAL ABSORPTION

GENERAL PHYSIOLOGY OF INTESTINAL ABSORPTION

Intestinal Villi and Microvilli

The small intestine is the interface between ingested foodstuffs and assimilation of nutrients. Although the physical length of the small intestine is approximately 6 meters, the presence of villi (luminal projections of the intestinal mucosa) greatly enhances the surface area for digestion and absorption (Fig. 6-8). Each villus has a central lacteal, the lymphatic vessel that runs in the core of the villus and connects with the intestinal lymphatics in the submucosa (Fig. 6-9). Each villus also has a rich plexus of capillaries that ultimately flow into the portal vein. In opposite polarity to the villi are the crypts of Lieberkühn, invaginations of the mucosa that contain relatively undifferentiated cells. These cells replace sloughed-off cells of the villi by migration and maturation from the crypts to the villus tips (Fig. 6-10). Although villi also contain goblet cells and immune cells, the main cell type for digestion and absorption is the enterocyte. Each enterocyte has microvilli at its apical surface, further enhancing the total digestive and absorptive area of the small intestine. Enterocytes live only 3 to 7 days before being renewed. As maturation occurs from the undifferentiated crypt cell to the enterocyte, these cells acquire many enzymes, such as disaccharidases and peptidases necessary for final digestion prior to absorption of nutrients through the apical microvilli. Many receptors and carriers are also acquired. These are essential for the absorption of monosaccharides, amino acids, and lipids. The enterocytes are attached to each other by tight junctions, such that nearly all absorption takes place at the entero-

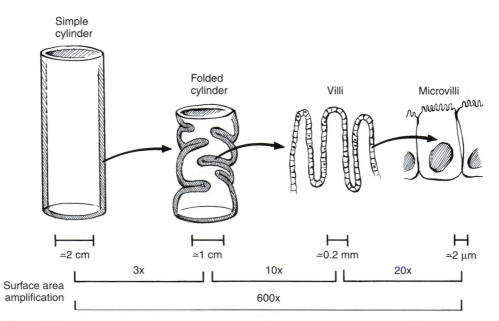

Figure 6-8. Amplification of the intestinal surface area by intestinal folds (plicae conniventes) villi, and microvilli. The numbers indicate the factor by which the surface area is amplified over a flat surface. Together, the folds, villi, and microvilli amplify the surface area by approximately 600-fold. (Adapted from Yamada T, Alpers DH, Owyang C, Powell DW, Silverstein FE, eds. Textbook of Gastroenterology, 2nd ed. Philadelphia: JB Lippincott, 1995;1:327.)

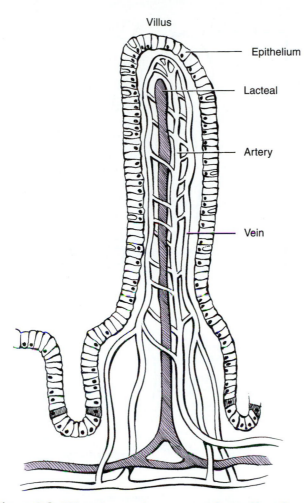

Villus

Epithelium

Lacteal

Artery

Vein

Figure 6-9. Villus microvascular anatomy and central lacteal
lymphatic vessel. (Adapted from Lundgren O. Studies on blood flow
distribution and countercurrent exchange in the small intestine.
Acta Physiol Scand 303:1, 1967; and from Yamada T, Alpers DH,
Owyang C, Powell DH, Silverstein FE, eds. Textbook of
Gastroenterology, 2nd ed. Philadelphia: JB Lippincott, 1995;2:
2497.)

cyte microvilli rather than through the intercellular spaces. The concentration of
enzymes and carriers tends to be greater in the proximal small intestine (duodenum and jejunum) than in the ileum; however, specific receptors for vitamin B_{12}
occur only in the ileum.

General Mechanisms of Absorption and Transport

Chyme must be transported from the duodenum down the full length of the
small intestine to the ileum for full exposure to the surface area provided by the
villi and microvilli. The muscularis externa of the small intestine consists of an
inner circular and outer longitudinal layer of smooth muscle and is responsible for
at least two important types of contractions: segmentation and peristalsis. Segmentation causes the mixing of chyme by forcing luminal contents orally and aborally
as alternating segments of the small intestine contract. Peristalsis is the propulsive

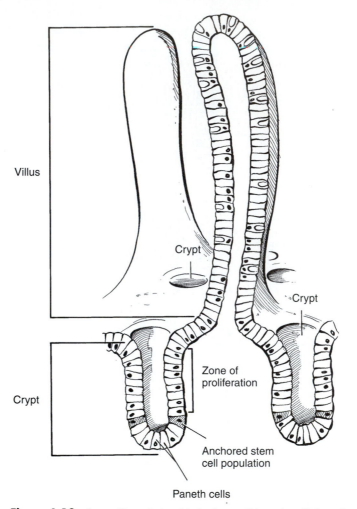

Villus

Crypt

Crypt

Zone of
proliferation

Crypt

Anchored stem
cell population

Paneth cells

Figure 6-10. Crypt-villus relationship in the small intestine. (Adapted from Yamada T, Alpers DH, Owyang C, Powell DH, Silverstein FE, eds. Textbook of Gastroenterology, 2nd ed. Philadelphia: JB Lippincott, 1995;1:562.)

action that moves the digested material toward the colon (aborally). These muscle movements are primarily controlled by the enteric nervous system with modulation by parasympathetic input and hormones.

For digestion and absorption to occur, the intestinal contents must be fluid, with water serving as a diffusion medium from the luminal contents to the entero-cyte surface. Ingestion of fluid and secretion from organs of the gastrointestinal tract provides water, with 1.5 L contributed by the small intestine itself. The small intestine reabsorbs most of the nearly 8500 ml of water presented to it daily and delivers only 500 to 2000 ml to the colon for final water absorption (Fig. 6-11).

Once electrolytes, peptides, carbohydrates, and lipids reach the enterocyte, other processes must occur for each nutrient to be absorbed. This may include further digestion by the enterocyte, as in the case of carbohydrates and peptides, or active transport from the lumen, as in the case of some electrolytes. The plasma membrane of the enterocyte provides little solubility for polar groups to transgress; thus there is the necessity for proteins in the plasma membrane to "carry" mole-

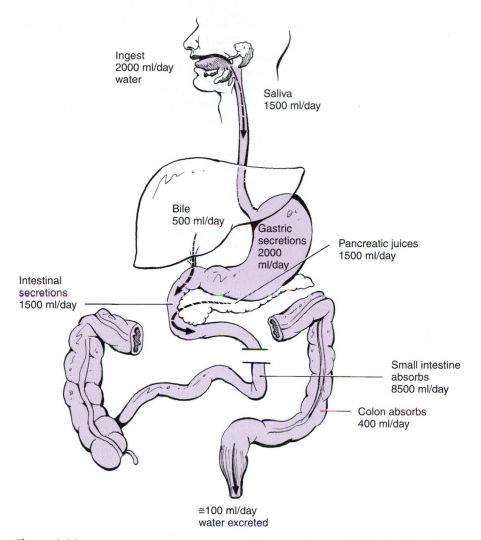

Figure 6-11. Overall fluid balance in the human gastrointestinal tract. (Adapted from Berne RM, Levy MN, eds. Physiology. St. Louis: CV Mosby, 1983:802.)

cules into the enterocyte. Active transport requires adenosine triphosphate, which provides energy for molecules to move against a concentration gradient. The Na^+/K^+-ATPase, located on the basolateral membrane of enterocytes, pumps potassium into the cell and sodium out of the cell; both ions are against their concentration gradient. Proteins in the plasma membrane are transport channels, permitting bidirectional movement of ions, with actual ion movement occurring down a concentration gradient. Channels can be in an "open" or "closed" state. The chloride channel on the apical membrane of enterocytes is an example. Secondary active transport is a mixture of active and passive processes; it uses ions moved by active (adenosine triphosphate requiring) pumps that form a concentration gradient for that ion and link the transport of energetically unfavorable molecules to movement of that ion down its concentration gradient. An example is the Na^+/glucose transporter, located on the apical surface of enterocytes. The Na^+/K^+-ATPase sets up a large sodium gradient, with the intracellular milieu having a low concentration of sodium. Sodium tends to move into the cell, and via the Na^+/glucose transporter can also carry glucose intracellularly against its concentration gradient (Fig. 6-12). This process itself is passive but would not be possible without the Na^+/K^+-ATPase. The Na^+/glucose transporter is an example of cotransport (symport) because both sodium and glucose move in the same direction. Exchangers (antiport) are secondary active transporters that move same-charged molecules in opposite directions. Amino acids, peptides, bile acids and vitamin B_{12} are absorbed into the enterocyte by a sodium cotransport mechanism similar to that of glucose. Water moves passively toward hyperosmolar compartments. After water has diffused, both compartments (i.e., lumen and enterocyte or enterocyte and lamina propria) are iso-osmolar. Because electrolytes are the major osmotic species, water movement is indirectly regulated by electrolyte transport. In fact, sodium is the major ion that drives water absorption. However, glucose and other molecules are also osmotic and once they are absorbed, water follows passively.

SPECIFIC PHYSIOLOGY OF INTESTINAL ABSORPTION

Absorption of Water and Electrolytes

The contents of the small intestine are first made iso-osmotic through bidirectional fluxes of both ions and water. This is usually accomplished in the duodenum provided that the emptying function of the stomach is normal and the volume arriving in the duodenum is not too great. If stomach emptying is not normal and the volume of a hyperosmotic meal reaching the duodenum is large, then the iso-osmotic condition is not achieved until the jejunum. Since water passively flows

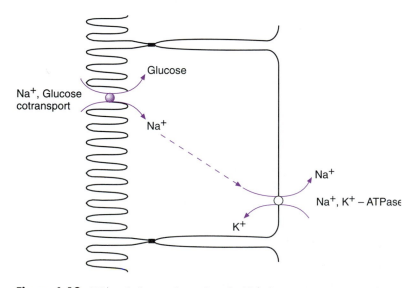

Figure 6-12. NA^+ and glucose absorption. An Na^+ glucose cotransport carrier on the apical membrane serves to bring glucose and Na^+ into the cell. Sodium is then pumped out by way of Na^+, K^+-ATPase; glucose proceeds across the basolateral membrane by way of a specific facilitated transport carrier. Similar Na^+ cotransport mechanisms exist for many amino acids, dipeptides, tripeptides, certain B vitamins, and bile salts. (Adapted from Yamada T, Alpers DH, Owyang C, Powell DH, Silverstein FE, eds. Textbook of Gastroenterology, 2nd ed. Philadelphia: JB Lippincott, 1995;1:334.)

toward hyperosmolarity, water exits the plasma at the level of the villi and flows into the lumen. Significant flux of water can lead to systemic hypovolemia and a sympathetic response of tachycardia and perspiration, called the dumping syndrome.

The ultimate driving force for absorption of water, electrolytes, and many organic molecules is the Na^+/K^+-ATPase, located on the basolateral surface of all enterocytes. This pump requires adenosine triphosphate and magnesium to operate and removes three sodium ions out in exchange for two potassium ions into the cell. Because the net positive charge is removed, the electrical potential is negative intracellularly with respect to the extracellular environment. The Na^+/K^+-ATPase creates a sodium gradient that tends to drive sodium toward the inside of the cell. There are many cotransporters on the enterocyte microvilli that are coupled with sodium: glucose, amino acids, di- and tripeptides, and bile salts. Each one of these transporters is a different individual protein. The presence of sodium ions in the lumen greatly enhances, for example, glucose absorption; conversely, the presence of glucose facilitates sodium absorption. Also on the apical surface is a Na^+/H^+ antiport and a Cl^-/HCO_3^- antiport (Fig. 6-13). With both transporters considered, sodium and chloride ions are moved into the cell while hydrogen and bicarbonate ions are placed outside the cell. Bicarbonate and hydrogen ions are produced by carbonic anhydrase intracellularly and rid the cell of the products of metabolism (CO_2). Water can follow sodium passively when absorbed into the cell, ultimately entering the plasma compartment.

Enterocytes also secrete electrolytes, mainly bicarbonate and chloride ions. Bicarbonate secretion occurs predominantly in the proximal intestine but is also important in other regions of the small bowel. Secretion of bicarbonate can occur via the Cl^-/HCO_3^- exchanger, but other mechanisms may exist. Chloride secretion is brought about by the basolateral presence of a $Na^+/K^+/Cl^-$ cotransporter (Fig. 6-14), which brings all three ions into the cell; it is a secondary active transport process. Once chloride accumulates intracellularly from actions of the

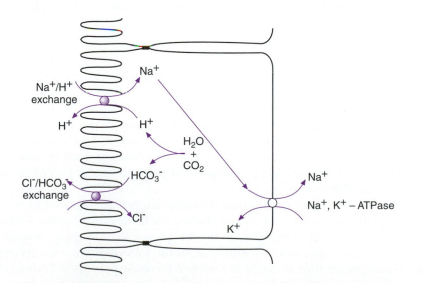

Figure 6-13. Small intestinal sodium and water absorption. (Adapted from Yamada T, Alpers DH, Owyang C, Powell DH, Silverstein FE, eds. Textbook of Gastroenterology, 2nd ed. Philadelphia: JB Lippincott, 1995;1:333.)

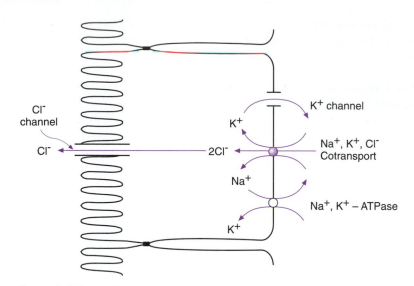

Figure 6-14. Small intestinal chloride secretion. (Adapted from Yamada T, Alpers DH, Owyang C, Powell DH, Silverstein FE, eds. Textbook of Gastroenterology, 2nd ed. Philadelphia: JB Lippincott, 1995;1:339.)

$Na^+/K^+/Cl^-$ cotransporter and Cl^-/HCO_3^- exchanger, apical chloride channels open and chloride exits into the lumen of the small intestine. The significance of the absorptive and secretory mechanisms becomes apparent when a transport process fails to function. The toxin of *Vibrio cholerae* stimulates chloride secretion and inhibits sodium and chloride absorption in the enterocyte. Thus water moves into the intestinal lumen following sodium and produces voluminous watery diarrhea. Therapy includes oral administration of NaCl and glucose, since the Na^+/glucose cotransporter and Na^+/K^+-ATPase are unaffected by the toxin. This treatment greatly enhances intestinal water absorption even in the presence of the toxin.

Absorption of Amino Acids

Protein digestion begins with activation of pepsinogen to pepsin in the acid environment of the stomach, optimally at pH 1 to 3. Pepsin cleaves the peptide bond between aromatic amino acids and the neighboring carboxyl amino acid. Pepsin is inactivated in the more alkaline environment of the duodenum and is not essential for protein digestion judging from patients who have undergone gastrectomy or are taking long-term H^+/K^+-ATPase inhibitors such as omeprazole. Pepsin digestion of proteins leaves a mixture of polypeptides as part of the chyme entering the small intestine.

Polypeptides present in the small intestine are further digested by proteases present in pancreatic secretions and on the microvillous surface of the enterocyte. The majority of protein digestion is by the pancreatic proteases trypsin, chymotrypsin, elastase, and carboxypeptidase A and B. Enterokinase converts trypsinogen to trypsin, which then activates the other pancreatic proteases. Trypsin cleaves polypeptides adjacent to the basic amino acids lysine and arginine, whereas chymotrypsins cleave bonds at aromatic amino acids (e.g., phenylalanine, tryptophan, tyrosine) and elastase cleaves aliphatic peptide bonds (Fig. 6-15). These three en-

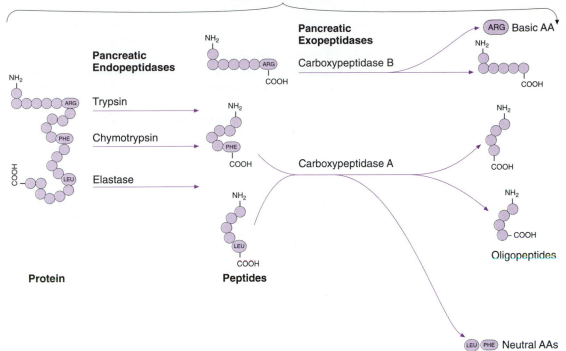

Figure 6-15. Intraluminal protein digestion by pancreatic proteases. (Adapted from Yamada T, Alpers DH, Owyang C, Powell DH, Silverstein FE, eds. Textbook of Gastroenterology, 2nd ed. Philadelphia: JB Lippincott, 1995;1:457.)

zymes are endopeptidases because they hydrolyze an internal peptide bond. Carboxypeptidase A and B are exopeptidases cleaving only at the carboxy-terminal end and preferentially cleave neutral and basic amino acids, respectively. The proteolysis performed by pancreatic enzymes leaves oligopeptides and some free amino acids. The microvilli of enterocytes contain endopeptidases and exopeptidases on their surface, which cleave oligopeptides to amino acids and di- and tripeptides.

Absorption of di- and tripeptides occurs probably via a secondary active transport process. These products are then hydrolyzed to amino acids by enterocyte intracellular peptidases. Amino acids are predominantly absorbed by coupling to sodium cotransport on the apical membrane. Subsequent diffusion through the basolateral membrane occurs down a concentration gradient, and the amino acids eventually enter the villus capillary plexus. There are at least five Na^+/amino acid symports, each with specificity based on the amino acid structure. There is a neutral transporter that transports neutral amino acids; similarly, there are basic (arginine, lysine, histidine), dicarboxylic (glutamate, aspartate), hydrophobic (phenylalanine, methionine), and imino (proline, hydroxyproline) transporters. Syndromes caused by congenital loss of a transporter have been described and can lead to specific amino acid deficiencies.

Absorption of Carbohydrates

Digestible carbohydrates are those for which enzymes are present in the gut for hydrolysis and subsequent absorption. Indigestible carbohydrates, or dietary fiber, cannot be catabolized because enzymes that hydrolyze them are absent from the gut; however, catabolism by colonic bacteria is possible and can produce flatulence. Dietary carbohydrate includes the disaccharides sucrose (table sugar) and lactose (milk sugar), the monosaccharides glucose and fructose, and the plant starches amylose, a large polymer of glucose linked by α1,4 bonds, and amylopectin, another glucose polymer linked by α1,4 bonds as well as α1,6 bonds. The animal starch glycogen, another glucose polymer linked by α1,4 bonds, is also a digestible carbohydrate.

The enterocyte is not capable of transporting carbohydrates larger than monosaccharides. Therefore carbohydrates larger than monosaccharides must be catabolized before absorption is possible. Salivary and pancreatic amylases hydrolyze internal α1,4 glucose-glucose bonds, but α1,6 linkages as well as terminal or branch α1,4 bonds are resistant to amylase digestion. When food is ingested, salivary amylase begins digestion of α1,4 linkages of amylose and amylopectin, yielding α1,6-branched α1,4-linked glucose polymers termed α-limit dextrans (Fig. 6-16). Salivary amylase also produces the di- and tripolymers of glucose, called maltose and maltotriose. Salivary amylase action is limited because of inactivation in the acid pH of the stomach; the optimal pH for activity is 6.7. Pancreatic amylase continues hydrolysis of carbohydrates to maltose, maltotriose, and α-limit dextrans in the lumen of the small intestine. The microvilli of the enterocyte contain the final enzymes that catabolize oligosaccharides and disaccharides to monosaccharides for absorption. Glucoamylase, or α-limit dextranase, cleaves α1,4 bonds on the nonreducing end of oligosaccharides formed by amylase digestion of amylopectin. This digestion generally leaves a tetrasaccharide with one α1,6 bond, and this bond is then more vulnerable to cleavage. The sucrase-isomaltase complex has two catalytic sites: one with sucrase activity and one with isomaltase activity. The isomaltase site is essential for α1,6 bond cleavage, and resulting digestion of the

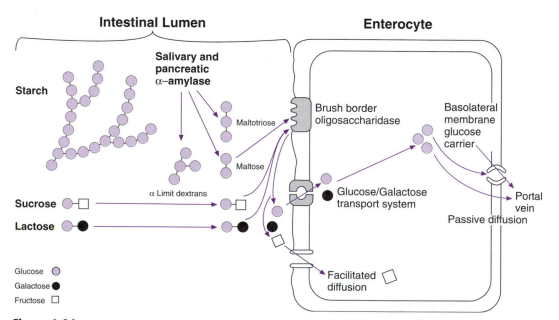

Figure 6-16. Digestion and absorption of carbohydrates. (Adapted from Kelley WN, ed. Textbook of Internal Medicine, 2nd ed. Philadelphia: JB Lippincott, 1992:407.)

tetrasaccharide forms maltotriose. Isomaltase, as well as sucrase, can sequentially remove glucose from the nonreducing ends of maltose, maltotriose, and α-limit dextrans; however, isomaltase cannot cleave sucrose. Sucrase can hydrolyze the disaccharide sucrose to fructose and glucose. Lactase is also present on the enterocyte microvilli and catabolizes lactose to galactose and glucose.

Once monosaccharides are formed by enzymatic digestion at the microvillus, the sugars are available for absorption. Glucose and galactose are transported into the enterocyte with sodium by the Na^+/glucose contransporter; absorption of glucose is greatly increased in the presence of sodium, and vice versa. Fructose uptake is by facilitated diffusion across the apical membrane. Galactose and glucose exit the basolateral membrane by a transporter; the mechanism of fructose exit from the enterocyte is less clear. The sugars enter the lamina propria and are taken into the capillary plexus in the villus and ultimately enter the portal vein.

Absorption of Lipids

Lipids in the diet are accounted for primarily by triglycerides and phospholipid (lecithin) as well as cholesterol (in the form of esters) (Fig. 6-17). Normal lipid digestion and absorption require the interaction of several components of the gastrointestinal tract: the liver and biliary tract, pancreatic enzymes, entero-

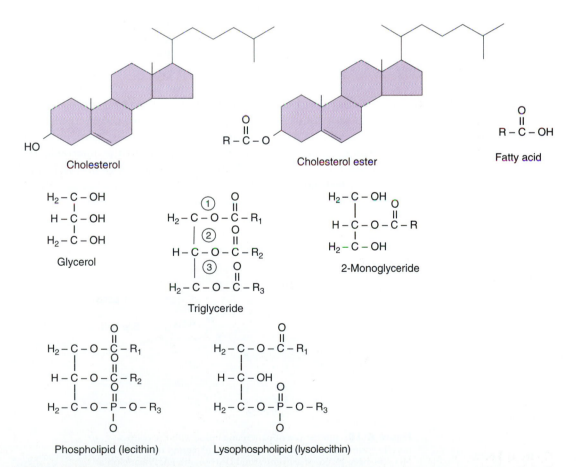

Figure 6-17. Structures of lipids in the diet (R = variable length alkyl chain).

cytes, an alkaline environment, patent lymphatics, and functional enterohepatic circulation. Perturbation of any one of these processes can lead to fat malabsorption and steatorrhea.

The bulk of digestion of lipids happens in the small intestine. However, some lipolysis may occur in the stomach by action of a fundically-secreted gastric lipase whose optimal activity is at pH 4 to 5. Gastric lipase hydrolyzes triglyceride to diglyceride and fatty acid, is resistant to pepsin but degraded by the pancreatic proteases in the alkaline duodenum, and is inhibited by the presence of bile salts. The contribution of gastric lipase is small, however, when compared to that of the lipolytic events in the small intestine. Finally, gastric antral grinding provides the shearing force to create minute lipid droplets and thus increases the surface area for digestion prior to entry into the duodenum.

With entry into the duodenum, lipolysis occurs only after several events unfold. First, triglycerides, cholesterol, and phospholipids as well as products of gastric lipase digestion form into micelles by the action of bile acids secreted from the biliary tract; the micelles are stabilized by phospholipids and monoglycerides in the alkaline lumen. Second, colipase, secreted by the pancreas, attaches to the micelle and serves as an anchor to which pancreatic lipase can attach. Pancreatic lipase has little lipolytic activity on micelles when acting without colipase. Colipase-micelle binding is enhanced by activity of pancreatic phospholipase A_2 (PL A_2) on lecithin in the micelle. PL A_2 requires calcium and bile salts for enzymatic activity and forms the products lysolecithin and fatty acid. With lecithin hydrolysis, triglycerides in the micelle become exposed. Third, pancreatic lipase anchors to the colipase-micelle structure (Fig. 6-18) and hydrolyzes the 1 and 3 bonds of triglycerides, forming 2-monoglyceride and fatty acid. Pancreatic lipase has its highest activity at pH 6 to 6.5 in the presence of colipase. Another enzyme, pancreatic esterase, hydrolyzes the fatty acid ester bonds of cholesterol and fat-soluble vitamins in the presence of bile salts. Thus the principal lipid digestive products of pancreatic lipase (PL A_2) and esterase are fatty acids, 2-monoglycerides, lysolecithin, and cholesterol (unesterified). The delivery of these products to the microvilli is dependent on solubilization of these hydrophobic compounds by continued association in micelles in the intestinal lumen.

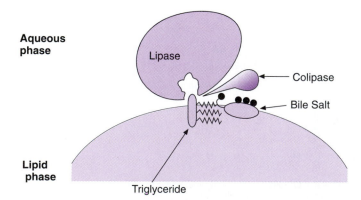

Figure 6-18. Interaction of pancreatic lipase with the colipase-micelle complex to hydrolyze triglycerides. (Adapted from Sleisenger MH, Fordtran JS, eds. Gastrointestinal Disease, 5th ed. Philadelphia: WB Saunders, 1993;1:984.)

Fatty acids, cholesterol, and monoglycerides enter the enterocyte from the micelle by passive diffusion (Fig. 6-19); however, a surface binding protein may exist for long-chain fatty acid uptake. Since these compounds are lipid-soluble and smaller than undigested triglycerides and cholesterol esters, they easily traverse the enterocyte plasma membrane. Once inside the cell, long-chain fatty acids and cholesterol are carried by binding proteins in the hydrophilic environment of the cytosol and are directed to the endoplasmic reticulum (ER) for further processing. Cholesterol and fat-soluble vitamins are carried by a sterol carrier protein to the smooth ER, where cholesterol is re-esterified by acyl-CoA:cholesterol acyltransferase. Long-chain fatty acids are carried through the cytoplasm by fatty acid binding proteins, and, depending on the presence or absence of dietary fat, are transported to the smooth or rough ER, respectively. In the fasting state (low fat), fatty acids combine with glycerol-3-phosphate from glucose metabolism to ultimately reform triglycerides in the rough ER. With the addition of fat in the diet, the synthetic pathway is switched and fatty acids and 2-monoglycerides recombine to form diglycerides and then triglycerides in the smooth ER. Lysolecithin, a water-soluble product from PL A$_2$ digestion, can reform lecithin in the enterocyte by combining with fatty acid in the fed (high-fat) state. However, like fatty acid metabolism, lysolecithin combines with glycerol-3-phosphate in the fasting state to ultimately form lecithin.

Once cholesterol esters, triglycerides, and lecithin are resynthesized in the ER, they form lipoproteins by associating with apolipoproteins made in the rough ER of the enterocyte. Apolipoproteins are the vehicles for lipid transport through the cytosol and out of the cell. Lipoproteins are subclassified by their size, lipid content, and apoprotein composition. Chylomicrons and very low-density lipopro-

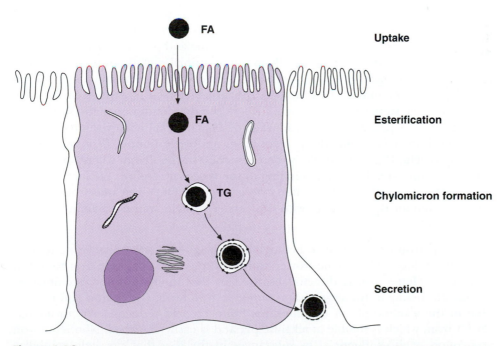

Figure 6-19. Lipid processing by the enterocyte. (Adapted from Isselbacher KJ. Biochemical reports of lipid malabsorption. Fed Proc 26:1420, 1967; and Johnson LR, ed. Physiology of the Gastrointestinal Tract, 2nd ed. New York: Raven Press, 1987:1530.)

teins are large in size and carry predominantly triglycerides and fat-soluble vitamins, whereas low-density lipoproteins are smaller and carry mostly cholesterol esters. The smallest are high-density lipoproteins, which contain mostly phospholipid (lecithin). Deficiency of an apolipoprotein leads to defective transport of lipid. Abetalipoproteinemia is a condition in which apo B, a protein necessary for the formation of chylomicrons and very low-density lipoproteins, is deficient and leads to fat-laden enterocytes, fat malabsorption, and neurologic sequelae of vitamin E deficiency. The assembled lipoproteins exit the enterocyte basolateral membrane in vesicles and enter the lamina propria, where they flow into the central lacteal (lymphatic vessel). Short-chain fatty acids (less than 12 carbons) can pass directly into the portal blood from the enterocyte without the need for reincorporation in triglycerides. The short-chain fatty acids that are present in the colon arise from bacterial action on unabsorbed carbohydrates and may represent an important energy source for the colonocyte.

Absorption of Vitamins and Minerals

Folate. Folate's biologic active form, tetrahydrofolate, is critical for "one-carbon" transfer reactions in the synthesis of the nucleic acid thymidine from deoxyuridine. Folate deficiency leads to macrocytic anemia. Folate is present in green vegetables and fruits and is consumed as pteroylpolyglutamate. Absorption occurs primarily in the jejunum (Fig. 6-20). Pteroylpolyglutamate is hydrolyzed to pteroylglutamate monomers by the microvillus enzyme conjugase, and is taken into the cell by a pteroylglutamate carrier that is active at pH 5.5 to 6. Inside the enterocyte, pteroylglutamate is reduced and methylated, producing 5-methyltetrahydrofolate, which is carried out of the basolateral membrane via a carrier into the villus capillary plexus and portal circulation.

Vitamin B_{12}. Vitamin B_{12} (cyanocobalamin) is a coenzyme in amino acid metabolism. Deficiency, which normally takes 1 to 3 years to develop because of reserves stored in the liver, leads to macrocytic anemia and potential degeneration of nerve fibers. Vitamin B_{12} is exclusively found in animal dietary sources and not in plants. In the stomach, vitamin B_{12} binds to R proteins found in saliva after the vitamin B_{12} is liberated from food by acid. Intrinsic factor (IF), secreted by the parietal cells in the stomach, binds vitamin B_{12} in the duodenum once the R proteins are degraded by pancreatic proteases (Fig. 6-21). The alkaline environment of the duodenal lumen facilitates IF-B_{12} association and once bound, IF is resistant to proteolysis. The IF-B_{12} molecule is then absorbed in the ileum, where specific receptors for the complex reside; binding to the receptor requires calcium. The uptake mechanism into the ileal enterocyte is unclear. Once released from the enterocyte, vitamin B_{12} associates with the carrier protein transcobalamin II in the portal blood.

Iron. Iron is a cofactor in hemoglobin, myoglobin, and porphyrin enzymes. Iron can be ingested as heme iron found in meats or as nonheme iron found in vegetables. Heme iron is directly absorbed in the duodenum and proximal jejunum. Nonheme iron is ingested predominantly as ferric (Fe^{3+}) iron and is insoluble in the alkaline pH of the intestine. Stomach acid reduces ferric to ferrous (Fe^{2+}) iron, which is soluble at alkaline pH and is easily absorbed. Nonheme iron absorption is also influenced by substances in the diet that can help solubilize (e.g., vitamin C) or precipitate (e.g., phosphates, vegetable phytates) intraluminal iron. The microvilli of the duodenal enterocyte have high-affinity receptors for

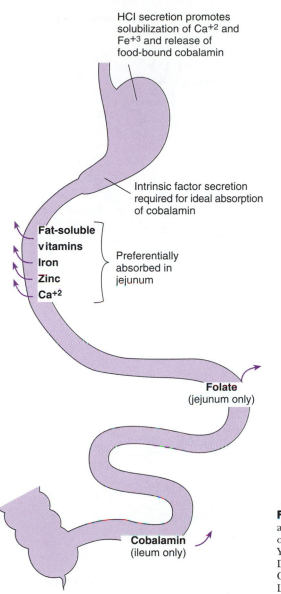

HCl secretion promotes
solubilization of Ca^{+2} and
Fe^{+3} and release of
food-bound cobalamin

Intrinsic factor secretion
required for ideal absorption
of cobalamin

**Fat-soluble
vitamins
Iron
Zinc
Ca^{+2}**

Preferentially
absorbed in
jejunum

Folate
(jejunum only)

Cobalamin
(ileum only)

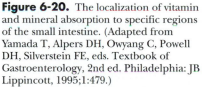

Figure 6-20. The localization of vitamin
and mineral absorption to specific regions
of the small intestine. (Adapted from
Yamada T, Alpers DH, Owyang C, Powell
DH, Silverstein FE, eds. Textbook of
Gastroenterology, 2nd ed. Philadelphia: JB
Lippincott, 1995;1:479.)

iron that transport iron into the cell. Several intracellular binding proteins are
likely present but remain uncharacterized. Subsequently, iron is released from the
cell into the villus capillary plexus. In the circulation, iron is bound to transferrin,
a protein with two iron-binding sites. In tissue, iron is stored as ferritin, a molecule
that can bind as many as 4500 atoms of iron.

Vitamins A, D, E, and K. The vitamins A, D, E, and K are known as fat-
soluble vitamins and are absorbed in a similar manner as dietary lipids. Complete
uptake is dependent upon micellar formation, an alkaline intestinal lumen, and
patent lymphatics. Absorption primarily occurs in the jejunum.

Vitamin A is necessary for cellular growth and differentiation and is a precursor of the visual pigment rhodopsin. Deficiency leads to xerophthalmia, a syn-

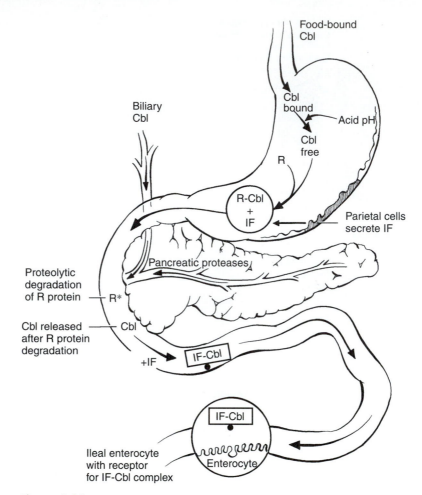

Figure 6-21. Sequential steps in the absorption of cobalamin (Cbl). R indicates R protein; IF, intrinsic factor. (Adapted from Yamada T, Alpers DH, Owyang C, Powell DH, Silverstein FE, eds. Textbook of Gastroenterology, 2nd ed. Philadelphia: JB Lippincott, 1995;1:470.)

drome that can produce irreversible blindness. β-carotene, a pigment found in vegetables, is the principal dietary source of vitamin A, along with retinyl esters found in meat. β-carotene enters the microvilli by passive diffusion; the enterocyte cleaves β-carotene into two molecules of retinaldehyde and reduces the retinaldehyde to retinol. Retinyl esters from animal origin are hydrolyzed to retinol by pancreatic esterase and enter the enterocyte by passive diffusion. Inside the cell, retinol binds to cellular retinol binding protein II and is re-esterified by acyl CoA:retinol acyl transferase to retinyl esters. This process is similar to that of cholesterol absorption. The retinyl esters are incorporated into chylomicron lipoproteins and are excreted into the lymphatics.

Vitamin D regulates calcium absorption by the small intestine. Deficiency leads to rickets and osteomalacia, defects in bone mineralization. Vitamin D is activated in the skin by action of ultraviolet light on 7-dehydrocholesterol stores but is also ingested in the diet from fortified dairy products. Dietary vitamin D (ergocalciferol) is absorbed by the enterocyte and processed into chylomicrons, which enter the lymphatics. Absorbed vitamin D is not biologically active until hydroxylation occurs in the liver and kidney.

Vitamin E is found in cell membranes and functions as an antioxidant, especially in neuronal tissues. Deficiency is associated with a progressive neurologic disorder characterized by cerebellar dysfunction. Vitamin E, of which α-tocopherol is the most active form, is found in vegetables and grains. In the small intestinal lumen, vitamin E is present as esters and is hydrolyzed to its nonesterified form by pancreatic esterase. Vitamin E is then absorbed by passive diffusion, packaged into chylomicrons, and excreted into the lymphatics.

Vitamin K is a cofactor in the liver for the γ-carboxylation of glutamic acid residues found in coagulation factors II, VII, IX, and X and proteins C and S. Deficiency of vitamin K causes a dysfunction of clotting, manifested by a prolonged prothrombin time. Vitamin K is synthesized in the intestine by bacteria as menaquinone but is also ingested in the diet from green leafy vegetables as phylloquinone. As with the other fat-soluble vitamins, vitamin K is absorbed by passive diffusion and delivered to the lymphatics in chylomicrons.

MECHANISMS OF SIGNS AND SYMPTOMS OF MALABSORPTION

Malabsorption is a syndrome with a constellation of symptoms including diarrhea, weight loss, protein loss, body wasting, and signs of vitamin deficiency. The degree of each sign or symptom varies and depends on the severity of the deficiency and the organ or biochemical process most affected. Clinical evidence of malabsorption can range from the virtual absence of symptoms (and noticeable only by subtle signs of vitamin deficiencies) to massive weight loss and steatorrhea.

Diarrhea

Diarrhea in malabsorption is classified as osmotic; however, some general mucosal diseases of the small intestine may additionally have a secretory component. Clinically, malabsorption of carbohydrates and fats is readily recognized by characteristic symptoms. Protein malabsorption is not as readily recognized unless severe, as in the case of congenital absence of an amino acid transporter. Malabsorptive diarrheas, unlike true secretory diarrheas, abate during fasting.

Osmotic diarrhea is the characteristic feature of carbohydrate malabsorption. Undigested and unabsorbed carbohydrates are osmotically active and draw water into the intestine in an attempt to make the luminal contents iso-osmotic. Furthermore, when the carbohydrate reaches the colon, it is metabolized by bacteria to short-chain fatty acids, which increases the osmolality of the colonic contents and further draws water into the lumen. Short-chain fatty acids are absorbed by colonocytes, and this reduces some of the intraluminal osmotic load; however, if the capacity of colonic bacteria to metabolize carbohydrate is exceeded, carbohydrate remains in the lumen as an osmotically active moiety. Short-chain fatty acids are organic anions that can attract cations into the lumen, further increasing the osmolality and drawing more water into the lumen. Flatulence often accompanies carbohydrate malabsorption because of gas produced by bacterial fermentation of unabsorbed carbohydrates.

Steatorrhea is a manifestation of dysfunctional lipid absorption and can be caused by decreased pancreatic or biliary secretions, faulty enterocyte processing, or lymphatic obstruction. Steatorrhea is the hallmark sign of a generalized malabsorptive process, and its presence overshadows signs of protein and carbohydrate malabsorption. In the colon, bacteria hydroxylate the undigested lipids, which cause an increase in the permeability of the cell and stimulates active anion secretion by the colonocyte. The resulting stools are bulky, pale, foul-smelling, and greasy and often float in the toilet. The stools float because of the gas produced by bacterial action on unabsorbed carbohydrates and not because of the fat malabsorption itself. Steatorrhea can occur if more than 100 cm of ileum is diseased or resected because the hepatic bile acid pool becomes diminished as a result of the loss of enterohepatic circulation and inability of the liver to keep up with fecal losses. If less than 100 cm of ileum is involved, new hepatic synthesis can usually replace the bile acid loss in the stool. However, the increased secondary bile acids in the stool can stimulate colonic secretion of electrolytes and water, producing "bile acid diarrhea."

Diseases that affect the mucosa of the small intestine can also cause diarrhea with a secretory component. For example, if the villus tips are destroyed, leaving only the crypts of Lieberkühn intact, the crypts become hyperplastic as a compensatory mechanism. The undifferentiated cells of the crypt have not acquired disaccharidases or peptidases or the sodium-coupled carriers for absorption. The cells also lack Na^+/H^+ and Cl^-/HCO_3^- antiports on their immature enterocyte apical surfaces. However, these cells retain the ability to secrete chloride because of the presence of Na^+/K^+-ATPase and $Na^+/K^+/Cl^-$ cotransporter. The net result is failure of sodium (and water) absorption as well as continued secretion of osmotically active chloride, causing the secretory diarrhea.

Weight Loss

The etiology of body weight loss in malabsorptive diseases is multifactorial. Longstanding mucosal disease as a cause of malabsorption ultimately causes anorexia, decreasing the appetite and contributing to a wasting syndrome. With the lack of intestinal processing of nutrients owing to disease, organs are forced to utilize body stores of fat and protein, which ultimately reduces body mass. The nutrients that replenish these stores are not available to organs because of malabsorption, and a negative balance exists between caloric intake and expenditure. The weight loss occurs despite initial hyperphagia by the patient.

Protein Loss

Normally there is little or no protein excreted into the gut lumen, and what little is present usually gets catabolized to its constitutive amino acids. In malabsorption, the normal mucosal barrier to proteins is diseased or lost, allowing protein to exit from the interstitial space through the enterocyte and into the gut lumen. Liver production of albumin, the major plasma protein, cannot maintain levels lost by leakage from the intestine. Furthermore, malabsorption of protein prevents uptake of precursors for the synthesis of albumin. Edema and ascites are consequences of hypoproteinemia. Obstruction of the lymphatics, independent of mucosal disease, can cause intestinal protein loss by increasing hydrostatic pressure and dilating the interstitial spaces. This pressure can overcome the enterocyte tight junction barrier, causing spillage of lymph (and protein) into the gut lumen.

Vitamin Deficiency

The fat-soluble vitamins A, D, E, and K are processed in a similar manner to that of dietary lipids. Interference with micellar formation, an alkaline lumen, enterocyte processing, and lymphatic flow leads to improper assimilation. Since the primary location of absorption is the jejunum, mucosal disease or jejunal bypass can prevent the uptake of these vitamins. Pancreatic lipase activity is not a full requirement for fat-soluble vitamin absorption, and complete vitamin deficiency occurs only rarely in pancreatic insufficiency.

Folate malabsorption can occur with mucosal disease of the jejunum, where the enzyme conjugase is present on the apical surface. Lack of healthy enterocytes prevents normal reduction and methylation to 5-methyltetrahydrofolate and thus inadequate absorption. Many drugs, such as methotrexate, can interfere with conversion to tetrahydrofolate.

Vitamin B_{12} absorption requires the presence of intrinsic factor and an intact ileum. Blockage of the IF-B_{12} association in the duodenum (pancreatic insufficiency, luminal acid pH, diminished IF levels) or IF-B_{12} binding in the ileum (ileal resection or inflammation) leads to vitamin B_{12} malabsorption.

Iron is absorbed as ferrous iron or heme iron. Blockage of the conversion of ferric to ferrous iron caused by decreased gastric acid or duodenal inflammation or bypass can lead to malabsorption. Ingestion of heme iron bypasses this defect.

CLINICAL CORRELATES

PANCREATIC EXOCRINE DEFICIENCY

The most common cause of pancreatic exocrine deficiency in Western societies is chronic pancreatitis, usually as a consequence of alcoholism. Chronic pancreatitis is insidious in onset; therefore early diagnosis is often delayed. By the time the disease is manifested, considerable damage has been done to the gland. Fat and protein malabsorption become apparent when 90% of the pancreatic exocrine function is lost. Protein malabsorption occurs because of the marked decrease in secretion of trypsinogen, chymotrypsinogens, proelastase, and procarboxypeptidases A and B. However, steatorrhea ensues as a result of the diminished lipase and colipase activity; secretion of lipase is reduced more rapidly than that of the proteases. Carbohydrate malabsorption is rare because of the reserves of amylase, requiring 97% loss in secretion before malabsorption ensues. Diminished bicarbonate secretion by the pancreas further hampers lipid digestion by inactivating the minute amount of lipase secreted and by precipitating bile salts, preventing micelle formation. Vitamin B_{12} may be malabsorbed in pancreatic exocrine insufficiency. The R-B_{12} association in the stomach normally separates in the alkaline bowel lumen, allowing IF to bind vitamin B_{12}. Trypsin hydrolyzes the R protein, and bicarbonate secreted by the pancreas facilitates the IF-B_{12} binding. In the absence or diminished presence of enzymes coupled with the decreased bicarbonate secretion, vitamin B_{12} absorption is diminished.

BILE ACID INSUFFICIENCY

Liver Disease

Intrinsic chronic liver disease of any cause affects hepatocyte number and function. Since bile is synthesized by hepatocytes, the amount of bile made is compromised in conditions of cirrhosis or chronic hepatitis. Although decreased production diminishes the total circulating bile salt pool, it is rare for steatorrhea to occur. Milder degrees of fat malabsorption may still take place.

Biliary Obstruction

Gallstones and cancer of the head of the pancreas can obstruct the bile duct, preventing bile secretion into the duodenal lumen and causing jaundice. As in chronic liver disease, the degree of fat malabsorption is usually mild and does not result in steatorrhea.

Bacterial Overgrowth

In this syndrome, the low count (10^5 organisms/ml) of normal gram-positive aerobic organisms is replaced by a high count of gram-negative organisms, such as *Escherichia coli,* and anaerobic organisms from the colon such as *Clostridia* and *Bacteroides* species. Bacterial overgrowth occurs in conditions of hypomotility (e.g., scleroderma, diabetes mellitus), partial intestinal obstruction (e.g., Crohn's ileitis, postsurgical strictures), small bowel diverticula, and in reduced gastric acid secretory states. The absence of a normally low stomach pH markedly increases the amount of bacteria presented to the small intestine. Bacteria in this syndrome do not invade the mucosa but remain in the lumen. The hallmark feature of bacterial overgrowth is diarrhea. Fat malabsorption contributes to diarrhea because bacteria in the lumen deconjugate and dehydroxylate bile acids, thus preventing micelle formation. Some anaerobic bacteria directly catabolize the microvilli disaccharidases, causing carbohydrate malabsorption. Among these, lactase is the most sensitive to inactivation. The presence of bacteria reduces the effectiveness of enterokinase and thus the initial step in luminal protein digestion. The microorganisms in the gut also compete for proteins and amino acids that are ingested. Bacterial overgrowth characteristically leads to vitamin B_{12} deficiency by competing for uptake of the IF-B_{12} complex, reducing availability to the ileum for absorption. Vitamin A, D, E, and K absorption is decreased because of impaired micellar formation, which can lead to deficiency; however, vitamin K deficiency is rare because of synthesis of vitamin K by the luminal bacteria. Iron deficiency anemia is possible because of occult blood loss from the gut and usually is not due to malabsorption. However, if achlorohydria is the cause of bacterial overgrowth, the reduced acid inhibits non-heme iron absorption.

Ileal Disease/Resection

The ileum is specifically important for the enterohepatic circulation of bile acids and vitamin B_{12} absorption, along with continued nutrient and water absorption. Ileal inflammation is typical of Crohn's disease and if severe, or if stricture formation develops, it can lead to ileal resection to correct bowel obstruction. Enteroenteric or enterocolonic fistulas can develop owing to transmural inflammation, which can result in nutrients bypassing a large segment of bowel. Vitamin B_{12} deficiency occurs when more than 50 cm of ileum is affected because of the loss of IF-B_{12} complex receptors. The length of ileum affected or removed determines whether bile acids or unabsorbed lipids cause diarrhea. When more than 100 cm of ileum is involved, fat malabsorption and steatorrhea occur because of a diminished bile salt pool. If a lesser degree of ileum is involved, hepatic bile acid production can keep up with losses to prevent fat malabsorption. However, the presence of bile acids in the stool stimulates colonic electrolyte and water secretion, producing bile acid diarrhea. Both situations are a result of inefficient enterohepatic recirculation of bile.

GASTRIC DISORDERS

Postgastrectomy Syndrome

Dumping syndrome and nutritional deficiencies caused by malabsorption characterize postgastrectomy disorders. Gastrectomy refers to removal of part of the stomach (usually the antrum and part or all of the gastric body) with subsequent anastomosis to the duodenum (Billroth I) or jejunal loop (Billroth II) and is usually done as treatment for refractory peptic ulcer disease or gastric cancer (Fig. 6-22). Dumping syndrome occurs because there is a loss of sequential contraction from the antrum to the pylorus to the duodenum; a hyperosmolar meal is rapidly presented to the small intestine. Water, which moves passively from the plasma compartment, enters the hyperosmolar lumen, producing a significant fluid shift and resulting in systemic hypovolemia. The liquid contents stimulate hypermotility and the release of vasoactive peptides (serotonin and vasoactive intestinal peptide), which cause vasodilation. Orthostatic hypotension and syncope may ensue. The large load presented to the intestine is rapidly processed, producing hyperglycemia from absorbed carbohydrates and concomitant hyperinsulinemia. The hyperinsulinemia often outlasts the increased blood glucose, subsequently producing hypoglycemia. Thus patients with classic dumping syndrome typically complain of postprandial lightheadedness or fainting, tachycardia, and diaphoresis.

Malabsorption and maldigestion occur after gastrectomy. The reduction of stomach acid does not allow conversion of ferric to ferrous iron for absorption. Furthermore, Billroth II surgery bypasses the duodenum where most iron is absorbed; ingestion of heme iron would not correct the malabsorption. The lack of acid allows colonization of the upper gastrointestinal tract with bacteria and can

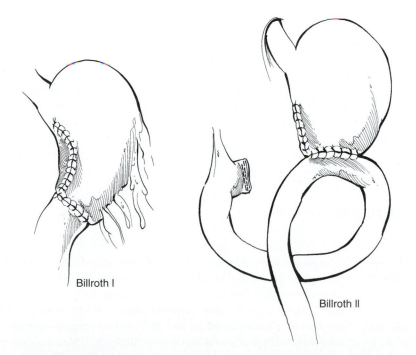

Billroth I

Billroth II

Figure 6-22. Billroth I (left) and Billroth II (right) anastomoses. (Adapted from Yamada T, Alpers DH, Owyang C, Powell DH, Silverstein FE, eds. Textbook of Gastroenterology, 2nd ed. Philadelphia: JB Lippincott, 1995;2:1524.)

lead to bacterial overgrowth. Bypass of the duodenum prevents the normal wall distention by chyme, thus prohibiting the CCK and secretin responses for biliary and pancreatic secretions. In patients with a gastrojejunostomy, the arrival of ingested food may precede the arrival of pancreatic enzymes and bile, leading to maldigestion. Intrinsic factor, secreted by parietal cells in the stomach body and fundus, is not lost as a result of the gastrectomy operation because usually only the distal stomach is removed. However, gastrectomy patients often develop chronic gastritis and gastric atrophy over a period of years, which leads to diminished IF production and thus diminished vitamin B_{12} absorption.

Pernicious Anemia/Achlorohydria

Pernicious anemia is a familial disease characterized by achlorohydria, atrophic gastritis, and macrocytic anemia caused by vitamin B_{12} deficiency. Fundic gland atrophy occurs, with loss of parietal cells; the antrum is usually spared. Autoantibodies to parietal cells and antibodies that block IF are characteristic, and patients afflicted with pernicious anemia are at risk for other autoimmune diseases. Achlorohydria causes a compensatory increase in gastrin secretion from the antrum. The lack of stomach acid can lead to iron deficiency; lack of IF leads to vitamin B_{12} malabsorption and the subsequent macrocytic anemia.

Vagotomy

Truncal vagotomy prevents vagal stimulation of acid in patients with severe refractory peptic ulcer disease, but it also denervates the entire stomach. The emptying of ingested liquids is accelerated but the movement of solids is slowed. Because of impairment of gastric emptying, a drainage procedure must be performed allowing satisfactory exit of food from the stomach. A highly selective vagotomy (Fig. 6-23) cuts only the branches of the vagus nerve that supply the fundus and stomach body, leaving the antral musculature intact. This reduces acid secretion only, and no drainage procedure is required. Solid emptying from the stomach is relatively spared.

Truncal vagotomy reduces basal acid secretion by 85% and maximal acid secretion by 50%. The response of the parietal cell to gastrin is attenuated after vagotomy. This reduction of acid output does not prevent iron absorption or permit bacterial overgrowth because some acid secretion is still achieved. The gastroparesis produced by truncal vagotomy in combination with a drainage procedure removes the grinding and sieving function of the antrum and can cause mild forms of malabsorption by delivery of larger than normal food particles to the intestine.

MUCOSAL DISEASES

Celiac Sprue

Celiac sprue (gluten-sensitive enteropathy) is an intestinal disease characterized by damage to the mucosal lining of the small intestine. Mucosal damage by the gliadin component of gluten, a protein found in wheat, rye, barley, and oats, appears to be the cause. Although it often appears after a child is weaned from breast milk and when cereal is introduced in the diet, celiac disease can also present in adulthood, when the diagnosis is often more difficult. The mucosal architecture is characterized pathologically by the loss of villi and the presence of excessive numbers of intraepithelial lymphocytes (Fig. 6-24). The enterocyte epithelial layer is flattened on microscopic examination, with hyperplasia of the crypts.

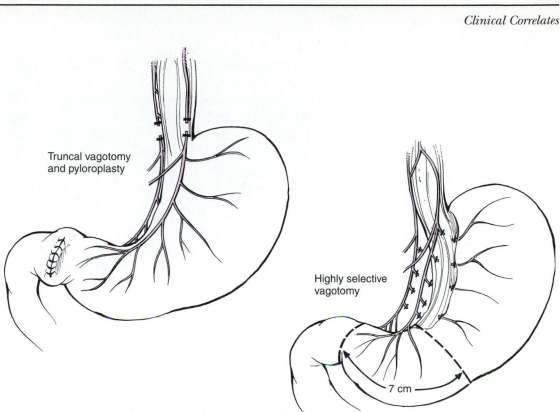

Figure 6-23. Types of vagotomy. (Adapted from Yamada T, Alpers DH, Owyang C, Powell DH, Silverstein FE, eds. Textbook of Gastroenterology, 2nd ed. Philadelphia: JB Lippincott, 1995;2:1526.)

Celiac disease activity begins first in the proximal intestine and extends distally, probably reflecting gluten exposure more proximally and subsequent digestion or absorption before reaching the distal bowel. Most patients have antigliadin antibodies that diminish serologically after treatment for celiac sprue.

Celiac sprue is the prototypical disease for malabsorption. The degree of malabsorption in celiac sprue may predict the severity of mucosal involvement. Patients exhibit abdominal distention, flatulence, progressive weight loss, and diarrhea. The diarrhea in celiac disease is multifactorial but is often steatorrhea. Carbohydrate, fat, and protein malabsorption happen because of villus destruction. Carbohydrate malabsorption is caused by loss of enterocyte hydrolases and produces flatulence and osmotic diarrhea. Fat malabsorption allows colonic bacteria to hydroxylate the undigested lipid, causing colonocyte secretion of water in addition to steatorrhea. In the small bowel, there is decreased water and electrolyte absorption with the loss of coupled sodium cotransporters, and chloride secretion takes place by the increased number of undifferentiated enterocytes. Since the disease affects the proximal small intestine primarily, absorption of iron and folate are compromised. Uptake of fat-soluble vitamins is reduced in severe mucosal disease. Removal of gluten from the diet reverses the villi flattening and restores normal intestinal absorption. Development of malignant lymphoma can be a late complication of this disease.

Tropical Sprue

Tropical sprue is a disease of adult travelers to tropical areas of the world, manifesting as diarrhea and later as nutritional deficiencies. The etiology is ob-

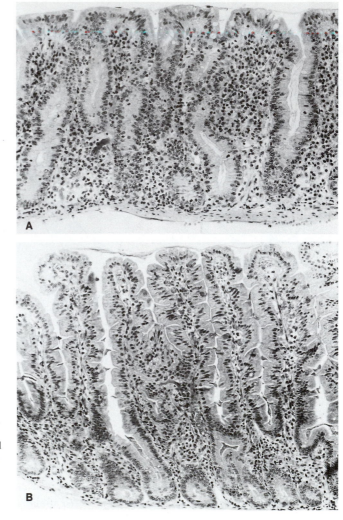

Figure 6-24. Celiac sprue. (**A**) Observe the flat mucosal surface in this biopsy specimen. The villi are effaced, and the crypts have become elongated. The lamina propria contains a prominent infiltrate of chronic inflammatory cell, and lymphocytes infiltrate the surface epithelium. (**B**) The appearance of this same patient's mucosa after an absolutely gluten-free period of 3 weeks, during which time total parenteral nutrition was administered. The villi have returned to a normal appearance, and the inflammatory infiltrate within the lamina propria and surface epithelium has receded. Compare the abnormal appearance of the surface epithelial cells in (**A**) with those seen in (**B**). (From Yamada T, Alpers DH, Owyang C, Powell DH, Silverstein FE, eds. Textbook of Gastroenterology, 2nd ed. Philadelphia: JB Lippincott, 1995;2:2863.)

scure but thought to be due to toxin secretion or colonization by aerobic coliform bacteria. Tropical sprue affects the entire small bowel; the microscopic picture shows elongated crypts, broadened or shortened villi, and infiltration of the lamina propria by chronic inflammatory cells. Full flattening of the villi is rare in tropical sprue.

The defective mucosa prevents proper processing of carbohydrates, fats, and proteins by the enterocyte, causing osmotic diarrhea and potentially steatorrhea. Folate is the most common deficiency in tropical sprue and is caused by the loss of conjugase digestion on the microvilli as well as malabsorption by the affected or absent enterocyte. Vitamin B_{12} deficiency can occur if the tropical sprue lesion involves the ileum and is longstanding enough to deplete stores. Folate and vitamin B_{12} depletion lead to the macrocytic anemia often observed in this disease. Complete fat-soluble vitamin deficiency is rare, but depleted levels occur. Net secretion of water and electrolytes ensues because of the loss of sodium coupled transporters and the increased number of immature enterocytes in the crypts. Bile acid diarrhea does not occur in tropical sprue because anaerobic bacteria are not present in the intestine to deconjugate bile salts. Even in the presence of ileal disease, the enterohepatic circulation of bile salts is only moderately affected. Treatment with folate and tetracycline antibiotics is the mainstay of therapy, in addition to vitamin B_{12} repletion if needed.

Ischemic Enteropathy

Chronic mesenteric ischemia occurs in patients with atherosclerotic disease in which two of three major visceral arteries (celiac, superior mesenteric, and inferior mesenteric) are severely narrowed or occluded. Its hallmark is abdominal angina, characterized by severe postprandial pain. Often there is considerable weight loss caused by anorexia and fear of eating. Some patients develop diarrhea, but malabsorption is usually mild. The degree of malabsorption depends on the amount of injury as the ischemic insult develops, producing a gradient of injury beginning from the tips of the villi to deeper layers of the bowel wall. Initially, the permeability barrier of the enterocyte to molecules breaks down, causing protein loss. Subsequently, the epithelium is shed causing malabsorption as a result of the loss of microvillus enzymes and nutrient uptake mechanisms. Reversal of the ischemia and removal of damaged bowel are the treatments of this disease.

Radiation Enteropathy

Radiation enteropathy is a condition caused by irradiation of the bowel and is most commonly seen after therapy in cervical cancer patients. Acutely (within 2 weeks of exposure), the small bowel mucosa becomes edematous, with villus atrophy and a decrease in mucosal thickness causing a watery diarrhea that abates with termination of radiation therapy. Damage to the bowel wall can be worsened by the presence of pancreatic proteases and bile. Short-term malabsorption of vitamin B_{12}, bile acids, and disaccharides occurs until the mucosa is replaced by crypt cell migration. Chronic effects of radiation enteropathy can take up to 30 years to manifest. Although obstruction from stricture development is the most common problem in chronic radiation enteropathy, varying degrees of malabsorption can occur. The ileum, particularly, can be affected or bypassed by fistula formation, causing deficiency in vitamin B_{12} absorption and compromising the enterohepatic circulation. Steatorrhea can be a manifestation of malabsorbed bile salts, or bile salt diarrhea can be caused by colonocyte water secretion. Therapy is usually symptomatic for the diarrhea plus repletion of nutrients.

OTHER DISORDERS

Lactose Intolerance

Lactase deficiency most commonly happens as a decline in lactase enzyme activity from birth to adulthood and is genetically predetermined. Populations in Africa, Asia, and the Mediterranean countries as well as the American black population have the highest prevalence of deficiency. Additionally, any disease affecting the mucosal lining of the small intestine causes lactase deficiency, and this enzyme appears to be the most sensitive to impairment of the disaccharidases. Lactose ingested in the diet is malabsorbed, allowing bacterial fermentation in the gut and producing flatulence, abdominal distention, and bloating. The increased osmotic load causes diarrhea. Withdrawal of lactose from the diet prevents symptomatic lactose intolerance.

Short Bowel Syndrome

Short bowel syndrome is the clinical consequence of extensive surgical small bowel resection as a result of a variety of catastrophes to the small intestine such as small bowel volvulus, vascular thromboembolism, or extensive Crohn's disease. The length of bowel remaining in the patient determines the severity of this syndrome; resection leaving 25% or less of small bowel invariably leads to malabsorption. Although the remaining segment may undergo adaptive changes, the amount and location of small bowel removed determine the specific deficiencies or malabsorptive conditions that develop. Gastric acid hypersecretion often occurs after small bowel resection and contributes to damage of the remaining mucosa, impairs micellar formation, and reduces pancreatic enzyme function. The effects may be mediated by the peptide hormone gastrin. Proximal bowel resection prohibits the normal distention-induced release of CCK and secretin, resulting in reduced biliary and pancreatic secretions for digestion. Iron and folate deficiencies also develop with proximal bowel resection. Ileal resection can result in vitamin B_{12} malabsorption. Reduced absorption of fat, protein, and carbohydrates also occurs owing to loss of mucosal surface area. In addition, severe fluid losses up to 5 L/day are common as a result of water and electrolyte malabsorption and secretion. Fat-soluble vitamin deficiency develops. If the ileocecal valve is resected, coliform bacteria may travel from the colon to the remaining small intestine, producing the bacterial overgrowth syndrome and further contributing to malabsorption. Ironically, vitamin K synthesized by bacteria may be available for absorption, limiting deficiency of this nutrient. Finally, there is decreased transit time for nutrients coursing through the shortened bowel, especially if the ileocecal valve is absent, reducing the contact time between nutrients and mucosa and thus impairing absorption. By these mechanisms, the most common clinical feature in this syndrome is diarrhea, followed by wasting and nutritional deficiencies. Management includes treatment of diarrhea and peroral or parenteral replacement of water and nutrients.

Protein-Losing Enteropathy

Protein-losing enteropathy is a generalized syndrome with many causes that leads to protein excretion into the gut with resultant hypoproteinemia and hypogammaglobulinemia. The excretion is without regard to the size of the protein. The clinical manifestation is edema caused by loss of albumin from the intravascular space. Protein loss can be seen in diseases of lymphatic obstruction (lymphangiectasia) in which increased hydrostatic pressure forces lymph (and therefore protein) into the lumen of the bowel. Mucosal diseases such as Crohn's disease or sprue can damage the enterocyte epithelial barrier and thus allow seepage of interstitial fluid containing protein. Correction and treatment of the underlying cause often improve the hypoproteinemia.

MOTILITY DISORDERS

Excessive circulating thyroid hormone in hyperthyroidism reduces small bowel and colonic transit time, producing diarrhea and steatorrhea if fat digestion and absorption times are limited. Treatment of the hyperthyroidism returns bowel motility to normal.

Small bowel involvement by diabetes mellitus usually causes diarrhea and is thought to be secondary to autonomic neuropathy. In those patients with both pancreatic exocrine and endocrine deficiency, steatorrhea is present. Commonly, gut motility is decreased and is manifested by gastroparesis and constipation. Poor gastric motility cannot provide antral grinding for initial lipid emulsification and can contribute to steatorrhea. Furthermore, small intestinal stasis caused by the autonomic neuropathy produces bacterial overgrowth and leads to deconjugation of bile acids and fat malabsorption. Specific therapy may include tetracycline for bacterial overgrowth but often treatment is for symptomatic relief of the diarrhea or improvement of motility.

Scleroderma, also called progressive systemic sclerosis, is a generalized disorder of connective tissue characterized by degenerative and inflammatory changes that subsequently lead to fibrosis. In the intestinal tract, hypomotility of the small intestine may occur due to smooth muscle loss. Luminal stasis can ensue and bacterial overgrowth will produce diarrhea. Treatment of bacterial overgrowth and improvement of motility are options for therapy.

Amyloidosis is a systemic disease that is a consequence of extracellular deposition of the abnormal protein amyloid. Many organs are often affected by infiltration of amyloid. In the gastrointestinal tract, a frequently involved organ system, amyloid infiltrates the smooth muscle and autonomic nerves as well as the mesenteric vasculature, causing dysmotility of the small bowel. Malabsorption often occurs through a combination of bacterial overgrowth, reduced motility, and mesenteric ischemia. Diarrhea is the major symptom with small bowel involvement. Treatment of the underlying condition in secondary causes of amyloidosis may lead to its regression.

CLINICAL TESTING

Clinical tests assist the physician in elucidating the etiology and degree of suspected malabsorption. The medical history is paramount and often directs the practitioner to specific tests that confirm a suspected diagnosis; it is the most important aspect in evaluating these patients. Physical examination of the patient gives clues to nutritional deficiencies; peripheral edema or wasting may be evident. The number and order of diagnostic studies depend on the history and clinical signs and symptoms of the patient.

Blood Tests

Albumin is quantitatively the major protein produced by the liver and has a half-life of about 20 days. Levels of serum albumin can therefore reflect hepatic synthetic dysfunction from chronic liver disease, nutritional deficiencies, and protein loss from the urinary or gastrointestinal tract. Excessive loss by the gastrointestinal tract will overwhelm normal hepatic synthesis and cause hypoalbuminemia, producing the syndrome of protein-losing enteropathy. Other factors such as availability of amino acid precursors, proteinuria, and vascular volume expansion as seen in cirrhosis also affect serum levels of albumin. Loss of albumin from the intravascular space reduces oncotic pressure although hydrostatic pressure is unchanged, thus producing edema from the imbalance between hydrostatic and oncotic forces. Normal levels of serum albumin are 3.5 to 5.5 g/dl.

Prealbumin (transthyretin) is a glycosylated serum protein produced by the liver that transports thyroid hormone. It is not the precursor to albumin as the name might imply but is named for its faster electrophoretic mobility relative to albumin. Prealbumin has a half-life of 1.9 days, and levels may be sensitive to acute liver diseases such as acetaminophen toxicity. It is also useful for assessment of more rapid changes in nutritional status. Normal serum levels in adults are 16 to 40 mg/dl.

Carotene levels in the serum are a useful measure of vitamin A absorption (and by inference, absorption of lipids and other fat-soluble vitamins). However carotene is not stored in the liver and does not assess vitamin A deficiency. Normal levels are 20 to 80 µg/dl.

Hemoglobin measurement may identify anemia present as a result of malabsorption. The mean corpuscular volume, a measure of the size of red cells, is decreased in iron deficiency (i.e., microcytic anemia) and increased in either folate or vitamin B_{12} deficiency (i.e., macrocytic anemia).

Vitamin B_{12} levels in the serum are normally 200 to 600 pg/ml. Reduction in this level may be a result of ileal disease, acidity in the proximal bowel lumen, or gastric atrophy and loss of IF. In patients who are known to have ileal Crohn's disease or pancreatic insufficiency, vitamin B_{12} levels should be assessed even in the absence of macrocytic anemia.

Folate serum level depression can indicate any general mucosal disease with resultant malabsorption but is particularly seen in tropical sprue. Normal levels are 6 to 15 ng/ml. In macrocytic anemia, folate as well as vitamin B_{12} levels should be assessed. Correction of macrocytic anemia using folate in patients with vitamin B_{12} deficiency is possible but puts the patient at risk for neurologic sequelae. Replacement therapy should be specific for the deficiency.

The term "liver function tests," as it is commonly used, refers to serum transaminases (aspartate and alanine aminotransferases), alkaline phosphatase, and bilirubin measurements. Abnormalities of these tests usually indicate acute or chronic hepatocellular disease or biliary obstructive disease. Strictly speaking, transaminases and alkaline phosphatase are not "functions" of the liver. Measurement of serum proteins and prothrombin time better assesses liver function. Aspartate aminotransferase and alanine aminotransferase elevations are sensitive indicators of hepatocyte cell death such as is caused by viral hepatitis or acetaminophen toxicity. Normal levels of both transaminases are less than 40 U/ml. In chronic liver disease, increases in aspartate aminotransferase and alanine aminotransferase may be subtle, an indication that very few functional hepatocytes are left because of longstanding destruction and dropout of cells. Alkaline phosphatase levels are elevated in diseases in which there is intrahepatic or extrahepatic biliary obstruction. Parenchymal diseases of the liver that produce rises in aspartate aminotransferase and alanine aminotransferase may also exhibit elevations in serum alkaline phosphatase; however the main value of alkaline phosphatase measurements is in differentiation of hepatocellular disease from obstructive biliary disease. Bilirubin is the end product of heme degradation by hepatocytes and is passed into the stool via bile. Serum elevations of bilirubin may indicate defective processing because of injured hepatocytes or obstruction to bile flow.

Calcium levels that are depressed in the serum may indicate vitamin D deficiency, since this fat-soluble vitamin regulates calcium absorption in the gut. Calcium is actively absorbed in the duodenum and passively in the rest of the small intestine. Generalized mucosal disease can prevent adequate absorption. In addition, unabsorbed fatty acids can bind ionized calcium, preventing absorption and decreasing serum levels.

Cholesterol levels in the serum may be depressed in malabsorption despite intrinsic hepatic synthesis. Cholesterol esters are not assimilated by enterocytes in mucosal disease of the small intestine and exit unabsorbed in the stool.

Fecal Fat Determination

The qualitative fecal fat test is a screening test for fat malabsorption. Patients should ingest at least 100 g of fat for the test to be reliable. Furthermore, a negative test does not rule out malabsorption. Fresh stool is mixed with normal saline on a glass slide, glacial acetic acid is added followed by Sudan stain, and the slide is heated under a flame to hydrolyze fatty acids from triglycerides. In patients with fat malabsorption, multiple (≥100) large fat droplets are seen under the microscope at medium power (Fig. 6-25).

The quantitative fecal fat test measures the amount of fat present in collected stool and the volume of the stool. A patient must ingest at least 100 g of fat in the diet for reliable interpretation. Stool is collected over a 72-hour period; this is because a patient's bowel movements may vary and give inaccurate impressions of stool fat excretion with shorter collections. Normal levels of 5 g/24 hours, or less than 6% of ingested fat, are exceeded in fat malabsorption. Stool volume of more than 1 L/day may indicate a secretory component or rapid transit or severe mucosal disease.

Hydrogen Breath Test

The hydrogen breath test is most often used to detect disaccharide enzyme deficiency or to determine the presence of bacterial overgrowth. For lactase deficiency, 50 g of lactose is ingested orally. If the microvillus enzymes are impaired, the high dose of lactose reaches the colon, where bacterial fermentation of lactose can take place. Hydrogen gas is one of the products of fermentation and rapidly passes into the circulation and is excreted through the lungs. Breath hydrogen is measured at 30-minute intervals over a period of 3 hours, and a rise of 20 ppm from baseline is diagnostic for lactase deficiency. To test for bacterial overgrowth, glucose is ingested and hydrogen is measured in the breath. Patients with bacterial overgrowth often have a high resting hydrogen breath level. Characteristically, after a glucose load there is an early rise of hydrogen excretion, indicating fermen-

A   B

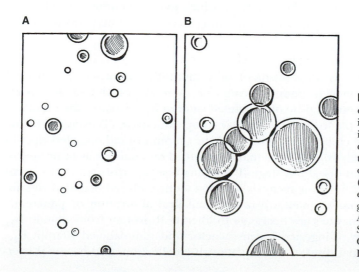

Figure 6-25. The hallmark of a positive qualitative stool fecal fat examination is an increase in the number, and more important, an increase in the size of fat droplets. **(A)** This specimen has 1% triglyceride and is equivalent to a quantitative stool fat of 5 to 6 g/24 hours. **(B)** This specimen has 5% triglyceride and is equivalent to a quantitative stool fat of 10 g/24 hours. (Adapted from Yamada T, Alpers DH, Owyang C, Powell DH, Silverstein FE, eds. Atlas of Gastroenterology. Philadelphia: JB Lippincott, 1992:55.)

tation in the small bowel. Sometimes there may be a second rise once the remaining glucose enters the colon.

D-Xylose Test

The D-xylose test is the classic method for assessment of absorption by the small bowel; it is a test of mucosal integrity. D-xylose is a pentose sugar that is largely absorbed passively and intact across the mucosa. The sugar then enters the bloodstream and is excreted by the kidneys. The patient ingests 25 g of xylose in 500 ml of water, and the urine is collected for the following 5 hours. Those undergoing testing are encouraged to drink plenty of water. Normally, at least 5 g of xylose is excreted into the urine over 5 hours. In the case of renal disease when accurate urine collection is not possible, a blood level of 25 mg/dl of D-xylose indicates adequate absorption and is reached in 1 hour. In malabsorptive conditions, most of the xylose is lost in the stool and thus does not enter the circulation.

Small Bowel Follow-Through X-Ray

The small bowel follow-through x-ray is a series of x-ray films taken after ingestion of radiopaque contrast material (barium sulfate) to visualize the loops of the small intestine. This is a dynamic study with films taken at regular intervals as the barium progresses down the intestine. It can provide information on intestinal transit time and mucosal irregularities, strictures, or masses. If an abnormality is suspected by the radiologist, fluoroscopic examination may be performed to give a closer view of the area. The terminal ileum is often closely scrutinized because of its frequent involvement in Crohn's disease.

Small Bowel Biopsy

Biopsy of small intestinal mucosa can be done with forceps at the time of upper endoscopic examination or by special biopsy instruments passed orally into the small bowel (i.e., Crosby-Kugler capsule, Rubin-Quentin multipurpose tube, or the Carey capsule). Microscopic examination of the biopsy may be diagnostic in diffuse mucosal diseases such as celiac sprue, but other diseases may not yield specific abnormal histologic findings; or if the disease is patchy in distribution, biopsy may miss the lesion when blind biopsies (e.g., Crosby-Kugler capsule) are used or when there is no grossly visible abnormality at which to direct endoscopic biopsies. However, the test is often very useful in narrowing the causes of malabsorption.

Schilling Test

The Schilling test is an assessment of vitamin B_{12} absorption. A stage I Schilling test is performed by administering oral radiolabeled vitamin B_{12}. After 2 hours, a 1000-µg parenteral dose of unlabeled vitamin B_{12} displaces the absorbed radiolabeled B_{12} from tissue into the vascular compartment and is excreted by the urine. A 24-hour urine collection is done, and the amount of radiolabeled vitamin B_{12} is counted (normally 10 to 20% of that ingested). Low counts may indicate gastric disease and/or ileal disease. A stage II Schilling test is performed in the event of an abnormal stage I; intrinsic factor is ingested along with radiolabeled vitamin B_{12}, and the test becomes a measure of terminal ileal absorption or pancreatic function. Pancreatic enzymes are necessary to liberate R protein from vitamin B_{12} and allow the binding of ingested intrinsic factor and radiolabeled vitamin B_{12}. Conditions such as renal disease, inadequate urine collection, and bacterial overgrowth can predispose to low urinary excretion of the radiolabeled vitamin B_{12} and cause false interpretation of the test. When the stage II Schilling test is abnormal in the absence of renal disease (or with an adequate urine collection), it can be repeated after a trial of antibiotics to treat possible bacterial overgrowth.

Bile Acid Breath Test

The bile acid breath test measures bile acid deficiency states, such as ileal disease or bacterial overgrowth. Normally, 95% of conjugated bile acids secreted by the liver into the intestine enter the ileum, where active uptake transports the bile acids back to the liver for reutilization. In this test, ^{14}C glycocholate (glycine-conjugated cholic acid) is ingested; normally only 5% reaches the colon, where bacteria deconjugate the glycocholate and metabolize the glycine to $^{14}CO_2$, which is collected in expired air. Bacterial overgrowth hydrolyzes more glycocholate producing increased levels of $^{14}CO_2$. Similarly, diminished enterohepatic circulation in ileal disease or resection allows more glycocholate to enter the colon, where bacterial action liberates increased $^{14}CO_2$.

Bentiromide Test

The bentiromide test measures pancreatic exocrine function. An oral dose of 500 mg of bentiromide (*N*-benzoyl-L-tyrosyl-para-aminobenzoic acid) is ingested. Subsequently, chymotrypsin secreted by the pancreas cleaves bentiromide and allows para-aminobenzoic acid (PABA) to be absorbed from the intestine, conjugated by the liver, and excreted in the urine. Pancreatic insufficiency is suspect when less than 60% of the ingested dose is excreted during a 6-hour collection of urine. Liver disease, renal disease, and mucosal disease can give falsely low values.

Fecal α_1-Antitrypsin

Alpha$_1$-antitrypsin is a serine protease inhibitor synthesized by the liver. In protein-losing enteropathy, α_1-antitrypsin, albumin, and other proteins are leaked into the intestinal lumen. Unlike albumin, α_1-antitrypsin is stable in the presence of pancreatic and intestinal enzymes that contain serine proteases and therefore is excreted in the stool intact. It is used as a measure of protein loss from the gut. Stool is collected for 24 hours and frozen until assayed. Normal values are less than 54 mg/dl.

CASE PRESENTATION

A 48-year-old woman complains of crampy abdominal pain, bloating, watery diarrhea, and fatigue for the past 15 months. She has lost 18 lb without dieting over this time period. She passes three to four loose stools daily, which occasionally are malodorous and float in the toilet. She had previously been in good health and required no prior hospitalization aside from childbirth.

This patient has a progressive, chronic illness involving the gastrointestinal tract. The presence of bloating, watery diarrhea, and floating stools suggests carbohydrate malabsorption. Malodorous stools may represent a degree of fat malabsorption. Weight loss also signals malabsorption in this context.

Her appearance is somewhat malnourished. An abdominal examination is unremarkable, and the stool is negative for occult blood. Routine laboratory tests show normal electrolytes and renal function and normal liver function tests. However, her serum albumin level is 2.6 g/dl. A decreased hemoglobin (11 g/dl) and mean corpuscular volume (72 fl) are noted, as well as a low serum iron concentration (42 μg/dl) with a normal total iron-binding capacity (340 μg/dl).

The reader should recognize a reduction in albumin concentration, indicating reduced hepatic synthesis and/or protein loss from the gastrointestinal tract. Since liver function tests are normal, reduced liver production would be caused by low availability of precursors from malabsorption. Iron-deficiency anemia has developed. The percent saturation of iron is low, indicating malabsorption from the proximal small intestine, since there is no evidence for occult fecal blood loss.

Because of your concern for malabsorption, you order a D-xylose test. The patient's urinary output was 2.2 g in 5 hours. You order a dedicated small bowel follow-through x-ray (Fig. 6-26) and arrange an upper endoscopic examination to obtain duodenal mucosal biopsies (Fig. 6-27).

D-xylose is a test of mucosal integrity and the patient's malabsorptive process is caused by small intestinal mucosal disease. The x-ray reveals a decrease in mucosal folds, indicating diffuse mucosal involvement with disease. Her duodenal biopsy shows loss of villi with an intraepithelial lymphocytic infiltrate and elongation of the intestinal crypts. These findings suggest the presence of celiac sprue.

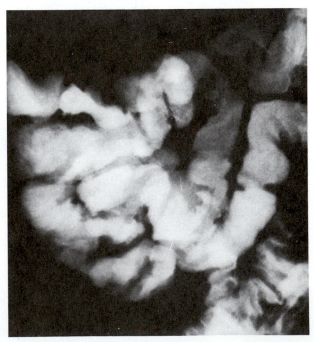

Figure 6-26. Our patient's dedicated small bowel follow-through x-ray. (From Juhl JH and Crummy AB, eds. Paul and Juhl's Essentials of Radiologic Imaging, 6th ed. Philadelphia: JB Lippincott, 1993:611.)

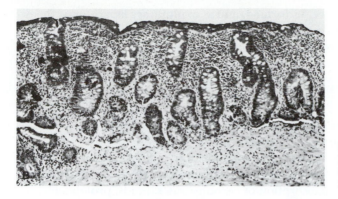

Figure 6-27. Our patient's small bowel biopsy. In: Yamada T, Alpers DH, Owyang C, Powell DH, Silverstein FE, eds. Textbook of Gastroenterology. 2nd ed. Philadelphia: JB Lippincott, 1995;2:1648.)

You prescribe a gluten-free diet. The patient's diarrhea and bloating gradually disappear over the next several weeks, and her weight improves. Two years later, she reports a return of her diarrhea and vague diffuse abdominal pain, despite adherance to her gluten-free diet. She experiences a loss of 10 lbs over the preceding 2 months. You repeat her dedicated small bowel follow-through x-ray (Fig. 6-28).

Although noncompliance with a gluten-free diet can cause a return of symptoms, the new symptom of diffuse abdominal pain and the return of malabsorption and weight loss may signify a complication of celiac sprue. The repeat x-ray study shows a disorganized bowel pattern with variable dilatation and narrowing of the lumen, separation and displacement of the bowel loops, and mucosal irregularity suggestive of infiltrative disease. This is consistent with lymphoma, which can develop in patients with celiac sprue.

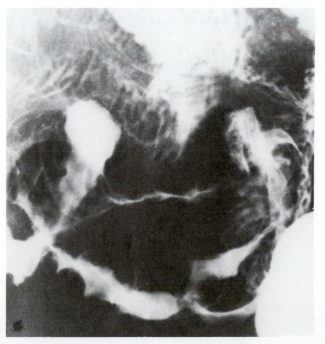

Figure 6-28. Dedicated small bowel follow-through x-ray of our patient 2 years after presentation. (From Juhl JH and Crummy AB, eds. Paul and Juhl's Essentials of Radiologic Imaging, 6th ed. Philadelphia: JB Lippincott, 1993:611.)

Staging radiologic tests are performed, and at exploratory laparotomy, the diagnosis of T-cell lymphoma is made on biopsy. Your oncologist recommends radiation therapy and combination chemotherapy, and the patient agrees to treatment.

SUMMARY

The processes of digestion and absorption require the coordinated response of all aspects of the alimentary tract: mastication and salivary secretion, gastric acid and grinding, pancreatic and biliary secretion, intestinal motility, and an intact microvillus border on enterocytes. Interference with normal digestion and absorption by disease can lead to malabsorption of carbohydrates, lipids, protein, and vitamins and their consequences of diarrhea, weight loss, and vitamin deficiency. Recognition of malabsorption by the health care professional is paramount in order to supplement the patient with nutrients. History and physical examination of the patient can provide clues to malabsorption, and specific tests for malabsorption aid the physician in identifying its cause and often can lead to a proper diagnosis and correction of the underlying illness.

SELECTED READING

Ahnen DJ. Nutrient assimilation. In: Kelly WN, ed. Textbook of Internal Medicine, 2nd ed. Philadelphia: JB Lippincott, 1992:404–411.

Kagnoff MP. Celiac disease. In: Yamada T, Alpers DH, Owyang C, Powell DW, Silverstein FE, eds. Textbook of Gastroenterology, 2nd ed. Philadelphia: JB Lippincott, 1995;2:1643–1661.

Kaunitz JD, Barrett KE, McRoberts JA. Electrolyte secretion and absorption: Small intestine and colon. In: Yamada T, Alpers DH, Owyang C, Powell DW, Silverstein FE, eds. Textbook of Gastroenterology, 2nd ed. Philadelphia: JB Lippincott, 1995;1:326–361.

Olsen WA. A pathophysiological approach to diagnosis of malabsorption. Am J Med 67:1007, 1979.

Riley SA, Turnberg LA. Maldigestion and malabsorption. In: Sleisenger MH, Fordtran JS, eds. Gastrointestinal Disease, 5th ed. Philadelphia: W B Saunders, 1993;1:1009–1027.

Trier JS. Intestinal malabsorption: Differentiation of cause. Hosp Pract 23:195, 1988.

Lippincott's Pathophysiology Series: Gastrointestinal Pathophysiology, edited by Joseph M. Henderson. Lippincott–Raven Publishers. Philadelphia © 1996.

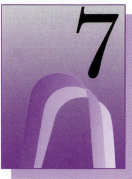

CHAPTER

7

Jaundice and Abnormal Liver Chemistries

D. Kim Turgeon and Richard H. Moseley

INTRODUCTION

Most forms of liver disease are heralded by the appearance of jaundice or by elevations in the serum values of liver chemistries or both. This chapter provides an integrated approach to the understanding and diagnosis of disorders associated with jaundice and/or abnormal liver chemistries. The first part provides essential background on normal hepatic anatomy and physiology. The laboratory tests used in the approach to the patient with liver disease are then introduced, followed by a classification of liver disease in which the causes are divided into major pathophysiologic categories. Within each category, selected diseases are discussed. In the final section, a clinical problem is presented that incorporates a detailed discussion of the clinical and laboratory evaluations of a jaundiced patient.

PATHOPHYSIOLOGY

STRUCTURE AND FUNCTION OF THE LIVER

Critical to an understanding of hepatobiliary disease is a familiarity with the anatomy and ultrastructure of the liver and biliary tree (Fig. 7-1). Neighboring hepatocytes, typically arranged in single-cell thick plates, are joined by junctional complexes that serve to demarcate the canalicular space from the basolateral, or sinusoidal, domain. Differences in the structure and function of the sinusoidal and canalicular membrane define the hepatocyte as a polarized cell. Adjacent plates of hepatocytes are separated by the hepatic sinusoids, which are lined by endothelial cells. Processes extending from the endothelial cell body contain pores (fenestrae)

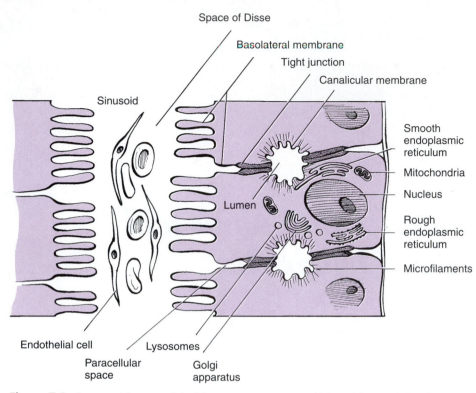

Figure 7-1. Structural features of the bile secretory apparatus. (Adapted by permission from Moseley RH. Bile secretion. In: Yamada T, Alpers DH, Owyang C, Powell DW, Silverstein FE, eds. Textbook of Gastroenterology, 2nd ed. Philadelphia: JB Lippincott, 1995:386.)

that allow direct contact between plasma and the sinusoidal membrane of the hepatocyte. Thus, unlike other endothelial, sinusoidal endothelial cells lack an underlying basement membrane. This feature is thought to facilitate the transfer of protein-bound solutes, such as bilirubin and bile acids, from the sinusoid to the space of Disse and, subsequently, to the hepatocyte; it also promotes the excretion of solutes, e.g., lipoproteins, from the hepatocyte to the sinusoid. In alcoholic liver disease a decrease in the number of fenestrations may occur that results in disturbances in the exchange of substances between hepatocytes and sinusoidal blood.

Functionally, the sinusoidal membrane is primarily involved in the bidirectional exchange of solutes. Transport processes for the uptake of amino acids, glucose, and organic anions such as bile acids, fatty acids, and bilirubin, and for the receptor-mediated endocytotic processes are present on this membrane domain. Domain-specific enzymes, particularly sodium potassium adenosine triphosphatase (Na^+/K^+-ATPase), and the export processes for albumin, lipoproteins, and clotting factors are also found on the sinusoidal membrane. In contrast, the predominant function at the canalicular membrane surface is bile secretion, although limited reabsorptive capacity has also been demonstrated. Certain membrane enzymes are selectively localized to the canalicular domain, including alkaline phosphatase, leucine aminopeptidase, and γ-glutamyl transpeptidase.

From adjacent canaliculi, bile enters small terminal bile ductules, the canals of Hering, consisting of fusiform cells in close association with neighboring hepatocytes. These short channels, in turn, traverse the limiting plate to form, successively, larger ductules and intralobular bile ducts, composed of cuboidal epithelial cells. Interlobular bile ducts, ranging in size from 30 to 40 µm, convey bile eventually to the extrahepatic bile duct, the gallbladder (if present), and the duodenum.

The major physiologic functions of the gallbladder are (1) concentration and storage of bile during interdigestive periods; (2) evacuation of gallbladder bile by smooth muscle contraction in response to cholecystokinin; and (3) moderation of hydrostatic pressure within the biliary tract. Although it is not essential for bile secretion, the gallbladder serves to concentrate bile up to 10-fold. The result of this concentrative process is the formation of gallbladder bile, isotonic to plasma and composed of higher concentrations of sodium, bile salts, potassium, and calcium and lower concentrations of chloride and bicarbonate than hepatic bile.

A unique feature of hepatic architecture is the organization of hepatocytes within a hepatic acinus that is arbitrarily divided into three functional zones (Fig. 7-2). Zone 1 hepatocytes abut the portal tract and are exposed to sinusoidal blood containing the highest concentration of solutes and oxygen. In contrast, zone 3 hepatocytes, present in the pericentral region around the terminal hepatic venule, are exposed to a relatively oxygen-poor environment. As a result, ischemic hepatitis preferentially causes centrizonal hepatocyte necrosis. In addition, zone 3 hepatocytes actively participate in drug metabolism and disposition. Consequently, most drugs in clinical use, if they are hepatotoxic, induce zone 3 necrosis.

DRUG METABOLISM

Approximately 2% of all cases of jaundice in hospitalized patients are drug-induced, underscoring the importance of the liver as a site for drug metabolism. Two phases of hepatic drug metabolism are recognized: phase 1 reactions, involving oxidation and reduction, largely mediated by the cytochromes P450 that result in minor modifications of the parent compound; and phase 2 reactions, consisting of conjugation of water-soluble moieties, such as glucuronic acid, sulfate, and glutathione, to the parent compound. Drugs may be metabolized by phase 1 and phase 2 reactions in sequence or directly metabolized by a phase 2 conjugation. In

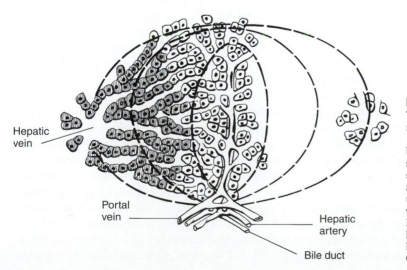

Figure 7-2. The hepatic acinus. The acinar axis is formed by the terminal branch of the portal vein (TPV), hepatic artery (HA), and bile ductule (BD). Blood enters the sinusoids in zone 1 and flows sequentially through zone 2 and zone 3, where it exits the acinus via the terminal branch of the hepatic vein (HV). (Adapted from Traber PG, Chianale J, Gumucio JJ. Physiologic significance and regulation of hepatocellular heterogeneity. Gastroenterology 95:1131, 1988.)

Hepatic vein

Portal vein

Hepatic artery

Bile duct

advanced liver disease, phase 1 reactions may be impaired by relative preservation of phase 2 reactions.

The cytochromes P450 are a family of hemoproteins situated predominantly in the endoplasmic reticulum of the hepatocyte in a membrane-bound form. Drug metabolism by the P450 system, although typically detoxifying, occasionally produces toxic intermediates such as electrophiles and free radicals which, if not further metabolized, can lead to covalent binding to cellular proteins and membrane lipid peroxidation, respectively. Conjugation with glutathione is mediated by cytosolic enzymes, the glutathione S transferases, and plays an important role in the detoxification of electrophiles produced by the P450 system. However, glucuronidation and sulfation are more frequently employed in hepatic biotransformation and are mediated by microsomal uridine diphosphate (UDP)-glucuronyl transferases and cytosolic sulfotransferases, respectively.

Exposure to specific substrates of a hepatic drug-metabolizing enzyme may induce the activity of that enzyme. Such induction may be clinically relevant if the enzyme induced produces a toxic intermediate. For example, chronic alcohol exposure induces a form of cytochrome P450 that oxidizes acetaminophen to a toxic electrophilic product, providing an explanation for the enhanced susceptibility of chronic alcoholics to acetaminophen hepatotoxicity.

BILIRUBIN METABOLISM

Jaundice, or icterus, is the yellow discoloration of the skin, mucous membranes, and body fluids produced by bilirubin. The ability to develop a differential diagnosis of jaundice requires a familiarity with certain fundamental aspects of the normal physiology of bilirubin production and excretion.

Bilirubin is formed by the breakdown of heme (Fig. 7-3). Approximately 80% of bilirubin is derived from heme released by senescent erythrocytes, whereas the remainder comes from the heme moieties of other hemoproteins, such as myoglobin and tissue cytochromes. The microsomal enzyme, heme oxygenase, converts heme to biliverdin, which is then converted to bilirubin by biliverdin reductase. The unconjugated bilirubin produced by these enzymatic reactions is transported in the plasma tightly bound to albumin. Competition for albumin binding by certain drugs displaces unconjugated bilirubin and, in the neonate, may result in the diffusion of bilirubin across the blood-brain barrier and bilirubin encephalopathy or kernicterus. Unconjugated bilirubin is avidly taken up by the liver, where it is converted to a water-soluble form by conjugation as a diglucuronide. This process facilitates its excretion into bile and is mediated by the microsomal enzyme, bilirubin UDP-glucuronyl transferase (UDP-GT).

Pathophysiologically, jaundice can be classified as the result of either an unconjugated or a conjugated hyperbilirubinemia (Table 7-1). Unconjugated hyperbilirubinemia results from increased bilirubin production, impaired hepatic uptake, or impaired conjugation. Increased red blood cell destruction in disorders associated with ineffective erythropoiesis and in hemolytic disorders results in increased bilirubin production and a mild unconjugated hyperbilirubinemia. Reductions in hepatic blood flow caused by congestive heart failure or portosystemic shunting impair the delivery of bilirubin to hepatocytes, resulting in a mild unconjugated hyperbilirubinemia. Impaired hepatic uptake at the sinusoidal membrane occurs in Gilbert's syndrome and following the administration of certain drugs, such as rifampin. Reduced activity of UDP-GT leads to impaired bilirubin conjuga-

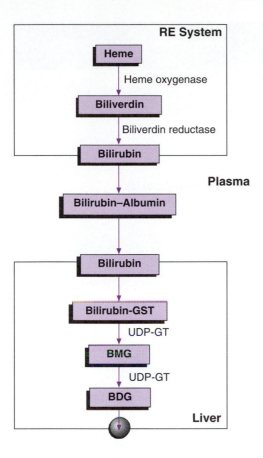

Figure 7-3. Bilirubin metabolism. The conversion of heme to biliverdin by microsomal heme oxygenase occurs predominantly in the reticuloendothelial cells of the spleen. Biliverdin undergoes further oxidation by cytosolic biliverdin reductase to form bilirubin. Unconjugated bilirubin circulates in plasma largely bound to albumin. After dissociation from albumin, bilirubin is taken up by the liver, where it is bound to the cytosolic proteins, glutathione S-transferases (GST). Glucuronidation of bilirubin is catalyzed by microsomal UDP-glucuronosyl transferase (UDP-GT), resulting in the formation of bilirubin monoglucuronide (BMG) and diglucuronide (BDG). Conjugated bilirubin is then excreted into bile. See text for additional details.

tion and is observed in the neonate and in patients with Gilbert's and Crigler-Najjar types I and II syndrome. UDP-GT activity can be induced by phenobarbital, effectively reducing the jaundice in Crigler-Najjar type II syndrome.

Hepatic bilirubin uptake and conjugating activity are preserved in most forms of liver disease, and canalicular excretion represents the rate-limiting step in overall bilirubin metabolism. Accordingly, conjugated hyperbilirubinemias can occur in a wide spectrum of hepatic diseases, including disorders associated with acute and/or chronic hepatocellular and cholestatic injury, extrahepatic biliary obstruction, and the familial abnormalities of bilirubin excretion, Dubin-Johnson and Rotor's syndrome.

BILE FORMATION AND CHOLESTASIS

Bile is a complex fluid, iso-osmotic with plasma, composed primarily of water, inorganic electrolytes, and organic solutes such as bile acids, phospholipids, cholesterol, and bilirubin. Bile acids (or bile salts) are the major organic solutes in bile. Bile acids present in bile are derived from two sources: (1) primary bile acids (cholic and chenodeoxycholic acid in humans) are synthesized from cholesterol in the liver; and (2) secondary bile acids (deoxycholic, lithocholic, and ursodeoxycholic acid in humans) are produced from primary bile acids by intestinal bacteria. Bile acids consist of two components that determine their physiologic and physicochemical properties: (1) a steroid nucleus with hydroxyl substituents; and (2) an

TABLE 7-1. *PATHOPHYSIOLOGIC CLASSIFICATION OF JAUNDICE*

Unconjugated Hyperbilirubinemia

Increased bilirubin production
  Hemolysis
  Ineffective erythropoiesis

Impaired bilirubin uptake
  Gilbert's syndrome
  Drugs (e.g., rifampin, radiographic contrast agents, flavispidic acid)
  Congestive heart failure
  Surgical or spontaneous portasystemic shunts
  Neonatal jaundice

Impaired bilirubin conjugation
  Gilbert's syndrome
  Crigler-Najjar syndromes
  Neonatal jaundice

Conjugated Hyperbilirubinemia*

Impaired canalicular excretion
  Hepatocellular injury (e.g., viral hepatitis, alcoholic hepatitis, cirrhosis)
  Intrahepatic cholestasis (e.g., intrahepatic cholestasis of pregnancy, TPN-induced jaundice)
  Familial disorders of conjugated bilirubin transport (Dubin-Johnson and Rotor's syndrome)

Disorders of the intrahepatic bile ducts
  Primary biliary cirrhosis
  Primary sclerosing cholangitis
  Liver allograft rejection
  Graft versus host disease
  Neoplasms

Disorders of the extrahepatic bile ducts
  Choledocholithiasis
  Neoplasms
  Primary sclerosing cholangitis
  Biliary strictures

*See also Table 7-2.

aliphatic side chain (Fig. 7-4). All of the major mammalian primary bile acids contain a 3 and a 7 hydroxyl substituent that greatly increase water solubility, or hydrophilicity. The terminal carboxylic acid group of the side chain is modified following the synthesis of the primary bile acids, and during the hepatic phase of the enterohepatic cycling of the secondary bile acids by enzymatic conjugation to glycine or taurine. The presence of hydrophilic (the hydroxyl substituents and the amide linkage on the aliphatic side chain) and lipid-soluble or hydrophobic (the steroid nucleus) regions allows conjugated bile salts to act as amphiphilic molecules that form micelles (or polymolecular aggregates) above a critical micellar concentration. Bile salt micelles can, in turn, solubilize other biologically important amphiphilic solutes, such as cholesterol and phospholipids, to form mixed mi-

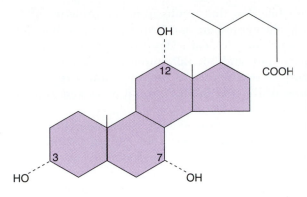

Figure 7-4. Bile acid structure. Bile acids consist of two components: a steroid nucleus with hydroxyl substituents and an aliphatic side chain. The trihydroxy bile acid shown is cholic acid (3α-, 7α-, 12α-OH). Additional bile acids include deoxycholate (3α-, 12α-OH), chenodeoxycholate (3α-, 7α-OH), ursodeoxycholate (3α-, 7β-OH), and lithocholate (3α-OH).

celles. Thus, this detergent-like property of bile acids is important in stabilizing the physical state of bile and in promoting fat digestion and absorption.

Bile acid synthesis from cholesterol is an example of a negative feedback system, although the nature of the regulation at a molecular and biochemical level is not well understood. Microsomal 7α-hydroxylation of cholesterol is thought to be the rate-limiting enzymatic step in bile acid synthesis. Gallstone dissolution therapy with chenodeoxycholate suppresses bile acid synthesis and, therefore, increases plasma cholesterol levels. In contrast, ursodeoxycholate does not suppress bile acid synthesis and plasma cholesterol levels are unchanged during chronic therapy with this bile acid.

Hepatic bile formation results from coordinated events at the sinusoidal and canalicular membranes as well as from intracellular and paracellular processes. In contrast to the passive, hydrostatic forces governing glomerular filtration by the kidney, bile formation by hepatocytes is considered to be an osmotic process involving the active secretion of inorganic and organic solutes into the canalicular lumen, followed by passive water movement. In this important respect, hepatic bile secretion can be characterized by the same processes found in more conventional secretory epithelia, such as the pancreatic acinar cell and the renal tubular cell. Canalicular bile formation has been traditionally divided into two components (Fig. 7-5): (1) bile acid–dependent bile flow (BADBF), defined as the slope of the line relating canalicular bile flow to bile salt excretion; and (2) bile acid–independent bile flow (BAIBF), attributed to the active secretion of inorganic electrolytes and other solutes and defined as the extrapolated *y*-intercept of this line.

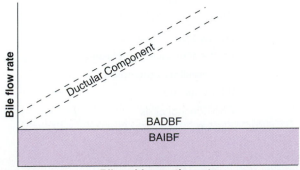

Figure 7-5. Schematic representation of the components of bile flow. BADBF: bile acid–dependent bile flow; BAIBF: bile acid–independent bile flow. (Adapted by permission from Moseley RH. Bile secretion. In: Yamada T, Alpers DH, Owyang C, Powell DW, Silverstein FE, eds. Textbook of Gastroenterology, 2nd ed. Philadelphia: JB Lippincott, 1995:387.)

In other words, BADBF represents bile flow that results from the presence of osmotically active bile acids in the canalicular lumen, and BAIBF represents bile flow that occurs in the theoretical absence of bile acids. However, in some if not all species the relationship between bile flow and bile salt output is curvilinear at low bile acid excretion rates and cannot be represented by the single linear regression illustrated in Figure 7-5. Therefore, BAIBF and BADBF should be viewed as interrelated rather than independent components of bile flow.

Impaired bile formation is termed cholestasis. Within this broad definition, a characteristic constellation of pathologic, physiologic, and clinical features has been described that merely represents selective consequences of this primary underlying defect. In morphologic terms, bile can be identified within the canalicular space of pericentral hepatocytes in liver biopsy specimens, and canalicular dilatation and a reduction in the number of canalicular microvilli can be demonstrated on ultrastructural examination. In pathophysiologic terms, reduction in biliary excretion of inorganic and organic solutes and of water can be measured. Cholestasis is further categorized as either a functional defect in bile formation at the level of the hepatocyte (intrahepatic cholestasis) or a structural or mechanical impairment in bile secretion and flow (extrahepatic cholestasis). The most frequent causes of intrahepatic and extrahepatic cholestasis are listed in Table 7-2. Several mechanisms can be identified that may play a role in the pathogenesis of intrahepatic cholestasis, including alterations in sinusoidal membrane function and/or composition, alterations in cytoskeletal organization and/or function, alterations in tight junction permeability, and impairment of canalicular membrane structure and/or function. Clearly, there is no single mechanism that can explain the development of cholestasis in all clinical settings, and multiple mechanisms may be involved in any given disorder. Clinically, cholestasis is reflected by the appearance in blood of several of these solutes, including bilirubin, bile acids, and cholesterol, that are preferentially excreted into bile under normal conditions. Biochemically, cholesta-

TABLE 7-2. DIFFERENTIAL DIAGNOSIS OF CHOLESTATIC SYNDROMES

INTRAHEPATIC	EXTRAHEPATIC
Acute hepatocellular injury	Choledocholithiasis
Viral hepatitis	Biliary strictures
Alcoholic fatty liver and/or hepatitis	Sclerosing cholangitis
Drugs	Cholangiocarcinoma
Chronic hepatocellular injury	Pancreatic carcinoma
Primary biliary cirrhosis	Pancreatitis (acute or chronic)
Sclerosing cholangitis	Periampullary carcinoma
Drugs	Biliary atresia
Total parenteral nutrition	Choledochal cysts
Systemic infection	Miscellaneous disorders
Postoperative state	
Benign recurrent causes	
Miscellaneous conditions	

sis is characterized by disproportionate elevations in serum alkaline phosphatase activity and/or serum bilirubin concentration relative to serum aminotransferase elevations, as discussed below.

GALLSTONE FORMATION

There are two general types of gallstones: cholesterol stones, accounting for approximately 80% of gallstones in the United States, and pigment stones (Table 7-3). Pigment stones are usually divided into two subtypes. Black or mulberry stones are almost exclusively found in the gallbladder and are largely composed of calcium bilirubinate. Brown or earthy stones tend to form in the bile duct and contain, in addition to calcium bilirubinate, free fatty acids derived from the action of bacterial phospholipases on biliary lecithin, reflecting their underlying etiology.

Altered hepatic bile composition, enhanced cholesterol nucleation, and gallbladder dysfunction are all factors that determine cholesterol gallstone formation. Cholesterol, insoluble in water, is secreted into the canalicular lumen as unilamellar phospholipid vesicles which, in the presence of a sufficient concentration of bile acids, are solubilized into mixed lipid micelles. In bile supersaturated with cholesterol or containing low concentrations of bile acids, excess cholesterol in unilamellar phospholipid vesicles aggregates to form large multilamellar vesicles, from which cholesterol monohydrate crystals may nucleate. Although cholesterol supersaturation appears to be a prerequisite for cholesterol gallstone formation, factors inhibiting or promoting nucleation may be critical since bile supersaturated with cholesterol frequently occurs in individuals without cholesterol gallstones.

TABLE 7-3. *CLASSIFICATION OF GALLSTONES*

| | | PIGMENT | |
	CHOLESTEROL	BLACK	BROWN
Location	Gallbladder, ducts	Gallbladder, ducts	Ducts
Composition	Cholesterol	Ca^{2+} bilirubinate	Ca^{2+} bilirubinate and free fatty acids
Etiologic factors	Age	Age	Age
	Race	Chronic hemolysis	Chronic biliary infection
	Female gender	Cirrhosis	Biliary stasis
	Obesity		
	Rapid and/or prolonged weight loss		
	Diseases of the terminal ileum		
	Drugs (e.g., oral contraceptives, clofibrate)		

Increasing age is a risk factor for the development of cholesterol stones. Native Americans are much more prone to cholesterol stones than caucasians, and the incidence of cholesterol gallstones is higher in caucasians than in blacks or Asians. A female:male ratio of approximately 2:1 is observed for cholesterol stones, with multiparous women having a higher risk than nulliparous women. Obesity, associated with excessive hepatic secretion of cholesterol, and rapid weight loss are strongly associated with cholesterol gallstone disease. Disorders such as Crohn's disease or surgical resection of the terminal ileum may result in depletion of the bile salt pool and predisposition to cholesterol gallstone formation. Clofibrate, used in the treatment of hypercholesterolemia, increases cholesterol output into bile, thereby predisposing to cholesterol gallstone formation. The risk of cholesterol gallstones is also higher with estrogen replacement therapy and oral contraceptive use.

There are several recognized risk factors for the development of pigment stones. Hemolytic conditions, in which an increased bilirubin load is presented to the liver for biliary excretion, cirrhosis, and advancing age are all associated with black pigment stone formation. Chronic infection and/or parasitic infestation of the biliary tract and anatomic abnormalities that promote biliary stasis, such as Caroli's disease, as well as advancing age are predisposing factors in brown pigment stone formation.

LABORATORY TESTS

Most clinical laboratories include aspartate aminotransferase (AST; formerly serum glutamic-oxaloacetic transferase or SGOT), alanine aminotransferase (ALT; formerly serum glutamic-pyruvic transferase or SGPT), gamma-glutamyl transepeptidase (GGT or GGTP), lactate dehydrogenase (LDH), and alkaline phosphatase in a panel of tests termed liver function tests. This is really a misnomer since none of these tests measure or reflect hepatic function. Instead, these tests serve only as markers of hepatic injury.

MARKERS OF HEPATOCELLULAR INJURY

AST and ALT are enzymes found within a variety of tissues. AST is predominantly found in the liver, cardiac and skeletal muscle, and the kidney. In the liver, AST is located in both the cytosol and the mitochondria. In contrast, ALT is largely found in the cytosol of the liver and, to a lesser extent, in muscle. Consequently, serum levels of these enzymes can be elevated not only in disorders associated with hepatocellular injury but also in conditions such as endocarditis, myocardial infarction, and musculoskeletal trauma. When liver disease accounts for the observed enzyme elevations, the degree of the elevation can help in narrowing the differential diagnosis. For example, the highest enzyme elevations are seen in toxin- or drug-induced, viral, or ischemic hepatitis. The height of the elevation of the transaminases is proportional to the extent of acute liver damage. It is not uncommon to see transaminase elevations higher than 10,000 IU in cases of acute hepatic necrosis from either acetaminophen overdose or hepatic ischemia. Elevations in the 500 to 3000 IU range, with an ALT elevation greater than the AST elevation, are characteristic of viral hepatitis. An AST:ALT ratio of less than 1 is typically seen in viral hepatitis, both acute and chronic forms, as well as in extrahepatic biliary obstruction. In contrast, elevations of less than 300 IU and an AST:ALT ratio greater than 2 are characteristic of alcoholic hepatitis.

LDH is an enzyme found in cardiac and skeletal muscle, liver, lung, and red blood cells. Although it is commonly included in laboratory profiles, the diagnostic specificity and clinical utility of serum LDH values are relatively limited. Modest elevations of serum LDH levels are seen in hepatocellular diseases and are less common in cholestatic diseases. The isoenzyme LDH 5 suggests hepatic origin. Myocardial infarction and hemolysis represent nonhepatic causes of serum LDH elevations.

MARKERS OF CHOLESTATIC INJURY

Alkaline phosphatase is an enzyme found in bone, liver, placenta, intestine, and leukocytes. More than 80% of alkaline phosphatase is derived from liver and bone. As discussed above, in the liver alkaline phosphatase is associated with the exterior surface of the bile canalicular membrane. Although significant hepatocellular injury results in some elevation in alkaline phosphatase activity, elevation of alkaline phosphatase to a degree greater than transaminase elevation is consistent with cholestatic liver injury.

Fractionation of alkaline phosphatase isoenzymes is available to confirm the origin of an elevated serum alkaline phosphatase level. Other clinically useful approaches to support a hepatic origin of an elevated serum alkaline phosphatase level include serum γ-glutamyl transpeptidase (GGT or GGTP), serum 5′ nucleotidase (5′NT), and serum leucine aminopeptidase (SLAP). All of these enzymes are also present on the bile canalicular membrane. In addition to in the liver, GGT is found in kidney, pancreas, intestine, and to a lesser extent cardiac tissue. GGT is induced by alcohol and, as a result, the finding of an isolated elevation of serum GGT has been considered a marker of chronic alcohol consumption with or without underlying liver disease. However, isolated elevations in serum GGT levels can also be seen after recent alcohol consumption without chronic use, in patients taking antiseizure medications or warfarin, and in patients with normal liver biopsies and no discernible reason for this elevation. Elevations of these enzymes are specific for hepatobiliary disease and all correlate well with elevations in alkaline phosphatase activity.

ASSESSMENT OF HEPATIC SYNTHETIC FUNCTION

Hepatocytes are responsible for the synthesis of albumin, fibrinogen, prothrombin, factors V, VII, IX, and X, and most of the globulins (gamma globulins are an important exception). As a result, serum measurements of these proteins are clinically useful in the assessment of hepatic synthetic function.

Albumin is the single most abundant serum protein, and the liver synthesizes approximately 12 g of albumin per day. Normal serum albumin levels range from 3.5 to 4.5 g/dl and reflect the rate of synthesis, rate of degradation, and the volume of distribution. Albumin synthesis is regulated by changes in nutritional status, osmotic pressure, systemic inflammation, and corticosteroids. Serum albumin levels tend to be normal in liver diseases of acute onset such as acute viral hepatitis, drug-related hepatotoxicity, and biliary obstruction. Furthermore, hypoalbuminemia is not specific for liver disease since it occurs in severe protein malnutrition, states of chronic inflammation, protein-losing enteropathies, and the nephrotic syndrome. However, in the setting of liver disease, serum albumin levels of less than 3 g/dl support chronicity.

Clotting is the result of a complex series of enzymatic reactions. The liver is responsible for the synthesis of 11 of these clotting proteins, including fibrinogen, prothrombin, factor V, labile factor, factor VII, stable factor, factor IX, thromboplastin, factor X, factor XII, and factor XIII. The liver is also responsible for clearing some of these clotting factors from the serum. As a result, the clotting cascade is often disturbed in liver disease. This can be assessed by measuring individual factors or by tests that measure the interplay of a number of factors. The prothrombin time is the most useful assay to assess this aspect of hepatic synthetic function. Prothrombin time measures the rate at which prothrombin is converted to thrombin, which results in the polymerization of fibrinogen to fibrin. In addition to prothrombin and fibrinogen, the prothrombin time is influenced by factors I, II, V, VII, and X. The prothrombin time is prolonged if any of these proteins are deficient. The hepatic synthesis of factors II, VII, IX, and X requires vitamin K. Therefore, prolongation of the prothrombin time can be seen in hepatic dysfunction, vitamin K deficiency, ingestion of vitamin K antagonists, congenital deficiencies of coagulation factors, or consumption of coagulation factors. Hypovitaminosis K and severe parenchymal liver disease can be differentiated by parenteral administration of vitamin K. When prothrombin time returns to normal or at least improves by 30% within 24 hours after a single dose of vitamin K, hepatic synthetic function is intact and hypovitaminosis K was responsible for the prothrombin time prolongation. Hypovitaminosis K can be seen in prolonged obstructive jaundice secondary to steatorrhea in dietary deficiency, or as a consequence of antibiotic therapy that alters the gut flora. In contrast, no response to parenteral vitamin K is seen in patients with a prolonged prothrombin time secondary to parenchymal liver disease. Unlike hypoalbuminemia, which is a reflection of the chronicity of hepatic dysfunction, prolongation of the prothrombin time can serve as a marker for the severity of acute liver dysfunction. For example, in acute viral hepatitis prolongation of the prothrombin time by 5 to 6 seconds suggests fulminant hepatic necrosis. The ability to assess acute hepatic dysfunction using the prothrombin time is because of the short half-life of factor VII.

IMAGING STUDIES

Plain films of the abdomen can suggest the presence of hepatomegaly or ascites, although a physical examination is more informative. Gallstones that contain calcium may be seen on plain abdominal films; approximately 15% of cholesterol or mixed stones and 50% of pigment stones are radio-opaque.

Oral cholecystography may be useful in the diagnosis of gallstones. Oral agents (e.g., iopanoic acid) given the day before the study are absorbed from the intestine and undergo hepatobiliary excretion and concentration within the gallbladder. Abdominal radiographs demonstrate gallstones as filling defects within an opacified gallbladder (Fig. 7-6). Nausea, vomiting, and diarrhea are extremely common side effects of the oral agents used, necessitating a second dose. Nonvisualization of the gallbladder after a second dose suggests a defect in gallbladder concentration such as chronic cholecystitis.

Ultrasonography of the gallbladder (Fig. 7-7) has almost completely replaced oral cholecystography as a diagnostic tool for the detection of gallstones, since it is better tolerated, equally or more accurate, and independent of liver function. Ab-

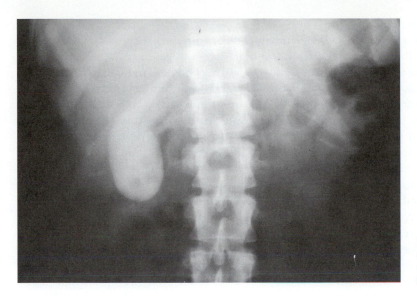

Figure 7-6. Oral cholecystogram with gallstones seen as filling defects within the gallbladder.

dominal ultrasonography also allows evaluation of the biliary tree, liver, spleen, pancreas, and kidney. Dilatation of the common bile duct may, for example, be observed with choledocholithiasis. Ultrasound is particularly useful in differentiating cystic from solid hepatic lesions. Abdominal ultrasonography is more sensitive than physical examination in the detection of ascites and can detect as little as 200 ml of fluid. Doppler-assisted ultrasonography is used to evaluate blood flow in the hepatic, portal, and splenic veins in the diagnosis of hepatic (Budd-Chiari syndrome), portal, or splenic vein thrombosis, respectively.

Radioisotope liver scans are performed using injections of gamma-emitting isotopes that are selectively taken up by the liver followed by external radiation scanning. There are several variations of this type of scan. The liver-spleen scan uses ^{99m}Tc-labeled sulfur colloid, which is taken up by Kuppfer's cells. Abnormali-

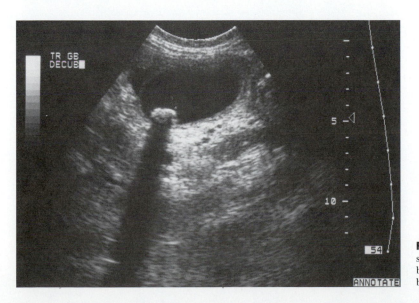

Figure 7-7. Ultrasound scan showing gallstones within the gallbladder. Note the shadowing below the stone.

ties, such as metastases or liver abscesses, are seen as areas of decreased uptake or "cold" lesions (Fig. 7-8). Diffuse hepatocellular disease, such as hepatitis, fatty change, or cirrhosis, may lead to inhomogeneous uptake and "colloid shift" (increased splenic and bone marrow uptake relative to hepatic uptake). ^{99m}Tc-tagged red blood cells are used to confirm suspected liver hemangiomas. Gallium-67 (^{67}Ga^{3+}) is concentrated in neoplastic and inflammatory cells to a greater degree than in normal hepatocytes and may be useful in the diagnosis of hepatocellular carcinoma and pyogenic liver abscess. Hepatobiliary scintigraphy employs ^{99m}Tc-labeled iminodiacetic acid, derivatives that undergo hepatic uptake and biliary excretion. Nonvisualization of the gallbladder, verified on delayed scans, is highly diagnostic of acute calculous and acalculous cholecystitis.

Computed tomography provides a visual image of the abdominal viscera in serial cross-sections. This technique is useful in the detection of mass lesions of the liver and pancreas and abdominal or retroperitoneal adenopathy (Fig. 7-9).

Direct injection of contrast material into the biliary system is achieved by either endoscopic retrograde cholangiopancreatography (ERCP) (Fig. 7-10) or percutaneous transhepatic cholangiography (PTC). ERCP is favored for distal biliary tract lesions, if sphincterotomy is anticipated, and in the presence of marked ascites or coagulopathy. PTC may be preferable in the setting of a proximal lesion or surgically distorted gastroduodenal anatomy. Both imaging modalities are useful in the diagnosis of obstructive jaundice.

LIVER BIOPSY

Percutaneous liver biopsy can be extremely useful in the diagnostic approach to the patient with liver disease and should be considered in any patients with chronic (longer than 6 months) elevations in liver chemistries. Major applications of liver biopsy other than in the evaluation of a patient with persistently abnormal liver chemistries include establishing the diagnosis in patients with (1) unexplained hepatomegaly; (2) suspected systemic disease, such as tuberculosis, sarcoidosis, or

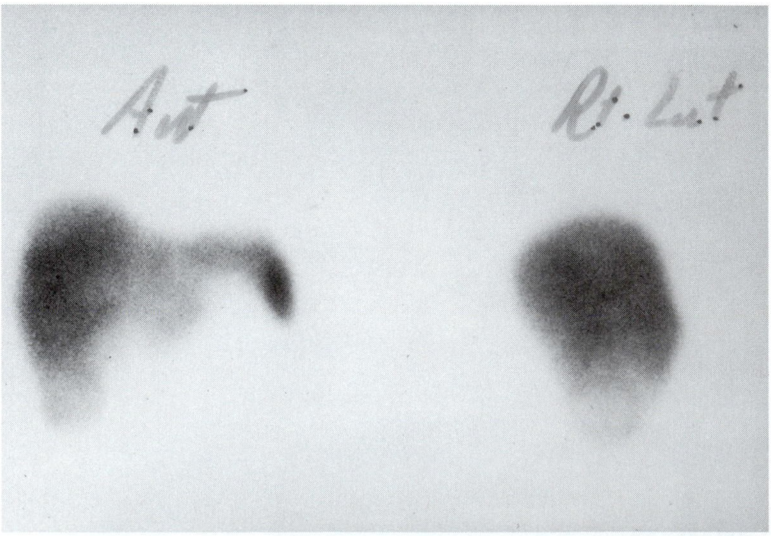

Figure 7-8. ^{99m}Tc-sulfur colloid scan showing decreased uptake ("cold spot") in a large right lobe hepatic adenoma.

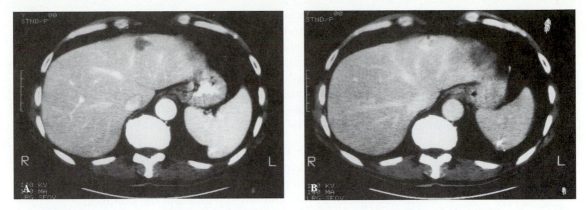

Figure 7-9. Computed tomographic scan of hepatic hemangioma. Note peripheral enhancement of the hemangioma in (**A**) and central enhancement of the lesion on delayed image in (**B**).

fever of unknown origin; and (3) suspected primary or metastatic carcinoma. Impaired coagulation, ascites, suspected hemangioma and suspected echinococcal cyst represent the major contraindications to needle biopsy of the liver.

CLINICAL CORRELATES

Liver disease is typically classified into three major types: hepatocellular, cholestatic, and infiltrative. These three forms of liver disease may result from immunologic and nonimmunologic mechanisms. Depending on the target of the im-

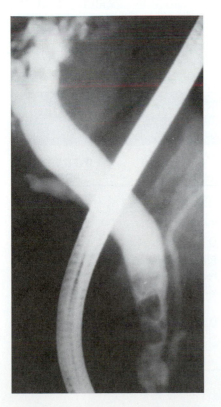

Figure 7-10. ERCP showing multiple common bile duct stones and biliary dilatation.

mune response, immunologic injury results in a hepatocellular form of injury (when the primary insult is to the hepatocyte membrane, as in viral and autoimmune hepatitis), a cholestatic picture (when the bile ducts are preferentially involved, as in primary biliary cirrhosis), or an infiltrative picture (when granulomas predominate). Evaluate of patients with suspected liver disease is aided by the presence of these relatively discrete patterns of liver injury and tests of discriminative value in the detection of these patterns. Routinely, the results of the following tests are determined:

1. Serum aminotransferase activity
2. Serum alkaline phosphatase
3. Serum total and direct bilirubin
4. Serum total protein, with albumin and globulin fractionation
5. Prothrombin time.

A pattern of typical abnormalities seen in the various forms of hepatobiliary injury emerges from this battery of tests, as outlined in Table 7-4. Further laboratory evaluation of most patients with evidence of chronic (> 6 months) hepatitis should, at the minimum, include the following tests:

1. Serum protein electrophoresis
2. Serum ferritin
3. Antinuclear antibody
4. Serum ceruloplasmin
5. Hepatitis B viral serology
6. Hepatitis C viral serology.

The rationale for such screening can be better understood by examining Table 7-5 and, in the following section, by reviewing the aspects of certain liver disorders.

TABLE 7-4. *ROUTINE BIOCHEMICAL TESTS IN THE PATIENT WITH IDEALIZED HEPATOBILIARY DISEASE*

TEST	HEPATOCELLULAR NECROSIS	CHOLESTASIS	INFILTRATIVE PROCESS
Aminotransferase	++ to +++	0 to +	0 to +
Alkaline phosphatase	0 to +	++ to +++	++ to +++
Total/direct bilirubin	0 to +++	0 to +++	0 to +
Prothrombin time	Prolonged	Prolonged; responsive to vitamin K	0
Albumin	Decreased in chronic disorders	0	0
Cholesterol	0	0 to +++	0
Bile acids	+ to +++	+ to +++	0

0, normal; + to +++, degrees of elevation.

TABLE 7-5. *DIAGNOSIS OF SELECTED HEPATOBILIARY DISORDERS*

FORM OF LIVER INJURY	SUPPORTING LABORATORY DATA
Hepatocellular	
Viral hepatitis	Viral serology
Drug-induced hepatitis	Eosinophil count
Autoimmune chronic active hepatitis	Immunoelectrophoresis
	Antinuclear antibody
	Anti–smooth muscle antibody
Wilson's disease	Serum ceruloplasmin
Hemochromatosis	Serum iron/total non-binding capacity
	Serum ferritin
α_1-antitrypsin deficiency	Protein electrophoresis
	Serum α_1-antitrypsin
	Pi typing
Cholestatic	
Primary biliary cirrhosis	Antimitochondrial antibody
	Immunoelectrophoresis
Infiltrative	
Hepatocellular carcinoma	α-fetoprotein

DISEASES ASSOCIATED WITH HEPATOCELLULAR INJURY

Viral Hepatitis

Viral hepatitis is a generic term that refers to an inflammatory process of the liver caused by at least five different viruses. These viruses include hepatitis A (HAV), hepatitis B (HBV), hepatitis C (HCV), delta hepatitis (HDV), and hepatitis E (HEV) (Table 7-6). The clinical manifestations of viral hepatitis show dramatic variation, ranging from an asymptomatic illness to fulminant hepatic failure. In its mildest form, viral hepatitis is asymptomatic or associated with flulike symptoms and is marked only by a rise in serum transaminase levels. Jaundice from viral hepatitis usually follows a prodromal period of days to weeks during which malaise, anorexia, nausea, headache, right upper quadrant abdominal discomfort, and low-grade fevers may be reported. During this icteric phase, the liver is usually palpable with a smooth but tender edge.

Hepatitis A is frequently a mild self-limited disease. Fulminant hepatic failure is rare and progression to chronic liver disease does not occur. Spread by the fecal-oral route, the average incubation period for this disease is 30 days. Serologic detection of hepatitis A virus–specific IgM antibody (anti-HAV IgM) supports the diagnosis of acute or recent hepatitis A infection. Seropositivity first becomes detectable at the onset of clinical illness and is always present at the onset of jaundice (Fig. 7-11). This marker persists in the serum for at least 120 days, far exceed-

TABLE 7-6. *BASIS FOR THE DIFFERENTIATION OF THE FIVE FORMS OF VIRAL HEPATITIS*

FEATURE	HEPATITIS A	HEPATITIS B	HEPATITIS C	DELTA HEPATITIS	HEPATITIS E
Viral Characteristic					
Size	28 nm	42 nm	38–50 nm	43 nm	32 nm
Nucleic acid	RNA	DNA	RNA	RNA	RNA
Serologic Features					
Markers of hepatitis A	Yes	No	No	No	No
Markers of hepatitis B	No	Yes	No	Yes	No
Markers of hepatitis C	No	No	Yes	No	No
Markers of delta hepatitis	No	No	No	Yes	No
Markers of HEV	No	No	No	No	Yes
Viral RNA		Yes		Yes	Yes
Incubation Period					
Mean	30 days	75 days	50 days	75 days	40 days
Range	15–45 days	30–180 days	15–160 days	30–180 days	14–60 days
Transmission					
Fecal-oral	Yes	No	No	No	Yes
Parenteral	Rare	Yes	Yes	Yes	No
Sexual	No	Yes	Possible	Yes	No
Clinical Features					
Peak ALT concentrations in acute disease	800–1000	1000–2000	300–800	1000–1500	800–1000
Fulminant hepatic failure	∽0.1%	∽2%	∽0.1%	∽5% in coinfection ∽70–90% in superinfection	∽2% ∽20% in pregnancy
Chronic hepatitis	No	∽5–10% ∽90% in neonates	∽50–80%	∽2–5% in coinfection ∽70–90% in superinfection	No
Hepatocellular carcinoma	No	Yes	Yes	Yes	No

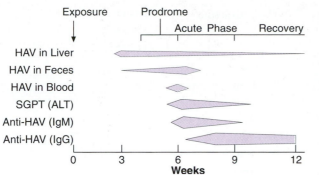

Figure 7-11. Schema of the seroimmunologic events observed during the course of typical hepatitis A infection. In some patients, anti-HAV of the IgM class may persist longer and fecal shedding of HAV may be briefer than indicated (Adapted from Schiff L, Schiff ER, eds. Diseases of the Liver, 6th ed. Philadelphia: JB Lippincott, 1987:465.)

ing the period of illness. Virus-specific IgG antibody to hepatitis A is clinically less useful, since this marker is present in sera of convalescent patients and persists for years.

Hepatitis B infection is associated with both acute and chronic disease. Spread by a parenteral route, there are a number of possible modes of transmission for HBV, including intravenous drug use, sexual activity, and rarely through blood transfusion or household contacts. The mean incubation period is 10 weeks. Approximately 2% of patients who are acutely infected develop fulminant hepatic failure and 5 to 10% progress to chronic hepatitis. Chronicity is defined by the presence of hepatitis B surface antigen (HBsAg; Fig. 7-12) for longer than 6 months and appears to be related to the age at the time of infection and the immune status of the host. Chronic hepatitis B is a major risk factor for the development of hepatocellular carcinoma. Several serologic markers are available to establish a diagnosis of hepatitis B infection. HBsAg is the first marker detectable in the serum. Its presence precedes the elevation of aminotransferases, and it persists for 1 to 3 months in acute self-limited infections (Fig. 7-13). Approximately 10% of patients do not manifest detectable levels of HBsAg in their serum during an acute infection. Antibody to the core antigen (HBcAb) appears in the serum 2 to 4 weeks following the appearance of HBsAg. Between the disappearance of HBsAg and the appearance of specific antibody to HBsAg (HBsAb) at approximately 3 to 5

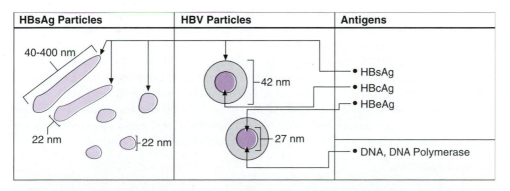

Figure 7-12. Diagram of the three morphologic forms of the HBV-associated particles, the antigens of HBV, and their interrelationships. DNA and DNA polymerase in the core of the 42-nm HBV particle are shown. (Adapted from Koff RS: In Sanyord JP, ed. The Science and Clinical Practice of Medicine, Vol 8. New York: Grune & Stratton, 1981.)

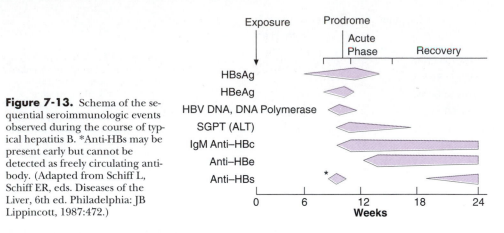

Figure 7-13. Schema of the sequential seroimmunologic events observed during the course of typical hepatitis B. *Anti-HBs may be present early but cannot be detected as freely circulating antibody. (Adapted from Schiff L, Schiff ER, eds. Diseases of the Liver, 6th ed. Philadelphia: JB Lippincott, 1987:472.)

months into acute self-limited infection, HBcAb is the only detectable serologic marker of recent or acute infection. Hepatitis B virus DNA (HBV-DNA) and hepatitis B e antigen (HBeAg) can be detected in the sera in acute hepatitis B infection. However, these markers are clinically applied in the setting of chronic infection, where their presence correlates with ongoing viral replication and infectivity.

HDV (delta agent) is an incomplete RNA virus that requires a helper function of HBV to replicate. Therefore, delta hepatitis only occurs in individuals who are either acutely (coinfection) or chronically (superinfection) infected with HBV. Coinfection of delta agent and HBV usually resolves. Superinfection with delta agent in chronic hepatitis B is associated with an increased frequency of chronic delta hepatitis and acceleration toward cirrhosis. HDV infection can be diagnosed serologically by detection of the antibody to the hepatitis D antigen (anti-HD) in a HBsAg-positive patient.

Hepatitis C virus (HCV), formerly described as non-A, non-B hepatitis, accounts for >90% of all transfusion-related hepatitis. Additional risk factors include intravenous drug use and exposure to blood and/or blood products, although a significant proportion of patients have no identifiable risk factor. The majority of patients with HCV progress to chronic infection and approximately 25% progress to cirrhosis. Serologic tests for HCV detect antibodies to viral antigens, either by enzyme linked immunosorbent assay (ELISA) or recombinant immunoblot assay (RIBA). Antibody response to HCV may be delayed for more than 6 months after infection. The most sensitive assay for hepatitis C infection is HCV RNA titers assayed by the polymerase chain reaction.

Hepatitis E (HEV) formerly called epidemic non-A, non-B hepatitis, is a disease that has been reported to occur only in developing countries. It is rarely seen in the United States, and when seen it is invariably found in visitors to endemic areas. Transmission, similar to that of hepatitis A, is by the fecal-oral route. Epidemics of HEV are associated with high mortality rates, especially in pregnant women. As with hepatitis A, there is no associated chronic liver disease.

Hemochromatosis

The autosomal recessive disorder, hereditary hemochromatosis, is characterized by increased intestinal absorption of iron leading to parenchymal cell iron overload (Table 7-7). Since the liver is the primary storage organ for excess iron, hepatic damage eventually leading to micronodular cirrhosis is a common and

TABLE 7-7. *COMPARISON OF MARKERS IN SYMPTOMATIC PRIMARY HEMOCHROMATOSIS AND ALCOHOLIC LIVER DISEASE*

	NORMAL RANGE	ALCOHOLIC LIVER DISEASE	HEMOCHROMATOSIS
Transferrin-iron saturation (%)	20–50	50–60	>62
Serum ferritin (ng/ml)	15–300	300–100	500–6000
Hepatic iron concentration (μg/g dry weight)	300–1800	1800–5000	10,000–30,000
Iron index (μmol Fe/g dry weight)/age	<1.1	<1.6	>1.8

early finding in hereditary hemochromatosis (Fig. 7-14). Congestive heart failure, secondary to a dilated cardiomyopathy, is the most common sequelae of iron deposition in the heart. Endocrine manifestations of hereditary hemochromatosis include hypogonadism, resulting from a combination of selective anterior pituitary dysfunction and primary testicular failure, and diabetes mellitus. Arthropathy and abnormal skin pigmentation are also frequent manifestations. Screening tests suggestive of hereditary hemochromatosis include an elevated serum iron level, an elevated transferrin saturation (serum iron divided by total iron-binding capacity), and an elevated serum ferritin; diagnosis, however, requires quantitative iron determination of liver biopsy specimens.

Secondary hemochromatosis can result from (1) iron-loading anemias (e.g., β-thalassemia, sideroblastic anemia); (2) increased oral intake (e.g., prolonged ingestion of medicinal iron, dietary iron overload as in Bantu siderosis); and (3) liver disease (e.g., alcoholic cirrhosis, porphyria cutanea tarda, postportocaval shunt).

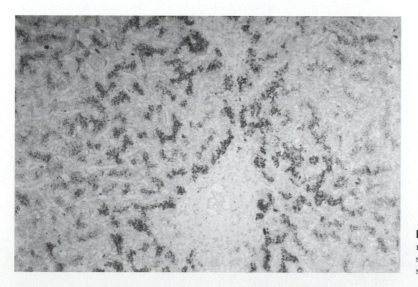

Figure 7-14. Liver biopsy in hemochromatosis. Increased iron stores are seen with Prussian blue staining.

Wilson's Disease

Wilson's disease (hepatolenticular degeneration) is a rare autosomal recessive disorder of copper storage that can lead to cirrhosis, degeneration of the basal ganglia, and greenish-brown pigmentation of the periphery of the cornea (Kayser-Fleischer rings) (Fig. 7-15). Most patients develop symptoms between the ages of 5 and 30 years. Hepatic presentation occurs in one of four ways: acute hepatitis, fulminant hepatitis, chronic active hepatitis, or the insidious development of cirrhosis. Rapid release of copper from the liver in fulminant hepatitis accounts for the hemolytic anemia characteristic of this disorder. Movement disorders typify the neurologic symptoms of Wilson's disease; in contrast, the psychiatric manifestations may be diverse, including antisocial behavior, schizophrenia, neuroses, and dementia. Diagnostic tests for Wilson's disease include a low serum ceruloplasmin level, an elevated 24-hour urinary copper excretion, and increased quantitative copper on liver biopsy (Table 7-8). Treatment consists of copper chelation with D-penicillamine or triethylene tetramine dihydrochloride (trientine). Orthotopic liver transplantation may be necessary in cases of fulminant Wilson's disease.

Alpha$_1$-Antitrypsin Deficiency

Alpha$_1$-antitrypsin (AAT) is synthesized by the liver and to a much lesser extent by monocytes and macrophages and functions as an inhibitor of leukocyte elastase. This glycoprotein migrates with the α_1-globulin fraction on serum protein electrophoresis and accounts for 80 to 90% of this fraction. The normal phenotype for this protease inhibitor (Pi) system is designated Pi MM by electophoretic mobility. Homozygous individuals for the slowest electrophoretic mobility pattern are designated Pi ZZ. These individuals have markedly decreased AAT levels and are predisposed to early-onset chronic active hepatitis and cryptogenic cirrhosis. The diagnosis of AAT deficiency should be considered in patients with a hepatocellular injury pattern who also show an absent α_1-globulin peak on serum protein electrophoresis. AAT levels and genetic Pi typing are used to confirm the diagnosis. Liver biopsy demonstrates characteristic periodic acid–Schiff-positive globules in periportal hepatocytes owing to the inability of the hepatocyte to process and secrete the Z protein (Fig. 7-16).

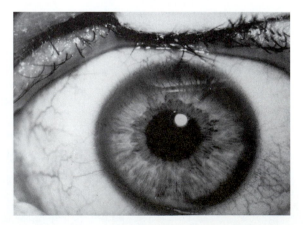

Figure 7-15. Kayser-Fleischer rings.

TABLE 7-8. *COMPARATIVE COPPER STATUS FOR PATIENTS WITH WILSON'S DISEASE AND VARIOUS CONTROL GROUPS*

GROUP	SERUM CERULOPLASMIN (MG/DL ± SE)	SERUM CU (µG/DL)	URINE CU (µG/24 HR)	LIVER CU (µG/G WET WEIGHT)	PLASMA ^{64}CU (24 HR/2-HR RATIO)	RADIOACTIVE COPPER (^{64}CU) ^{64}CU–% INTRAVENOUS DOSE EXCRETED IN URINE PER PERIOD		
						0–8 HR (MEAN ± SE)	8–24 HR (MEAN ± SE)	24–30 HR AFTER PENICILLAMINE (MEAN ± SE)
Wilson's disease								
Presymptomatic	6.3 ± 1.0	<60	>50	>50	<0.4	0.92 ± 0.17	0.17 ± 0.04	0.84 ± 0.11
Symptomatic	6.3 ± 1.0	<60	>50	>50	<0.4	1.22 ± 0.21	0.70 ± 0.16	3.45 ± 0.45
Heterozygote	25.4 ± 1.1	>60	<50	<50	>0.4	0.10 ± 0.01	0.05 ± 0.01	1.20 ± 0.17
Hepatic disease*	38.0 ± 2.9	>100	<50	<50	>0.6	0.20	0.17	1.94
Controls, male	33.3 ± 0.7	>80	<30	<10	>0.8	0.14 ± 0.02	0.07 ± 0.01	2.36 ± 0.33
Controls, female	36.6 ± 1.0	>80	<30	<10	>0.8	0.14 ± 0.02	0.07 ± 0.01	2.36 ± 0.33

*Excluding patients with primary biliary cirrhosis in whom figures for liver and urine copper may be found in the Wilson's disease range. (Data from Gibbs K, et al. The urinary excretion of radiocopper in presymptomatic and symptomatic Wilson's disease, heterozygotes and controls: Its significance in diagnosis and management. QJ Med 47:349, 1978, Gibbs K, Walshe JM: A study of ceruloplasmin concentration found in 75 patients with Wilson's disease, their kinships and various control groups. QJ Med 48:447, 1979, and Schiff L, Schiff ER, eds. Diseases of the Liver, 6th ed. Philadelphia: JB Lippincott, 1987:146.)

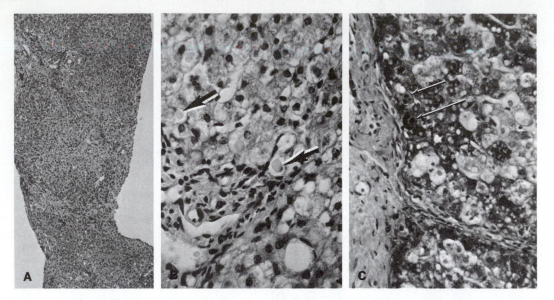

Figure 7-16. α_1-antitrypsin deficiency. (**A**) Biopsy at age 1 year shows early cirrhosis at low-power microscopy. (**B**) Spherical eosinophilic hyaline bodies resembling erythrocytes, but larger and not biconcave, are visible in periportal hepatocytes at high power (arrow). (**C**) Periodic–acid Schiff stain shows positive staining diastase-resistant globules adjacent to portal connective tissue. (From Schiff L, Schiff ER, eds. Diseases of the Liver, 7th ed. Philadelphia: JB Lippincott, 1993:1117.)

Autoimmune Chronic Active Hepatitis

This disease of disordered immunoregulation is associated with the presence of high titers of antinuclear antibody in homogenous patterns and with hypergammaglobulinemia. Features suggestive of this disorder are the absence of serologic evidence of viral hepatitis or metabolic liver disease, lack of exposure to hepatotoxic drugs or alcohol, the presence of associated autoimmune diseases, and a response to corticosteroid therapy. Variants of autoimmune hepatitis have been described in which antibodies to liver and kidney microsomes or smooth muscle antibodies may be present instead of antinuclear antibody.

Alcoholic Hepatitis

Common symptoms of alcoholic hepatitis include anorexia, nausea, vomiting, jaundice, abdominal pain, and fever, although the disease spectrum may range from the anicteric asymptomatic patient to the desperately ill patient with jaundice, ascites, and hepatic encephalopathy. As a result, the clinical manifestations of alcoholic liver disease frequently mimic those of other hepatobiliary diseases. In addition, it is important to recognize that alcoholics may have a variety of liver diseases other than alcoholic liver disease. Biochemically, AST is elevated disproportionately to ALT, although levels of less than 300 IU are the norm. Histopathologically, hepatocellular necrosis concentrated in pericentral areas, with alcoholic hyaline (Mallory's bodies) in damaged hepatocytes and a surrounding polymorphonuclear leukocyte infiltrate are observed (Fig. 7-17).

Drug-Induced Hepatotoxicity

Injury to the liver from drugs may take the form of hepatocellular necrosis, cholestatic injury, or a mixed pattern. Drug-induced hepatocellular injury clinically

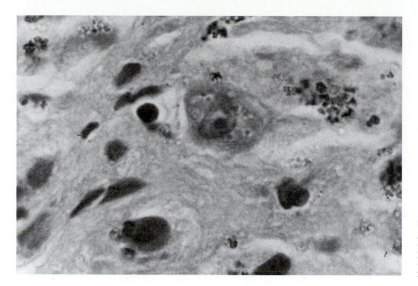

Figure 7-17. Liver biopsy in alcoholic hepatitis. A perinuclear Mallory body is present within the hepatocyte in the center of the figure.

resembles viral or ischemic hepatitis, and its severity can range from anicteric to fulminant hepatic failure. Drug-induced liver disease should be suspected when a patient has been exposed to a potentially hepatotoxic agent or a new medication within the preceding 3 months. A careful history of all prescription, over-the-counter, and herbal therapy must be taken. Occupational exposure should be considered and questioned. The additional presence of fever, rash, and eosinophilia should heighten suspicion, but these symptoms are not mandatory and are often absent.

Acetaminophen hepatotoxicity is probably the most commonly seen form of drug-induced liver injury. The mechanism of action of acetaminophen hepatotoxicity is via production of a toxic metabolite (*N*-acetyl-*p*-benzoquinoneimine) that interacts with essential hepatocyte macromolecules, resulting in cell death (Fig. 7-18). Doses of 10 to 15 g are known to produce hepatic necrosis in adults. Chronic use of alcohol prior to the ingestion enhances the hepatotoxicity of acetaminophen because of alcohol induction of certain P450 enzymatic pathways. In this situation as little as 3 to 4 g/day can produce significant hepatotoxicity.

CHOLESTATIC SYNDROMES

Primary Biliary Cirrhosis

Primary biliary cirrhosis (PBC) is a cholestatic liver disease of unknown etiology that predominantly affects women, usually between the ages of 40 and 60 years. The symptoms begin insidiously, most often as pruritus with or without jaundice. In PBC the small intrahepatic ductules are involved in a granulomatous reaction, becoming increasingly damaged until they ultimately disappear and cirrhosis intervenes (Fig. 7-19). Antimitochondrial antibodies are present in over 90% of patients with primary biliary cirrhosis (PBC) and in about 25% of patients with chronic active hepatitis and drug-induced liver injury (Fig. 7-20). In fact, an antimitochondrial antibody titer of greater than 1:40, even in the absence of serum alkaline phosphatase elevation or characteristic symptoms, may be strongly suggestive of PBC. In addition, a disproportionate elevation of IgM is a feature that differenti-

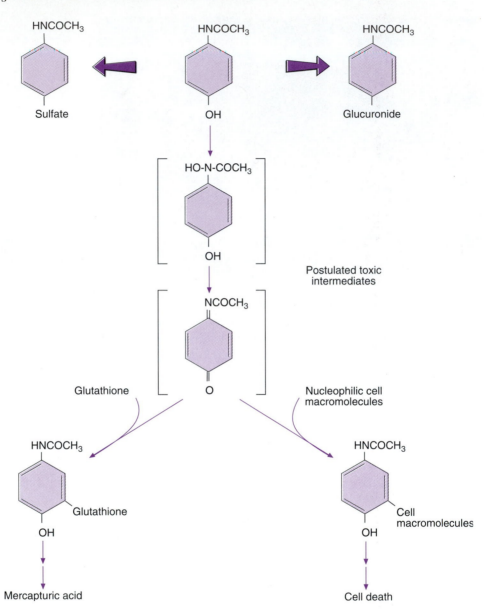

Figure 7-18. Schema of acetaminophen metabolism. Increased dose and blood levels provide the basis for increased amounts of active metabolite. Increased activity of mixed function oxidase leads to a higher proportion of active metabolite. Depletion of glutathione stores leads to a higher proportion of active metabolite that can bind to cytoplasmic proteins and produced necrosis. (Adapted from Zimmerman HJ: Hepatotoxicity. New York: Appleton-Century-Crofts, 1978.)

ates PBC from other liver diseases which are associated with prominent hypergammaglobulinemia and specifically from autoimmune chronic active hepatitis.

Primary Sclerosing Cholangitis

Primary sclerosing cholangitis (PSC) is another chronic cholestatic syndrome of unknown etiology, characterized by fibrosing inflammation of the biliary tract, commonly in association with ulcerative colitis. Unlike PBC, PSC occurs predomi-

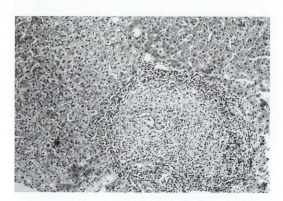

Figure 7-19. Stage I. Primary biliary cirrhosis. The portal zone shows a damaged bile duct with a surrounding lymphocytic granulomatous reaction. This appearance is diagnostic. (From Schiff L, Schiff ER, eds. Diseases of the Liver, 6th ed. Philadelphia: JB Lippincott, 1987:980.)

nantly in young adult males. Patients with PSC commonly present with progressive fatigue, pruritus, and jaundice. On serologic evaluation they have a cholestatic biochemical profile; autoimmune markers are not helpful. Visualization of the biliary tree is essential in making a diagnosis of PSC. Cholangiography shows multifocal stricturing and irregularity, generally involving both the intra- and extrahepatic biliary systems, producing a classic "beaded" appearance (Fig. 7-21). Cholelithiasis, choledocholithiasis, and cholangiocarcinoma occur with increased frequently in patients with PSC.

INFILTRATIVE PROCESSES

Isolated elevation of serum alkaline phosphatase levels, confirmed by serum leucine aminopeptidase, 5'-nucleotidase, or GGTP to be of hepatic origin, is strongly suggestive of an infiltrative process. The process can be localized to the liver (i.e., PBC), part of a systemic granulomatous disease (e.g., sarcoidosis, miliary tuberculosis, systemic fungal disease, or a drug reaction), or the first indication of metastatic carcinoma to the liver. A greater than threefold elevation in serum alkaline phosphatase levels in patients with cirrhosis should raise concern for the development of hepatocellular carcinoma. As noted above, the triad of an elevated

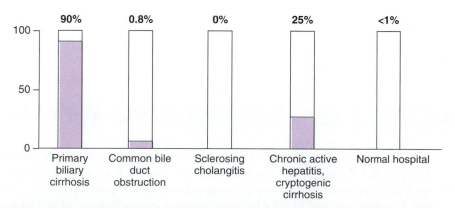

Figure 7-20. Percentage of positive serum mitochondrial antibodies in primary biliary cirrhosis and other diseases. (Adapted from Schiff L, Schiff ER, eds. Diseases of the Liver, 6th ed. Philadelphia: JB Lippincott, 1987:987.)

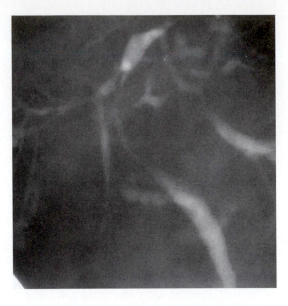

Figure 7-21. Endoscopic retrograde cholangiogram in primary sclerosing cholangitis.

serum alkaline phosphatase level, detectable titers of antimitochondrial antibody, and an elevated serum IgM level in a middle-aged woman is of considerable value in the diagnosis of PBC. Alternatively, in a patient with a history of malignancy, particularly of the breast or colon, the presence of an elevated serum alkaline phosphatase level warrants an evaluation for metastases. The absence of diagnostic findings on abdominal ultrasonography, computed tomography of the abdomen, technetium sulfur colloid nuclear imaging, and invasive tests such as ERCP, represents one of the major indications for percutaneous and/or laparoscopic liver biopsy.

In adults a sensitive radioimmunoassay for α-fetoprotein has been used in screening for primary hepatocellular carcinoma. More than 75% of patients with hepatocellular carcinoma have elevated α-fetoprotein levels. Significant elevations are also seen in patients with other gastrointestinal tract malignancies and with germ cell tumors and in non-neoplastic liver diseases such as chronic active hepatitis, viral hepatitis, alcoholic hepatitis, and PBC. In general, however, higher elevations of α-fetoprotein are seen in hepatocellular carcinoma than in non-neoplastic liver diseases. The specificity of this test in making the diagnosis of hepatocellular carcinoma is substantially increased when a cutoff of an α-fetoprotein higher than 400 ng/ml is used.

CASE PRESENTATION

A 47-year-old woman presented with new onset of pruritus over the previous 2 weeks. She reported that she otherwise felt well, with a normal appetite and no weight loss. She denied any episodes of abdominal pain, nausea, or vomiting. Her past medical history included only an appendectomy at age 14 years. Two months previously she had completed a course of trimethoprim-sulfamethoxazole prescribed for a urinary tract infection. There was no fam-

ily history of liver disease. There was no history of exposure to hepatitis, intravenous drug use, acupuncture, tattoos, or recent blood transfusion. In fact, she was a fairly regular blood donor and had last donated approximately 6 months ago.

Historically, there are several pertinent features to this patient's presenting illness. Generalized pruritus is a prominent and distressing symptom of various diseases, including cholestatic liver disease, uremia, diabetes mellitus, thyroid disease, polycythemia vera, and Hodgkin's disease. The pruritus of cholestasis is a particularly vexing problem, since the etiology is unknown at present and conventional therapy is largely ineffective. Assuming that this patient suffers from pruritus secondary to an underlying cholestatic liver disease, additional clues to a possible diagnosis are provided. The absence of abdominal pain, nausea, and vomiting makes the diagnosis of choledocholithiasis less likely, and the absence of weight loss and anorexia lessens the likelihood that cholestasis is the result of malignant extrahepatic obstruction. There is no history of previous biliary tract surgery to account for the possibility of a biliary stricture. Trimethoprim-sulfamethoxazole–induced cholestasis is well described, but the temporal association between drug use and symptoms is not met in this patient. The negative family history of liver disease is an important detail in any patient who has symptoms or laboratory test results suggestive of liver disease. The negative exposure history and blood donor status makes the diagnosis of chronic hepatitis unlikely.

On physical examination, there was mild scleral icterus. Scattered excoriations were present on the patient's legs, arms, back, and chest. There was no adenopathy. Lungs were clear to auscultation, and heart sounds were normal and without murmurs. On abdominal examination, liver span was 8 cm by percussion, with a nontender edge palpable at the right costal margin. A splenic tip was palpated in the left lateral decubitus position. The remainder of her abdomen was soft, nontender, and without masses. On rectal examination there were no masses and Hemoccult-positive stool was present. There was no peripheral edema.

Physical findings of some discriminative value include stigmata of chronic liver disease (e.g., spider angiomata, palmar erythema, parotid gland enlargement, gynecomastia, Dupuytren's contracture, and testicular atrophy), hepatomegaly and liver consistency, splenomegaly, gallbladder distention, and abdominal tenderness. Although the degree of hepatomegaly can be quite variable in all forms of hepatobiliary disease, a liver span greater than 15 cm is more often associated with passive congestion from right-sided heart failure or neoplastic and infiltrative processes (e.g., amyloidosis, myeloproliferative disorders, hepatic steatosis, and the glycogen and lipid-storage disorders). Splenomegaly in a patient with suspected liver disease is consistent with the present of portal hypertension. Jaundice, manifested by yellow pigmentation of the skin, mucous membranes, and sclerae, typically requires a serum bilirubin concentration of higher than 3 mg/dl for detection. Artificial light makes detection at low levels more difficult.

Laboratory work demonstrated the following findings: total protein 8.5 g/dl, albumin 3.7 g/dl, AST 212 IU/l, ALT 184 IU/l, LDH 199 IU/l, alkaline phos-

phatase 833 IU/l, total bilirubin 3.8 mg/dl, cholesterol 260 mg/dl, white blood cells $3.2 \times 10^3/mm^3$, hemoglobin 12.1 g/dl, hematocrit 35.2%, platelets $128 \times 10^3/mm^3$, and prothrombin time 12.8 seconds.

The disproportionate elevation in the serum alkaline phosphatase level relative to the serum transaminase elevations is most consistent with cholestatic liver injury. The elevated serum cholesterol level and slightly prolonged prothrombin time may also be secondary to cholestasis-induced decreased cholesterol excretion into bile and decreased absorption of fat-soluble vitamin K, respectively, although other causes are also possible. The mild pancytopenia may be a reflection of hypersplenism.

An abdominal ultrasound scan demonstrated a normal liver without intrahepatic or extrahepatic biliary dilatation. The common bile duct measured 0.5 cm; gallstones were present. There was moderate splenomegaly. The pancreas and kidneys were normal.

Although there is little suspicion from the history for extrahepatic obstruction, an abdominal ultrasound scan should be the initial diagnostic test in most patients presenting with cholestatic jaundice. The absence of ductal dilatation makes obstruction less likely, although intermittent or partial obstruction, which is a frequent occurrence with common duct stones, may not cause detectable ductal dilatation. Even high-grade obstruction does not invariably result in ductal dilatation, particularly in the acute setting.

That night the patient awoke at 2 A.M. with severe constant right upper quadrant abdominal pain associated with nausea. The pain was so severe that she went to the emergency room. On physical examination she had a low-grade temperature of 100.4°F, her abdomen was soft but there was severe right upper quadrant tenderness on palpation and a positive Murphy's sign. Repeat laboratory work showed AST 350 IU/l, ALT 265 IU/l, alkaline phosphatase 1033 IU/l, total bilirubin 5.4 mg/dl, white blood cells $12.5 \times 10^3/mm^3$, hemoglobin 12.8 g/dl, and hematocrit 37.1%. Because of the concern of choledocholithiasis, an abdominal ultrasound study was repeated, demonstrating a common bile duct of 1.5 cm. The distal duct and the pancreatic head were not well visualized because of overlying bowel gas.

Biliary colic tends to be nocturnal in onset. Murphy's sign, or inspiratory arrest during deep palpation of the right upper abdominal quadrant, is highly suggestive of acute cholecystitis. In acute biliary obstruction serum transaminases can often reach high levels, resembling an acute hepatocellular injury pattern. Even in the absence of bowel gas, ultrasonography detects less than one third of all stones in the common duct.

The patient was begun on broad-spectrum antibiotic coverage for presumed ascending cholangitis and an emergency ERCP was performed. On ERCP the common bile duct measured 1.8 cm, and two stones, approximately 0.8 to 1 cm in size, were identified. A sphincterotomy and stone extraction were performed. A laparascopic cholecystectomy was performed later that day. During surgery the liver was observed to be dark green and small, with fine surface nodularity. A laparoscopic-guided liver biopsy was performed. The

patient had an uneventful postoperative course. The liver biopsy specimen demonstrated infiltration and expansion of the portal tracts with lymphocytes, plasma cells, eosinophils, and histiocytes. The portal tracts had a paucity of bile ductules and contained scattered granulomas. Bands of fibrosis extended between portal tracts, an appearance consistent with cirrhosis.

The patient had acute biliary obstruction from choledocholithiasis in the setting of chronic liver disease, in this case primary biliary cirrhosis. Laboratory confirmation of this diagnosis was achieved with an antimitochondrial antibody titer of 1:240.

SUMMARY

The approach to the patient with jaundice and abnormal liver chemistries is not governed by well-defined diagnostic algorithms. Instead, a systematic approach to patients with suspected underlying liver disease involves a basic understanding of hepatic physiology and pathophysiology and access to the panel of available measurements of liver function and serum markers of hepatobiliary disease. The approach is, however, facilitated by several distinct patterns of liver injury.

SELECTED READING

Kaplan MM. Laboratory tests. In: Schiff L, Schiff ER, eds. Diseases of the Liver, 6th ed. Philadelphia: JB Lippincott, 1987:219–260.

Moseley RH. Approach to the patient with abnormal liver chemistries. In: Kelley WN, ed. Textbook of Internal Medicine, 2nd ed. Philadelphia: JB Lippincott, 1992:646–652.

Moseley RH. Approach to the patient with abnormal liver chemistries. In: Yamada T, Alpers DH, Owyang C, Powell DW, Silverstein FE, eds. Textbook of Gastroenterology. Philadelphia: JB Lippincott, 1991:829–845.

Moseley RH, Gumucio JJ. Cholestatic syndromes. In: Kelley WN, ed. Textbook of Internal Medicine, 2nd ed. Philadelphia: JB Lippincott, 1992:560–569.

Schiff L. Jaundice: A clinical approach. In: Schiff L, Schiff ER, eds. Diseases of the Liver, 6th ed. Philadelphia: JB Lippincott, 1987:209–218.

Traber PG, Gumucio JJ. Approach to the patient with jaundice. In: Yamada T, Alpers DH, Owyang C, Powell DW, Silverstein FE, eds. Textbook of Gastroenterology. Philadelphia: JB Lippincott, 1991:810–828.

Van Dyke RW. Approach to the patient with jaundice. In: Kelley WN, ed. Textbook of Internal Medicine, 2nd ed. Philadelphia: JB Lippincott, 1992:639–645.

Lippincott's Pathophysiology Series: Gastrointestinal Pathophysiology, edited by Joseph M. Henderson. Lippincott–Raven Publishers. Philadelphia © 1996.

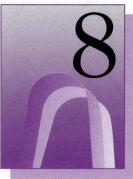

CHAPTER

8

Pancreatitis

Joseph M. Henderson

This chapter provides the reader with a thorough grounding in both normal and abnormal pancreatic physiology. A presentation of normal developmental anatomy and physiology lays the groundwork for helping the reader develop an understanding of and a rational approach to pancreatic disease. Common clinical situations are used to illustrate important pathophysiologic concepts encountered regularly by the practicing clinician.

ANATOMY

EMBRYOLOGY

The pancreas begins development during the fourth week of gestation by formation of ventral and dorsal buds off the duodenum. The ventral pancreatic bud actually arises from the primordial bile duct. The ventral bud rotates with the bile duct along the duodenal axis as it grows, and by the sixth week of gestation it becomes positioned adjacent and inferior to the dorsal pancreatic anlage. By the eighth week, fusion of the ventral and dorsal pancreas has occurred. The tail, body, and a portion of the head of the pancreas develop from the dorsal pancreatic bud, whereas the ventral pancreatic bud gives rise to the remainder of the head and to the uncinate process of the pancreas (Fig. 8-1).

Both the dorsal and ventral pancreatic anlagen contain an axial duct, and each duct maintains its separate opening into the duodenum. Fusion of the dorsal and ventral ducts near the head of the pancreas creates the main pancreatic duct of Wirsung. The main pancreatic duct drains the body, tail, and a portion of the head of the pancreas into the duodenum through the major papilla of Vater. The remaining portion of the dorsal pancreatic duct that lies within the head becomes the accessory duct of Santorini and drains primarily that portion of the head of the

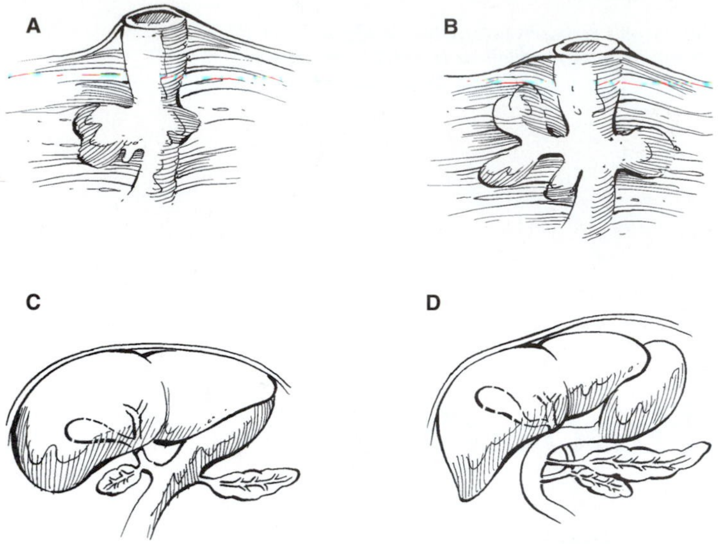

Figure 8-1. *Embryologic* development of the pancreas. Dorsal and ventral buds develop along the midgut at about the fourth week. The ventral bud divides into cranial and caudal buds, and the ventral pancreas arises as a smaller caudad bud from what will become the common bile duct (**A, B**). By the sixth week, the ventral pancreas rotates along the duodenal axis to reach the dorsal pancreas, pulling the end of the common bile duct along with it (**C, D**). The parenchyma of the dorsal and ventral pancreas fuse by the eighth week. Now, fusion of dorsal and ventral ducts can begin. (From Yamada T, Alpers DH, Owyang C, Powell DH, Silverstein FE, eds. Textbook of Gastroenterology, 2nd ed. Philadelphia: JB Lippincott, 1995;2:2181.)

pancreas directly into the duodenum through the minor (accessory) papilla (Fig. 8-2). The ducts of Santorini and Wirsung are usually connected through a small communicating branch. Since the ventral pancreas, and hence the ventral pancreatic duct, arises from the primitive bile duct, the main pancreatic duct and the common bile duct usually join near the papilla of Vater to form a common ampulla in the duodenal wall (Fig. 8-3). Occasionally these two ducts are found to maintain separate orifices, without a common channel, at the papilla of Vater.

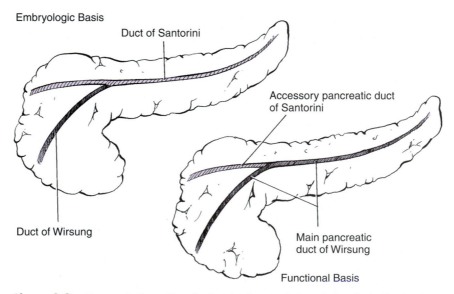

Figure 8-2. Pancreatic ducts. Terminology is often confusing. Embryologically, the dorsal duct or duct of Santorini drains the largest portion of the pancreas before duct fusion occurs. Clinically and functionally, however, the duct of Santorini is the smaller accessory pancreatic duct. The duct of Wirsung, embryologically confined to the ventral pancreas, becomes functionally the main pancreatic duct after duct fusion occurs. It drains the bulk of pancreatic secretion through the major papilla. (From Yamada T, Alpers DH, Owyang C, Powell DH, Silverstein FE, eds. Textbook of Gastroenterology, 2nd ed. Philadelphia: JB Lippincott, 1995;2:2058.)

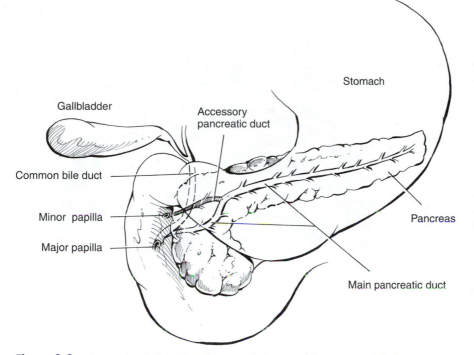

Gallbladder

Accessory
pancreatic duct

Stomach

Common bile duct

Minor papilla

Major papilla

Pancreas

Main pancreatic duct

Figure 8-3. Anatomic relationships of pancreatic ducts and the common bile duct.

The acini of the exocrine pancreas develop as branches off the primordial dorsal and ventral ducts between the third and fifth weeks of gestation. The islets of the endocrine pancreas develop as buds from the same ducts between the 10th and 14th weeks of gestation, but by 16 weeks they have become separated from the ducts and have acquired their own capillaries to become independent of the ductal system of the pancreas.

ANATOMIC RELATIONSHIPS

The adult pancreas is approximately 15 cm long, weighs around 90 g, and lies behind the parietal peritoneum of the posterior abdominal wall. The gland is oriented obliquely upward from head to tail, with the head nestled into the medial aspect of the C-loop of the duodenum and the tail projecting toward the splenic hilum (Fig. 8-4). Anteriorly, the pancreas is covered with parietal peritoneum, the gastric antrum, liver, transverse colon, and distal duodenum. Grossly the pancreas is divided into the head, neck, body, and tail, and the head has an inferior component derived from the ventral pancreas known as the uncinate process. Because of the fusion of the dorsal and ventral pancreas as previously discussed, the distal common bile duct passes through a groove within the parenchyma of the head of the adult pancreas to join the ventral pancreatic duct before terminating at the papilla of Vater. The slightly constricted portion of the pancreas is called the neck, which bends slightly anteriorly, upward, and to the left to connect the head and body of the pancreas. Just beyond the neck, the body arches over the spine as it

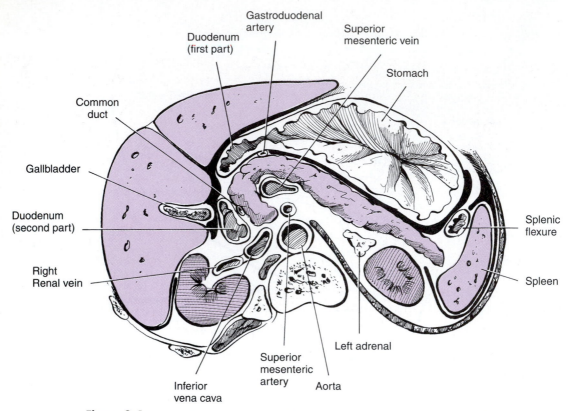

Figure 8-4. Stylized representation of oblique cross-section through the upper abdomen, viewed from below, showing anatomic relationships of the pancreas to other organs. (From Yamada T, Alpers DH, Owyang C, Powell DH, Silverstein FE, eds. Textbook of Gastroenterology, 2nd ed. Philadelphia: JB Lippincott, 1995;2:2053.)

continues its path rostral and to the left to terminate in the tail near the splenic hilum.

ANATOMY OF THE EXOCRINE PANCREAS

As we discuss the pancreatic or bile ducts, the terms *distal* and *proximal* are used to describe relationships along the duct. In this chapter, and in the minds of most clinicians when discussing biliary and pancreatic ducts, distal is the farthest point away from the origin of secretion and proximal is the point closest to the origin of secretion. Hence, the proximal pancreatic duct is that part of the duct in the tail of the pancreas, and the distal pancreatic duct is that part of the duct nearest the papilla of Vater (or the minor papilla when discussing the duct of Santorini). Likewise, the distal common bile duct is that part of the common bile duct nearest the papilla. Other textbooks, especially anatomy books, may use these terms in an opposite manner.

The ducts of the dorsal and ventral pancreas fuse completely in 90% of all specimens and this *main pancreatic duct* provides the major drainage of pancreatic exocrine secretions. The main pancreatic duct gradually increases in size as it courses through the pancreas from tail to head and picks up side branches originating from pancreatic lobules. Usually the duct of Wirsung and the common bile duct join to form a common ampulla of variable length. The ampulla is surrounded by a sphincter muscle called the sphincter of Oddi. This sphincter muscle has both pancreatic and bile duct components and is not a single common sphincter for both ducts (Fig. 8-5). Theoretically, the separate components of the sphincter help prevent reflux of duodenal contents into the biliary or pancreatic ducts, reflux of biliary secretions into the pancreatic duct, and reflux of pancreatic secretions into the biliary system. Pressure measurements (manometry) using small cannulas inserted into the common bile duct and the main pancreatic duct have shown higher pressures in the pancreatic duct than in the common bile duct. Whether this pressure differential has any physiologic significance is not known.

The duct of Santorini drains a portion of the head of the pancreas via the accessory or minor papilla located about 2 cm proximal and slightly ventral to the major papilla of Vater. In most people the majority of pancreatic secretions drain via the main pancreatic duct through the major papilla and duct of Wirsung. In about 10%, however, the main pancreatic duct and Wirsung's duct do not communicate, and the main pancreatic duct must then drain via the duct of Santorini and the minor papilla. This condition, known as pancreas divisum, has been implicated as a cause for recurrent pancreatitis in some patients in whom no other abnormality is found (Fig. 8-6). The ventral pancreas (inferior portion of the head and the uncinate process) still drains normally via Wirsung's duct because these structures have a common embryologic origin. Likewise, biliary drainage is not affected since the bile duct and ventral pancreas are of common origin, and so the common bile duct drains normally through the major papilla.

The pancreas consists primarily of exocrine tissue. The acinus is the basic element of the exocrine pancreas, and together with the various levels of pancreatic ducts accounts for more than 80% of the wet weight of the pancreas. Acini are subunits of lobules of the pancreas (Fig. 8-7). The acinus is composed of pyramidal cells whose apex is oriented toward a central lumen. This lumen is the origin of a secretory duct, and secretory ducts of adjacent acini coalesce to form intralobular ducts. Intralobular ducts, in turn, join to form interlobular ducts, which then join to form the main pancreatic duct. Acinar cells are the source for pancreatic en-

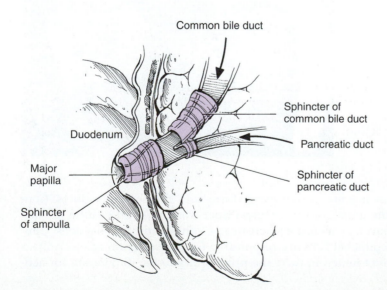

Figure 8-5. Sphincter of Oddi. Sphincter mechanisms at the terminus of the pancreatic and common bile ducts encompass not only the common area at the major papilla but extend up the separate ducts for a short distance. (From Yamada T, Alpers DH, Owyang C, Powell DH, Silverstein FE, eds. Textbook of Gastroenterology, 2nd ed. Philadelphia: JB Lippincott, 1995;2:2182.)

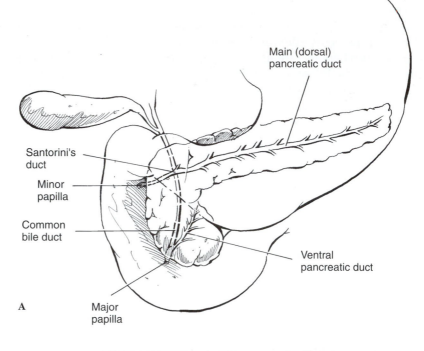

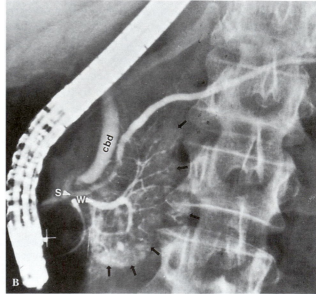

Figure 8-6. (**A**) Pancreas divisum. Failure of dorsal and ventral pancreatic ducts to fuse during development. The common bile duct and ventral pancreas (inferior portion of the pancreatic head) drain normally. The dorsal pancreas drains through the relatively small duct of Santorini and minor papilla. (**B**) ERCP film showing the duct of Santorini, duct of Wirsung, and common bile duct in pancreas divisum. (From Yamada T, Alpers DH, Owyang C, Powell DH, Silverstein FE, eds. Textbook of Gastroenterology, 2nd ed. Philadelphia: JB Lippincott, 1995;2:2596.)

zymes secreted in an inactive (proenzyme) form into the secretory ducts. Centroacinar cells line the lumen of the secretory duct adjacent to and within the acinus. Beyond this point the ducts are lined by low columnar epithelial cells. Centroacinar and duct epithelial cells are responsible for the secretion of electrolytes and water into the duct lumen to carry the proenzymes to the duodenum for activation.

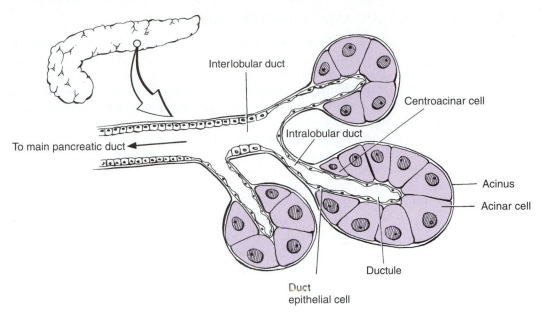

Figure 8-7.   Anatomy of the exocrine pancreas: pancreatic lobule, duct system, and acinus.

ANATOMY OF THE ENDOCRINE PANCREAS

The endocrine pancreas is composed of small islets of cells known as the islets of Langerhans. Islets are separated from adjacent acini by fine connective tissue. Islets are enveloped and penetrated by a rich capillary network that also conveys blood from the islet to the acinar cells. Afferent arterioles enter the islet, form a capillary glomerulus, then exit the islet as an efferent arteriole, which then enters adjacent exocrine pancreatic tissue. Although acini are also supplied by their own arterial system, the *insuloacinar portal system* permits the endocrine pancreas to locally affect the exocrine function of the gland (Fig. 8-8).

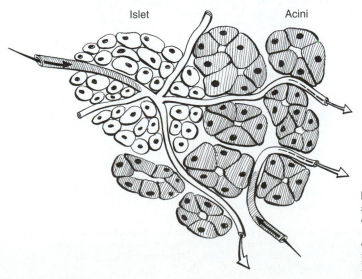

Figure 8-8.   Insuloacinar portal system and relationship of endocrine islets and exocrine acini within the pancreas. (Adapted from Goldfine ID, Williams JA. Receptors for insulin and CCK in the acinar pancreas: Relationship to hormone action. Int Rev Cytol 55:1, 1983.)

NERVE, VASCULAR, AND LYMPHATIC SUPPLY

The vascular supply of the pancreas is derived from branches of the celiac, superior mesenteric, and splenic arteries. Venous drainage is via the pancreaticoduodenal veins, the splenic vein, the superior mesenteric vein, and ultimately into the portal vein. Lymphatic drainage follows the vascular supply, mostly terminating in the pancreaticosplenic lymph nodes. Some lymph also enters the pancreaticoduodenal nodes and periaortic nodes near the origin of the superior mesenteric artery (Fig. 8-9). Innervation is provided by both the sympathetic and parasympathetic nervous systems via the celiac plexus and to a lesser extent via the superior mesenteric and hepatic plexuses (Fig. 8-10). Efferent parasympathetic (vagal) fibers pass through these plexuses without synapsing and then terminate in parasympathetic ganglia within fibrous septa separating pancreatic lobules. Postganglionic fibers supply the acini, ducts, and islets. Efferent sympathetic fibers are derived from neurons found in the lateral gray matter of the thoracic and lumbar spinal cord. These fibers synapse with neurons found in the sympathetic ganglia (celiac and superior mesenteric plexuses). Postganglionic sympathetic fibers then innervate blood vessels. Afferent pathways are not as well defined in the human pancreas but probably also travel along splanchnic and vagal pathways through the celiac plexus and then

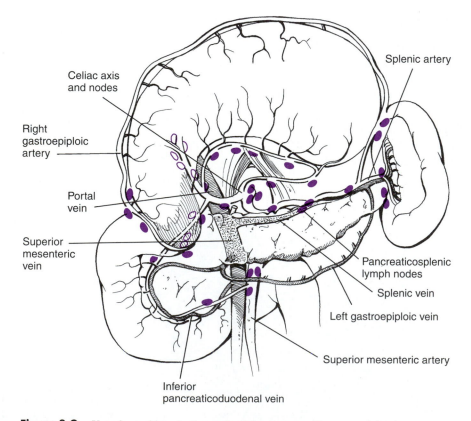

Figure 8-9. Vascular and lymphatic supply of the pancreas. The stomach has been reflected anterosuperiorly to better expose the pancreas. (Adapted from Yamada T, Alpers DH, Owyang C, Powell DH, Silverstein FE, eds. Textbook of Gastroenterology, 2nd ed. Philadelphia: JB Lippincott, 1995;2:2057.)

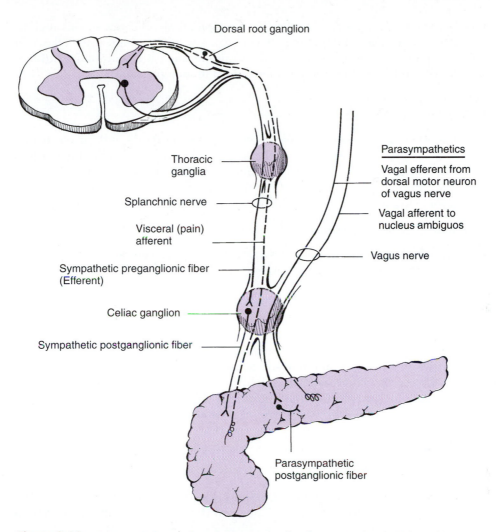

Figure 8-10. Autonomic innervation of the pancreas. See the text for details. (Adapted from Greenfield LJ, ed. Surgery. Scientific Principles and Practice. Philadelphia: JB Lippincott, 1993:780.)

to the sympathetic chain via the greater splanchnic nerves. All nerves to and from the pancreas travel through the celiac plexus.

PHYSIOLOGY

ENDOCRINE FUNCTION

There are four major cell types in the endocrine pancreas. The B (β) cells are the most numerous cells in the islet of Langerhans. They secrete insulin and are located in the center of the islet. Other cells of the islet are situated in the periphery around the B cells. The A (α) cells secrete glucagon, D cells secrete somatostatin, and F (PP) cells secrete pancreatic polypeptide. The proportions of A, D, and F cells distributed around the periphery vary in each acinus. In addition, there is some regional variation within the pancreas such that islets derived from the ventral pancreas have proportionately more F cells, whereas those derived from the dorsal pancreas are richer in A cells. The physiologic significance of this regional variation is not clear, but mixing of cell types within a single islet allows for paracrine regulation of the islet with one hormone, such as somatostatin, influencing release of other islet hormones, such as insulin and glucagon.

EXOCRINE FUNCTION

The exocrine pancreas secretes both digestive enzymes and an electrolyte-rich fluid. As previously mentioned, the acinar cells are responsible for synthesis and secretion of the digestive enzymes, and the centroacinar and duct epithelial cells are responsible for secretion of the fluid that carries the enzymes to the duodenum for activation. Each of these processes is discussed separately below.

Fluid and Electrolyte Secretion

The gastrointestinal hormone secretin stimulates secretion of water, bicarbonate, sodium, potassium, and chloride from the duct epithelium through activation of adenylate cyclase. The subsequent formation of cyclic adenosine monophosphate (cAMP) causes stimulation of a chloride channel on the luminal side of the epithelial cell, and chloride is released from the cytoplasm into the duct lumen. A chloride-bicarbonate exchange mechanism then exchanges the chloride for intracellular bicarbonate, thus producing a bicarbonate-rich fluid for transporting digestive enzymes. Cholinergic stimulation can achieve a similar effect independent of secretin. Whereas in the stimulated state the ductal fluid is rich in bicarbonate and low in chloride, the opposite is true in the resting (unstimulated) state. At rest, ductal fluid flows at a rate of about 0.2 ml/min, but during stimulation the flow rate is approximately 4 ml/min (Fig. 8-11). Altogether, the pancreas secretes about 2.5 L of fluid each day into the duodenum.

Enzyme Synthesis and Secretion

Pancreatic enzymes are synthesized and stored in the acinar cells. The basal region of acinar cells contains the nucleus and the rough endoplasmic reticulum

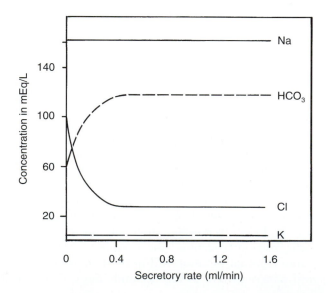

Figure 8-11. Relationship of secretory rate to electrolyte composition of pancreatic juice. (From Yamada T, Alpers DH, Owyang C, Powell DH, Silverstein FE, eds. Textbook of Gastroenterology, 2nd ed. Philadelphia: JB Lippincott, 1995;1:362.)

where protein synthesis occurs. Enzymes produced in the rough endoplasmic reticulum are then packaged into zymogen granules in the Golgi complex, located between the nucleus and apical portion of the cell (Fig. 8-12). These zymogen granules are then stored in the apical portion of the acinar cell until the cell is stimulated. Once stimulated, such as after a meal, zymogen granules are seen to decrease in both size and number within the acinar cell. This event corresponds to an increase in pancreatic enzyme secretion. Each zymogen granule contains all the enzymes of digestion the pancreas can secrete, although each granule may contain different proportions of the various enzymes. Enzymes within the granules are in solid rather than liquid form and become solubilized only after excretion from the cell into the alkaline fluid within the pancreatic ducts. However, even solubilized pancreatic enzymes are in an inactive proenzyme form. Conversion to the active form does not occur until the enzymes are in the duodenum. This provides a measure of protection for the pancreas from autodigestion. Furthermore, tight junctions between apical cells prevent reflux of secreted digestive enzymes from the ductular lumen into the intercellular space and thereby provide another layer of protection to the pancreas. Once secreted into the duodenum, the acid-labile pancreatic enzymes are protected from digestion by the bicarbonate-rich pancreatic fluid in which the proenzymes were transported. These precursor enzymes are then activated by enzymatic hydrolysis, discussed below.

The pancreas secretes a variety of digestive enzymes (Table 8-1). The majority of secreted enzymes are for digestion of the protein, starch, and fat we consume in our diet. Before these enzymes can become functional they must be activated within the duodenum. Trypsinogen is a proenzyme that undergoes enzymatic hydrolysis of its N-terminal fragment through the action of the brush border peptidase called enterokinase. The brush border is the lining of the small intestine consisting of villi, microvilli, and crypts. In addition to providing mechanisms to absorb digested nutrients, the cells of the brush border produce a variety of substances to facilitate digestion prior to absorption. Enterokinase is only one of those substances. Activated trypsin then catalyzes the activation of all the other precursor enzymes secreted by the pancreas as well as catalyzing the conversion of more

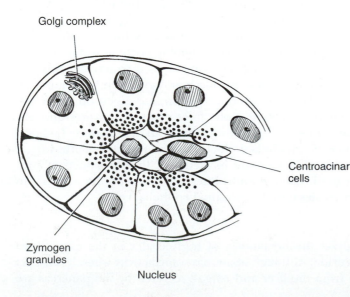

Golgi complex

Centroacinar cells

Zymogen granules

Nucleus

Figure 8-12. Architecture of a pancreatic acinus showing location of zymogen granules with respect to the lumen of the ductule. (Adapted from Bloom W, Fawcett DW. A Textbook of Histology, 11th ed. Philadelphia: WB Saunders, 1986.)

TABLE 8-1. *DIGESTIVE ENZYMES SECRETED BY THE PANCREAS*

ENZYME	TARGET
Amylase	α-1,4 Glycosidic links in starch, glycogen
Lipase	Triglyceride, producing fatty acids and 2-monoglycerides
Phospholipase A_2	Phosphotidylcholine, producing a free fatty acid and lysophosphotidylcholine
Carboxylesterase	Cholesterol esters, lipid-soluble vitamin esters, and glycerides (tri-, di-, monoglycerides)
Trypsin*	Interior peptide bonds involving basic amino acids
Chymotrypsin*	Interior peptide bonds involving aromatic amino acids, leucine, glutamine, and methionine
Elastase*	Interior peptide bonds involving neutral aliphatic amino acids
Carboxypeptidase A and B*	External peptide bonds involving aromatic and neutral aliphatic amino acids (A) and basic amino acids (B) at the carboxy-terminal end

*These enzymes are secreted by the pancreas as inactive proenzymes. They are activated within the duodenum.

typsinogen to trypsin. The pancreas also secretes a peptide known as pancreatic secretory trypsin inhibitor. This peptide inactivates trypsin by binding with the enzyme near its catalytic site and may serve as a back-up measure to protect the pancreas from itself. Feedback regulation of digestive events occurring within the duodenum is discussed below.

Amylase

Amylase is secreted not only by the pancreas but also by the salivary glands. Although the two isoforms have the same enzymatic activity, they can be identified separately by differences in electrophoretic mobility. Amylase digests dietary starch (from plant sources) and glycogen (from animal sources). Salivary amylase initiates the process and may in fact accomplish a considerable portion of starch digestion before the substrate reaches the small intestine to face pancreatic amylase. Amylase hydrolyzes α-1,4-glycosidic linkages of starch and glycogen but cannot digest the α-1,6-glycosidic links. Thus the products of amylase digestion are short-chain α-1,6-linked polysaccharides termed alpha limit dextrins. An intestinal enzyme then splits the 1,6-linked dextrins to allow amylase to attack more 1,4-links. Ultimately, maltose, a dimer of α-1,4-linked glucose molecules and maltotriose, a trimer of α-1,4-linked glucose molecules, are formed, and these products of amylase digestion are then further broken down by intestinal brush border enzymes to allow uptake of glucose molecules into the intestinal epithelial cells.

Lipase

Pancreatic lipase catalyzes the breakdown of triglycerides in the diet to two fatty acids and a monoglyceride. Although lipase has some activity when it must act alone, bile acids secreted from the liver and *colipase* secreted by the pancreas are required for the full activity of lipase. Bile acids act as an emulsifier to break up triglyceride droplets into smaller particles; thereby allowing lipase greater access, and colipase forms a complex between itself, lipase, and bile salts to further increase the surface area upon which lipase can act. The pancreas also secretes two other lipases. *Phospholipase* A_2 converts phosphatidylcholine to lysophosphatidylcholine and a free fatty acid. *Carboxylesterase* acts on a variety of substrates, including cholesterol esters, tri-, di-, and monoglycerides, and esters of lipid-soluble vitamins.

Proteases

A variety of proteases are secreted by the pancreas in a precursor form and are then activated in the duodenum. *Trypsin, chymotrypsin,* and *elastase* are endopeptidases that cleave proteins at specific sites adjacent to specific amino acids. *Carboxypeptidases* cleave peptide bonds at the carboxy-terminal ends of proteins. Oligopeptides and some free amino acids result from the combined action of these endopeptidases and carboxypeptidases, and the oligopeptides are then further digested by brush border enzymes or taken up by intestinal mucosal cells.

REGULATION OF SECRETION

A variety of agents regulate pancreatic enzyme secretion through contact with acinar cell membrane receptors. These receptors are located along the basolateral surface of the acinar cells. Receptors for cholecystokinin, acetylcholine, bombesin, substance P, vasoactive intestinal polypeptide, and secretin have been identified. Some of these agents are stimulatory, whereas others are inhibitory.

Stimulants of Pancreatic Secretion

Vasoactive intestinal polypeptide and secretin stimulate pancreatic secretion through activation of adenylate cyclase. As in other cells utilizing the adenylate cyclase pathway, cAMP is increased, resulting in activation of protein kinase A. Through mechanisms yet unknown, protein kinase A then causes increased secretion of bicarbonate-rich pancreatic juice.

The other agonists (cholecystokinin, acetylcholine, gastrin-releasing peptide, and substance P) act through specific receptors that use an alternate "second messenger" rather than cAMP. These agents cause an increase in intracellular cyclic guanosine monophosphate that results in intracellular increases of inositol triphosphate, diacylglycerol, arachadonic acid, and finally intracellular calcium (Fig. 8-13). These intermediates then activate various protein kinases, resulting in an increase in enzyme secretion. An interesting finding in animal studies has been that combining agonists that act through different membrane receptors results in a synergistic effect, not just an additive effect, in certain situations. For example, cholecystokinin augments secretin's bicarbonate response, but secretin does not seem to enhance cholecystokinin's enzyme secretory response.

Phases of Digestion

Pancreatic secretion can be divided into interdigestive and digestive phases. The interdigestive (fasting) phase closely follows the pattern of intestinal motor activity known as the migrating myoelectric complex (MMC). The MMC is divided into phase I, characterized by a lack of motor activity, and phases II and III, with progressively more motor activity. During phase I, pancreatic secretion of enzymes

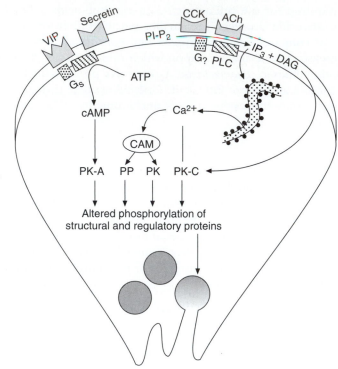

Figure 8-13. Schematic diagram of stimulus-secretion coupling of pancreatic acinar cell protein secretion. Abbreviations: VIP, vasoactive intestinal polypeptide; CCK, cholecystokinin; ACh, acetylcholine; PI = P_2, phosphatidyl inositol biphosphate; IP_3, inositol triphosphate; DAG, diacylglycerol; G_s, stimulatory guanine nucleotide-binding protein; PLC, phospholipase C; PK = A, PK = C, protein kinase A and C, respectively; PP, PK, calmodulin (CAM)-dependent protein kinases. (Adapted from Williams JA, Burnham DB, Hootman SR. Cellular regulation of pancreatic secretion. In Forte J, ed. Handbook of Physiology—The Gastrointestinal System, III. Bethesda, MD: American Physiological Society, 1989:419.)

and bicarbonate as well as secretion of bile from the liver and gallbladder is at its lowest level. During phases II and III, there is a progressive increase in pancreatic and biliary secretion and partial gallbladder contraction, in conjunction with increasing myoelectric activity. Motilin is an interdigestive hormone from the upper small intestine important in the MMC. In dogs it plays some role in the increase in pancreatic secretion seen in phase III, but its role if any in humans is not yet clear.

The digestive phase of pancreatic secretion is the most interesting and complex and is divided into three parts. The first phase, called the *cephalic phase,* is vagally mediated. It begins with the sensory portion of a meal, that is, with the sight, smell, and taste of food. This phase can account for a significant increase in secretion of both enzymes and bicarbonate. Sham feeding studies have been used to learn the physiology of this phase. Sham feeding studies, in which food is smelled, tasted, and chewed but not swallowed, suggest that this increase in pancreatic secretions may be attributable to both direct vagal cholinergic effects on the acinar cell and duodenal acidification related to the increase in gastric acid secretion that accompanies sham feeding. Duodenal acidification results in release of secretin from duodenal mucosa. Secretin then stimulates pancreatic bicarbonate secretion, allowing a buffering effect within the duodenum. This feedback mechanism (i.e., buffering) then subsequently reduces secretin release (because the acid stimulus for secretin release has been reduced) and thus reduces pancreatic secretion. Vagal stimulation by sham feeding results in more than just acetylcholine release, since blocking acetylcholine receptors with atropine does not completely abolish the secretory response to sham feeding. Peptide-containing (i.e., peptidergic) neurons have been identified within the pancreas, and there are data to suggest that vagal stimulation can also cause release of peptides like vasoactive intestinal polypeptide, gastrin-releasing peptide, cholecystokinin, and enkephalins. Data for vasoactive intestinal polypeptide and gastrin-releasing peptide are most convincing. Vasoactive intestinal polypeptide is known to stimulate both acinar cells (enzymes) and duct epithelial cells (water, bicarbonate).

The second (*gastric*) phase of the digestive period of pancreatic secretion begins when food enters the stomach. During this phase, pancreatic enzyme secretion increases, whereas secretion of water and bicarbonate does not substantially increase more than has occurred during the cephalic phase. This phase is neurally mediated through vagal afferents responding to stretching of the stomach (fundus, antrum). Plasma secretin and cholecystokinin levels rise within the first 10 minutes of meal ingestion. This constitutes the so-called vagovagal cholinergic reflex.

The final phase of the digestive period, the *intestinal phase,* begins when chyme enters the duodenum. Chyme is the product of gastric grinding, mixing, and sieving of ingested food. This phase is neurally (vagovagal) and hormonally mediated and results in the most profound secretion of enzymes of all the phases in the digestive period. Pancreatic water and bicarbonate secretion in this phase is primarily stimulated by duodenal acidification, but fatty acids and bile acids also contribute. Secretin seems to be the primary mediator of the response to duodenal acidification, but cholecystokinin and cholinergic influences are also important. As mentioned earlier, cholecystokinin alone causes no significant bicarbonate secretion but augments the secretin response. Enzyme secretion during the intestinal phase is stimulated by the presence within the duodenum of fatty acids of at least 8-carbon chain length, monoglycerides, peptides, amino acids, and calcium. Products of carbohydrate digestion have only a minor effect. In addition to fatty acids, peptides, and amino acids, the vagovagal reflex is important in the full response to meal-stimulated pancreatic enzyme secretion. Vagotomy and atropine cause a marked reduction in enzyme secretion in response to small loads of amino acids and fatty acids. However, large loads of these digestion products are potent stimuli for enzyme secretion despite interruption of the vagovagal reflex and appear to act through stimulation of cholecystokinin release in the upper small intestine.

Cholecystokinin-releasing peptide (CCKRP) is a peptide secreted by the enterocyte that is inactive during the basal, or interdigestive, period. CCKRP stimulates enterocytes to secrete cholecystokinin. During the interdigestive period, there is enough activated trypsin present in the gut lumen to degrade CCKRP, which is trypsin-sensitive. During the fed state, trypsin is busy with the protein load delivered to the duodenum and there is proportionally more CCKRP remaining undigested in the duodenal lumen. This results in stimulation of cholecystokinin release from enterocytes and subsequent pancreatic stimulation. Thus CCKRP "monitors" the duodenum for evidence of protein digestion and then causes the pancreas to increase its secretions to better handle the ingested food. A similar monitor peptide has been found in pancreatic juice, and there may also be a secretin-releasing peptide released from enterocytes with similar function.

In summary, duodenal acidification during all three phases of the digestive period of pancreatic secretion causes secretin release, and this release is augmented by the presence within the duodenum of bile and products of protein and fat digestion. Secretin causes release of pancreatic bicarbonate and water. Cholecystokinin, primarily secreted in response to products of protein and fat digestion within the duodenum, causes stimulation of pancreatic enzyme secretion. Cholecystokinin release occurs chiefly during the gastric and intestinal phases of the digestive period. Vagovagal reflexes and peptidergic responses are important in all three phases of the digestive period (Fig. 8-14).

Inhibitors of Pancreatic Secretion

A variety of agents are responsible for inhibiting pancreatic secretion, usually in a feedback fashion during or after a meal.

Pancreatic polypeptide is a peptide hormone present in the islets of Langerhans that acts to inhibit pancreatic secretion of water, bicarbonate, and enzymes. Pancreatic polypeptide is increased in plasma after sham feeding, consumption of a meal, or experimentally after duodenal acidification. In addition, vagal stimulation and hormones such as cholecystokinin, secretin, vasoactive intestinal polypeptide,

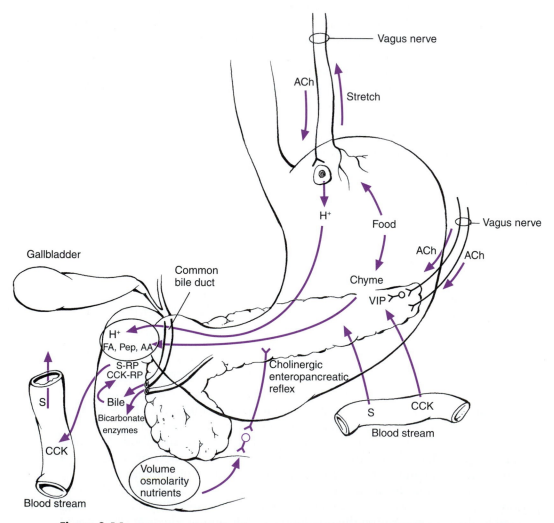

Figure 8-14. Summary of the digestive phase of pancreatic secretion. Elements of the cephalic, gastric, and intestinal phases are represented. See text for details. ACh: acetylcholine; H⁺: hydrochloric acid; FA: fatty acids; Pep: oligopeptides; AA: amino acids; S-RP: secretin-releasing peptide; CCK-RP: cholecystokinin-releasing peptide; VIP: vasoactive intestinal polypeptide. (Adapted from Yamada T, Alpers DH, Owyang C, Powell DH, Silverstein FE, eds. Textbook of Gastroenterology, 2nd ed. Philadelphia: JB Lippincott, 1995;1:376.)

and perhaps gastrin and gastrin-releasing peptide result in an increase in pancreatic polypeptide secretion by the pancreas. Pancreatic polypeptide may act as an antagonist for acetylcholine receptors and may also inhibit release of acetylcholine from postganglionic neurons within the pancreas; it acts at the level of the acinar cell.

Peptide YY is released from the distal ileum and colon in response to mixed meals, but intraluminal fat is the most potent stimulus for its secretion. This peptide decreases pancreatic responses to cholecystokinin and secretin, perhaps by inhibiting release of acetylcholine and norepinephrine and inhibiting release of mucosal cholecystokinin.

Somatostatin inhibits release of secretin from duodenal mucosa, and it competes with secretin at receptor sides. The ultimate effect is a decrease in pancreatic secretion of both bicarbonate and enzymes. Somatostatin is produced in gastric and duodenal mucosa as well as in pancreatic islets (D cells). However, only the form of somatostatin produced by the small intestine appears to be most involved in inhibiting pancreatic secretion. Somatostatin release is mediated by the autonomic nervous system in response to intake of fat and amino acids in meals.

Other inhibitors include the islet cell hormones *pancreatic glucagon* and *pancreastatin,* and the neuropeptides *calcitonin gene-related peptide* and *enkephalins.* Pancreatic glucagon inhibits pancreatic secretion stimulated by cholecystokinin, secretin, or a meal, in part by competing with cholecystokinin. The effect is a decrease in both bicarbonate/water and enzyme secretion. Pancreastatin inhibits pancreatic exocrine secretion by inhibiting acetylcholine release from vagal efferent nerve endings. Calcitonin gene-related peptide may act by stimulating somatostatin release. Enkephalins and similar opioids decrease mucosal secretin release and may also act by inhibiting acetylcholine release.

CLINICAL CORRELATES

ACUTE PANCREATITIS

Clinical Features

Nearly all patients experiencing an episode of acute pancreatitis complain of abdominal pain and have abdominal tenderness on examination. Pain is typically epigastric or in the left upper quadrant and sometimes radiates or "penetrates" toward the back. It reaches peak intensity after a few hours and is least bothersome when the torso is bent forward or when the patient lies on the side with knees drawn up toward the chest. In contrast to patients who have a perforated viscus and who prefer to lie perfectly still, the patient with pancreatic pain is often restless in an effort to find the most comfortable position. Most patients experience nausea and vomiting, and a low-grade fever is not uncommon.

The physical examination in severe cases of pancreatitis may reveal hypotension, shock, respiratory distress (hypoxia, adult respiratory distress syndrome), mental status changes, pulmonary edema, abdominal rigidity or guarding, and signs of retroperitoneal bleeding known as Cullen or Grey Turner signs. Cullen and Grey Turner signs are caused by blood dissecting from the retroperitoneum into the periumbilical region (Cullen) or the flanks (Grey Turner) and are identified by bluish discoloration in these regions.

Laboratory investigation often reveals a moderate increase in white blood cells, an elevated hematocrit due to hemoconcentration associated with intravascular volume contraction, and occasionally mild elevations of liver chemistry tests (aspartate aminotransferase, alanine aminotransferase, bilirubin, and alkaline phosphatase). Marked elevations of the liver chemistry tests should prompt evaluation for the possibility of gallstone pancreatitis. Serum amylase and lipase levels are almost always elevated at least twice the upper limit of normal values, but because amylase can fall rapidly, this enzyme may not be elevated in patients who present several days after onset of symptoms. Lipase values tend to remain elevated longer. Be wary of an isolated increase in amylase without a compatible clinical history and examination, since a variety of factors other than pancreatitis can result in an increased serum amylase concentration (see Clinical Testing section).

Most patients with mild or moderate cases of uncomplicated acute pancreatitis improve within a couple of days, and complete recovery can be expected within a week using conservative treatment consisting of vigorous volume replacement to correct tremendous volume loses caused by intense retroperitoneal inflammation, keeping the patient *nil per os* (NPO, no food or drink by mouth), and providing analgesia. It is thought that the NPO state helps to "rest" the pancreas and keep it in the basal, unstimulated state. Some clinicians also utilize nasogastric suction to aid in removal of normal gastric secretions to further reduce the chance of pancreatic stimulation, but such intervention has not been proved beneficial in the patient who is not experiencing vomiting.

Etiology and Pathophysiology

Most cases of acute pancreatitis, over 80%, are related to biliary stones (choledocholithiasis) or alcohol ingestion. In inner city populations, alcohol is the major cause, whereas in the more affluent suburban areas biliary tract stone disease is most common. In addition to these factors, other etiologies include pancreatic tumors, abdominal trauma (penetrating or blunt), drugs, infections, hyperlipidemia, operations (biliary tract, gastric, cardiac), idiopathic causes, and iatrogenic causes, such as endoscopic manipulation of the papilla of Vater through endoscopic retrograde cholangiopancreatography (ERCP) or after pancreatic biopsy.

Biliary tract disease was first attributed as a cause of acute pancreatitis in 1901 in a report by Opie. After observing a gallstone impacted at the papilla of Vater in a patient who had died of acute pancreatitis, Opie proposed what has come to be known as the "common channel theory" of the etiology of acute gallstone pancreatitis. Opie surmised that a long common channel allowed a gallstone to become impacted after the stone had passed the point of joining of the common bile duct and pancreatic duct. He proposed that this allowed both obstruction of pancreatic outflow as well as reflux of bile into the pancreatic duct, resulting in pancreatic injury caused in part by the detergent properties of bile. The common channel theory has been challenged on a number of points. One argument is that since most people have such a short common channel, a stone would obstruct both the common bile duct and the pancreatic duct and reflux could not occur. Furthermore, several studies have shown that the pressure within the pancreatic duct exceeds the pressure in the common bile duct, thus making reflux into the pancreatic duct physiologically unlikely. More likely, the role of biliary tract disease in gallstone pancreatitis centers on obstructing pancreatic outflow. Outflow obstruction could be caused by an impacted stone, as in Opie's case, or produced by periampullary inflammation, edema, or sphincter spasm occurring after passage of a stone through the papilla. Such stone passage through the papilla into the duodenum has been proposed as the most common cause of gallstone pancreatitis rather than a persistently impacted stone, based mostly on work of investigators who have found gallstones in the feces of most patients with intact gallbladders who are recovering from an episode of pancreatitis (in the absence of other likely causes). These studies found gallstones in the feces of the majority of patients with recent acute pancreatitis but in the minority of patients with gallbladder stones without a recent history of pancreatitis.

Ductal or ampullary obstruction presumably results in hypertension within the pancreatic ducts and subsequent rupture of smaller pancreatic ductules. This allows leakage of secretions into the pancreatic parenchyma, enzyme activation, and subsequent "autodigestion" of the pancreas. Alternatively, ductal obstruction could simply make release of enzymes from acinar cells impossible. Intracellular events as yet unknown could then allow enzyme activation within acinar cells. The exact mechanism is not known.

Alcohol is considered to be a cause of acute pancreatitis when patients give a history of either acute or chronic alcohol use and no other cause is apparent. Most cases of "acute" pancreatitis in the setting of alcoholism actually occur in a pancreas that has already been chronically damaged by alcohol, even in the absence of a clear clinical history of prior episodes of pancreatitis. In the absence of such a history or the presence of steatorrhea or pancreatic calcifications, the diagnosis of chronic pancreatitis is difficult to make without invasive methods. The mechanism by which alcohol induces pancreatitis is unknown. It is known that oral alcohol administration causes a transient stimulation of pancreatic secretion and a contraction of the sphincter of Oddi, theoretically resulting in ductal hypertension. In vitro studies suggest that alcohol can allow secretion of activated proteolytic enzymes as a result of an imbalance between proteolytic enzymes and protease inhibitors in pancreatic juice, but whether this occurs in vivo is not known.

Tumors of the pancreas or papilla, which are usually malignant, can result in acute pancreatitis based on ductal obstruction. Infections such as with *Clonorchis sinensis* and *Ascaris lumbricoides* can similarly cause pancreatitis, whereas viral infections and infections with *Mycoplasma pneumoniae* have been suggested to cause acute pancreatitis by direct infection of pancreatic acinar cells.

The mechanism or mechanisms of *drug-induced* pancreatitis are likely multifactorial, and controversy exists as to whether the association of certain drugs with pancreatitis is cause and effect or serendipitous. Common drugs generally considered capable of causing pancreatitis include thiazides, furosemide, estrogens, 6-mercaptopurine, azathioprine, L-asparaginase, α-methyldopa, tetracycline, pentamidine, procainamide, dideoxyinosine, valproic acid, and sulfonamides.

Hyperlipidemia, specifically hypertriglyceridemia, may be the result of pancreatitis more often than it is the cause. The mechanism by which hypertriglyeridemia causes acute pancreatitis is not clear, but speculation centers on ischemia of the pancreatic microcirculation related to liberation of free fatty acids in the pancreatic circulation by the action of lipase on triglycerides and the subsequent small vessel damage that occurs.

Postoperative acute pancreatitis most commonly results from operations on or near the pancreas, such as common bile duct explorations, sphincteroplasty or endoscopic sphincterotomy, distal gastrectomy, and splenectomy and from ERCP. Cardiopulmonary bypass and cardiac transplantation have frequently been associated with acute pancreatitis, but the etiology is unclear. Two theories center on hypoperfusion during surgery or atheromatous emboli, and a more recent suggestion relates to hypercalcemia, which often occurs during such operations owing to administration of high doses of calcium during cardiopulmonary bypass.

Pancreatic trauma from penetrating or blunt abdominal injury can result in disruption of the pancreatic duct and the development of pancreatitis acutely or months after the injury because of formation of a pseudocyst.

Other causes are less common or are more controversial in the etiology of acute pancreatitis. Pancreas divisum, where there is failure of fusion of the dorsal and ventral ducts during development, is a somewhat controversial cause of acute and chronic pancreatitis. This developmental anomaly results in the draining of the major portion of pancreatic secretion through the relatively smaller accessory duct and accessory papilla, theoretically with a build-up of pressure in the ductal system. There is not yet wide agreement as to the importance of this variant in the etiology of pancreatitis. Pregnancy in and of itself has in the past been thought to cause pancreatitis, but most documented cases have been associated with gallstones when stones have been sought out. Vascular insults, such as low-flow states (hypotension of any cause) and atheroembolic events, have also been associated with pancreatitis. Systemic autoimmune disorders, such as systemic lupus erythematosus, have also been implicated in acute and chronic pancreatitis on the basis of autoantibody attack on the pancreas and on the basis of an underlying vasculitis.

Despite the variety of possible inciting events, the underlying pathophysiology of the resulting pancreatitis is likely the same. Presumably, when activated pancreatic enzymes gain access to the parenchyma of the pancreas they result in damage to the pancreas, which is clinically manifest as acute or chronic pancreatitis. The exact mechanism whereby these enzymes become activated, or where such activation occurs, is not clear. Normally, inactive zymogens become activated by trypsin within the duodenum. One theory suggests that reflux of duodenal contents into the pancreatic duct results in the entry of activated enzymes into the pancreatic ductal system or that refluxed trypsin could allow activation of zymogens within the pancreatic ducts. Refluxed bile could alter duct permeability, thus allowing activated enzymes to enter the parenchyma. An alternate theory suggests that zymogen activation occurs within the acinar cell itself by the mixing of lysosomal hydrolases and zymogen granules, intracellular components normally separated from one another. Recall that the contents of zymogen granules normally never contact cell cytoplasm, being synthesized within rough endoplasmic reticulum, packaged into secretory granules in the Golgi complex, and then extruded by exocytosis into the duct lumen when acinar cell stimulation occurs. Finally, another possibility is that protease inhibitors normally secreted in acinar cells and cotransported with zymogens may be reduced in certain clinical situations and allow intrapancreatic activation of zymogen.

CHRONIC PANCREATITIS

Clinical Features

Chronic inflammation leading to fibrosis, loss of exocrine tissue, and occasionally endocrine pancreatic dysfunction defines the state of chronic pancreatitis. The Marseilles-Rome classification of chronic pancreatitis divides the condition into three categories. *Chronic calcifying pancreatitis* is caused by chronic alcohol use and is the most common type, accounting for up to 80% of all cases of chronic pancreatitis. It is characterized by formation of protein plugs or stones within the duct system. Stenosis and atrophy of the pancreatic ducts can also be seen. *Chronic obstructive pancreatitis* occurs from duct or papillary obstruction by tumor, stricture, or stenosis and is the next most common form. *Chronic inflammatory pancreatitis* is the least common form and its etiology is not well defined.

The clinical course of chronic pancreatitis can be summarized as follows. Typically the patient presents in the third or fourth decade of life with the first attack of pain, has a recurrent attack within the next couple of years, and then experiences more frequent attacks, especially if alcohol ingestion was the cause and the patient continues to drink. Finally, chronic pain, malabsorption, or diarrhea develops along with pancreatic calcifications, which can be seen on plain abdominal radiographs.

Etiology and Pathophysiology

Alcoholism is the leading cause of chronic pancreatitis worldwide. At autopsy, up to 45% of alcoholics *without* a prior history of clinical pancreatitis have morphologic changes of chronic pancreatitis. Such changes are rare in nondrinkers. In addition, one report found that just over 50% of asymptomatic alcoholics have abnormal pancreatic exocrine function or pancreatic stimulation tests. Although there is general agreement that alcohol plays a causative role in chronic pancreatitis, the mechanism is not known. There is not a well-defined threshold amount of alcohol consumption above which pancreatic damage can be predicted. Just as with alcoholic liver disease, there is considerable individual variation in susceptibility. The form of alcohol ingested does not appear to matter, nor does the presence of malnutrition, which was once thought important in the etiology of alcoholic pancreatitis.

Studies involving the collection of pure pancreatic juice from a catheter placed directly into the pancreatic duct show that after stimulation of pancreatic secretion with the hormones secretin and cholecystokinin, the pancreatic juice of patients with a history of heavy alcohol use contains a higher protein concentration and lower bicarbonate concentration than of patients with no history of alcohol use, even when there has been no history of alcohol-related clinical pancreatitis. Other studies show that the pancreatic juice of alcoholics has a markedly increased ratio of trypsinogen to trypsin inhibitor, thus potentially predisposing them to intraductal zymogen activation. Further studies find decreased amounts of a protein in pancreatic juice capable of inhibiting formation of insoluble calcium salts (stones). Deficiency of this inhibitor, called pancreatic stone protein, could thus allow the calculus formation so characteristic of chronic alcoholic pancreatitis. Furthermore, citrate, which can chelate calcium, has been shown to be secreted in smaller amounts in patients with heavy alcohol use, regardless of the presence of clinically identifiable chronic pancreatitis. Reduction of citrate secretion could also predispose to the development of intraductal protein plugs and stones. Ductal changes in chronic alcoholic pancreatitis begin in the smaller side branches of the main pancreatic duct rather than the main duct itself. Thus, damage to ducts begins peripherally and only later involves the larger main duct. This seems to be unique to alcoholic pancreatitis. Despite all these interesting observations, the mechanism by which these changes in pancreatic secretion occur, or which ones occur first, is not known.

Hereditary pancreatitis is an uncommon form of acute attacks of pancreatitis that ultimately develops into chronic pancreatitis, often with calcifications of the gland similar to what occurs in alcoholic pancreatitis. The disease is inherited in an autosomal dominant fashion, so males and females can be equally affected. There is variable penetrance however. This disease affects people at a young age, with 80% of patients experiencing their first episode of pancreatitis before the age of 20.

Cystic fibrosis is a pancreatic disease with widespread clinical findings, the most prominent of which is pulmonary disease. The disorder is autosomal recessive in inheritance and is characterized by defective chloride secretion owing to a defective gene coding for a membrane chloride channel called cystic fibrosis transmembrane conductance regulator. The membrane protein coded for by this defective gene results in markedly reduced chloride and bicarbonate secretion in the pancreas, intestine, and other organs. Within the pancreas, this results in obstruction of small ducts by inspissated secretions and cellular debris and thus begins the sequence leading to pancreatic exocrine failure. Interestingly, most cystic fibrosis patients have preserved endocrine pancreatic function for the most part. Hyperplasia and eventual necrosis of ductular and centroacinar cells occur, encroaching upon acini and resulting in the development of cystic spaces within the pancreas. Exocrine insufficiency and steatorrhea are hallmarks of the disease, and low concentrations of pancreatic enzymes and bicarbonate are found in the pancreatic juice of patients with cystic fibrosis.

The origin of pain in chronic pancreatitis is not fully elucidated. Afferent nerve fibers within the pancreas carry impulses to the celiac plexus. From there, the right and left splanchnic nerves carry impulses to the right and left paravertebral sympathetic ganglia. The etiology of those pain impulses in chronic pancreatitis is unclear. Ductal hypertension may be one mechanism, as it is known that pancreatic duct pressures are elevated and that some patients get pain relief with duct decompression procedures such as surgery or stent placements (stents are hollow plastic tubes placed within the main pancreatic duct to improve drainage, usually across strictured portions of the duct). Perineural inflammation and disruption of the perineural sheath owing to irritative substances produced in chronic pancreatitis are other potential mechanisms. The pain of chronic pancreatitis is typically steady and boring in nature; it penetrates to the back and lasts from days to weeks.

Malabsorption in chronic pancreatitis requires the loss of more than 90% of pancreatic exocrine function. Malabsorption of fat (steatorrhea) precedes malabsorption of protein (azotorrhea). Malabsorption of carbohydrate does not occur until there is near complete loss of pancreatic enzyme secretion, so this is rarely a clinical problem.

In contrast to patients with malabsorption based on intestinal mucosal diseases, patients with malabsorption associated with chronic pancreatic insufficiency have smaller volume stools (because fluid and electrolyte absorption is generally preserved), little or no carbohydrate malabsorption, and only rarely experience vitamin, iron, or calcium deficiency. However, malabsorption of cobalamin (vitamin B_{12}) can occur because pancreatic proteases are required to degrade the cobalamin–R protein complex so that cobalamin can bind intrinsic factor and be absorbed.

CLINICAL TESTING

STIMULATION TESTING

Secretin, or secretin and cholecystokinin given in combination, allows estimation of pancreatic exocrine functional reserve. In this test, secretin and/or cholecystokinin is administered intravenously followed by aspiration of duodenal juice though a catheter placed fluoroscopically. Pancreatic bicarbonate (and enzyme secretion if cholecystokinin is used) can then be estimated by measuring the amount of these products in duodenal juice. To collect pancreatic secretions, a catheter is placed through the esophagus and stomach into the duodenum. Another catheter is placed through the esophagus into the stomach to keep the stomach clear of secretions that could dilute the duodenal contents and affect the results. The duodenal tube has two openings or channels, one positioned in the proximal duodenum and the second positioned in the distal duodenum near the ligament of Treitz. A nonabsorbable marker such as polyethylene glycol is infused into the proximal port at a known rate and distal duodenal juices (plus polyethylene glycol) are aspirated from the distal port after administering secretin. Bicarbonate (and enzyme) secretion can thus be determined. Because the test is cumbersome and expensive, it is rarely used in most hospitals except perhaps in teaching hospitals. False-positive (i.e., falsely abnormal) test results can occur in the presence of mucosal diseases such as celiac sprue and in patients with prior gastric resection of the Billroth II variety.

BENTIROMIDE TEST

N-benzoyl-L-tyrosyl-p-aminobenzoic acid (NBT-PABA) is given orally in this test of pancreatic function, and PABA excretion in the urine is measured to assess pancreatic secretion of chymotrypsin, which is required to cleave the NBT-PABA bond. Released PABA is then absorbed, conjugated in the liver, and excreted in the urine. The sensitivity for severe chronic pancreatitis is about 80%, but it is far less reliable in the absence of advanced disease accompanied by steatorrhea. False-positive (abnormal) results can be found in cases of intestinal disease, where there is deficient secretion of secretin and cholecystokinin by enterocytes or simply malabsorption of appropriately cleaved PABA, in renal disease where clearance of PABA can be impaired, in liver disease (defective conjugation), and in diabetes.

DUAL LABEL SCHILLING'S TEST

In this test, patients ingest an oral cocktail that includes Co^{57}-labeled cobalamin/intrinsic factor complex and Co^{58}-labeled cobalamin/R-protein complex. Urine is collected for 24 hours and the amounts of Co^{57} and Co^{58} are determined. In pancreatic insufficiency, Co^{57}-labeled cobalamin is preferentially absorbed, since little of the Co^{58}-labeled cobalamin can be released from R-protein for absorption; therefore the ratio of Co^{58}/Co^{57} is low. This test may be more sensitive than the NBT-PABA test and does not seem to be affected by renal or hepatic disease. Furthermore, it correlates better with pancreatogram findings and results of pancreatic function (secretion) testing than does NBT-PABA.

FECAL FAT

This test is performed in the same manner as described in Chapter 6 on malabsorption. Chronic pancreatitis patients typically have very high values of fat excretion, but their total stool volume is usually less than that of patients with mucosal disease. Still, an abnormal fecal fat value alone cannot distinguish between pancreatic insufficiency and mucosal disease. Other clinical findings or tests are required to make the distinction.

RADIOGRAPHY

Plain films of the abdomen may reveal calcification in the pancreas. This finding is noted in about 30% of patients with chronic pancreatitis. Computed tomography (CT) scanning and ultrasonography can be of value in detection of pseudocysts or dilated pancreatic ducts and can also detect calcifications. The other important role of these imaging procedures is in trying to distinguish between chronic pancreatitis and a pancreatic mass.

ENDOSCOPIC RETROGRADE CHOLANGIOPANCREATOGRAPHY

This endoscopic examination, performed by passing an endoscope into the duodenum adjacent to the papilla of Vater and placing a catheter through the scope and into the pancreatic duct orifice, allows injection of radiographic contrast medium into the pancreatic duct so that an x-ray film of the ductal system of the pancreas can be obtained. This test is very sensitive for the ductal changes of chronic pancreatitis and is quite useful in the distinction of chronic pancreatitis from pancreatic cancer when the typical beaded appearance of chronic pancreatitis is seen (Fig. 8-15).

SERUM ENZYMES

Amylase and lipase are the most commonly used blood tests to diagnose or exclude acute pancreatitis. Both enzymes are released in large quantities into the circulation during acute inflammation of the pancreas. Amylase tends to be cleared most rapidly from the serum and is the first enzyme to fall during resolution of pancreatitis. If a patient presents more than a few days after onset of abdominal pain, serum amylase levels can be normal or only slightly elevated. Serum lipase is cleared less rapidly, so this enzyme is more likely to remain elevated in pa-

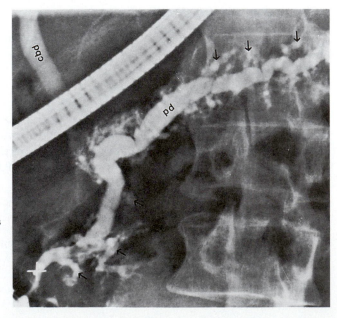

Figure 8-15. This pancreatogram shows changes of moderately severe chronic pancreatitis with a dilated main pancreatic duct (*pd*) and dilated side branches (*arrows*). The distal common bile duct (*cbd*) is also seen. (From Yamada T, Alpers DH, Owyang C, Powell DH, Silverstein FE, eds. Textbook of Gastroenterology, 2nd ed. Philadelphia: JB Lippincott, 1995;2:2597.)

tients whose onset of symptoms was several days earlier. Serum amylase concentrations can be elevated in nonpancreatic processes, such as those listed in Table 8-2. Fractionation into salivary and pancreatic amylase fractions is rarely done in clinical practice but can be useful. Macroamylasemia is another nonpancreatic cause of elevation of serum amylase levels. In this situation, serum amylase binds to an abnormal serum protein, forming a large complex that cannot be filtered by the kidney. Binding proteins may include immunoglobulins or other glycoproteins. In this condition, urinary amylase clearance is low or normal, and serum lipase is normal. Although lipase is more specific for pancreatic disease than amylase, both enzymes can be normal in patients with established chronic pancreatitis who have abdominal pain. Two possible explanations for lack of enzyme elevation in this setting are that the pancreas is "burned out" and does not have sufficient exocrine tissue to raise serum enzyme values or that the gland is so fibrotic that the enzymes have difficulty gaining access to the systemic circulation.

TABLE 8-2. *CAUSES OF HYPERAMYLASEMIA*

Pancreatic

Pancreatitis, pseudocyst, ascites, abscess

Pancreatic cancer

Pancreatic trauma

Pancreatic duct obstruction

Secretagogue stimulation

Endoscopic retrograde cholangiopancreatography

Nonpancreatic Intra-abdominal

Perforated viscus

Mesenteric infarction

Bowel obstruction

Cholangitis, cholecystitis

Appendicitis

Ruptured ectopic pregnancy

Ovarian cyst tumors

Renal failure

Extra-abdominal

Salivary gland trauma, tumors, duct obstruction, infection

Pneumonia

Lung cancer

Diabetic acidosis

Cerebral trauma

Thermal burns

From Yamada T, Alpers DH, Owyang C, Powell DH, Silverstein FE, eds. *Textbook of Gastroenterology.* Philadelphia: JB Lippincott, 1991:1864.

Serum immunoreactive trypsin levels are not commonly used in clinical practice, but the test appears to be a sensitive marker of pancreatitis. Utility of this assay over amylase and lipase assays remains to be established.

Urinary amylase measurement, or determination of the amylase creatinine clearance ratio, has been advocated as another means to diagnose or follow pancreatitis, but these measurements generally have little to offer over more easily obtained serum enzyme values.

CASE PRESENTATION

A 56-year-old man comes to your office with an 8-month history of loose stools associated with a 25-pound weight loss. The patient says he does not have any current abdominal pain but does recall an episode of upper abdominal and back pain occurring 2 months ago. The episode lasted for a week, resolved spontaneously, and was similar to other episodes of pain he has had about twice a year for the past 5 years. Stools are described as slightly loose and sometimes oily in appearance. No rectal bleeding, fever, or chills have occurred. His appetite is good, and he reports no dietary changes. His past medical history is only remarkable for a diagnosis of "borderline diabetes" given to him by his previous physician a few years ago. He is taking no medications and has no drug allergies. He is married and owns his own consulting firm. He smokes one pack of cigarettes a day and has a total 20 pack-year history. Alcohol intake consists of a daily glass of wine with dinner, and on weekends he usually consumes a six-pack of beer while golfing. Family history is positive only for heart disease affecting his father.

Weight loss is a significant but vague symptom that can be due to a variety of causes. Weight is simply a function of intake and output balance. Output is determined by energy expenditure in terms of calories burned by basal metabolism and activity and any losses of fluid or nutrients by the body (e.g., from sweat, vomiting, diarrhea, malabsorption, urination, respiration). Your patient gives a history of loose stools, which might be the source of his loss of weight. There is no rectal bleeding to suggest a colon malignancy, and his appetite is good. Therefore the main concern is increased basal metabolism (unlikely) or increased losses through diarrhea or malabsorption (very likely). Stools are oily and loose, suggesting undigested fat may be present. Mucosal disease or pancreatic disease could produce such maldigestion or malabsorption.

On physical examination, the patient is alert and not in distress. He appears slightly thin for his height. Head and neck examination reveals a loss of fat and muscle in the temple regions (bitemporal wasting), confirming significant weight loss. No lymphadenopathy can be found. Chest and heart examinations are normal. The abdominal examination reveals a soft, flat abdomen that is not tender to palpation. The liver is slightly enlarged on percussion, but the edge of the liver is smooth and does not suggest tumor or cirrhosis. The spleen tip is not palpable. No abdominal mass is palpated, and rectal examination is normal. The stool is negative for occult blood.

Unfortunately, the physical examination has given little clue to the cause for your patient's weight loss. It confirms that indeed a significant weight loss has occurred, and it does suggest an enlarged liver. Enlargement of the liver can be caused by infiltrating tumor or infiltrating fat, among other things. So-called "fatty liver" can be seen in diabetes and in alcohol abuse, among other conditions. So now you begin to wonder whether your patient might be overusing alcohol and replacing some of his nutritional calories with the empty calories of alcohol.

Laboratory evaluation shows normal electrolytes, a slightly elevated blood glucose level, and abnormal liver transaminases (aspartate aminotransferase [AST] 80 IU/dl, alanine aminotransferan [ALT] 20 IU/dl—normals <40). Bilirubin level is normal but serum amylase and lipase concentrations are slightly elevated. Serum albumin value is low at 3.0 g/dl. A complete blood count shows a borderline anemia (hemoglobin of 13 g/dl) with an elevated mean corpuscular volume. Platelet count is slightly low at 135,000/μl.

You decide correctly that it might be possible that your patient drinks more alcohol than he's told you. You find his transaminases are elevated, with an AST/ALT ratio >2, suggestive of alcohol-induced liver disease (alcoholic hepatitis or cirrhosis), and he has a macrocytic anemia. The mean corpuscular volume is a measure of red cell size, and enlarged red cells can be caused by vitamin deficiencies (vitamin B_{12} and folate) or the direct toxic effects of alcohol.

You order a 72-hour stool collection to measure fecal fat and find that on a 100-g fat diet your patient excretes an average of 600 g of stool per day containing 15 g of fecal fat. Normal fecal fat excretion is <7%, or 7 g on a 100-g fat diet. Still unclear is whether the problem is maldigestion (pancreatic insufficiency) or malabsorption (mucosal disease). You order a plain abdominal radiograph to look for pancreatic calcifications but find none. An ultrasound examination finds a normal-appearing liver, except for a diffuse echo pattern suggesting fatty infiltration, but the pancreas is not well seen because of overlying bowel gas. To try and confirm your suspicion of chronic pancreatitis and to rule out a bile duct stone or pancreatic tumor as a cause for your patient's clinical presentation and abnormal pancreatic enzymes, you refer him to a gastroenterologist for an ERCP. This reveals no stones and no sign of pancreatic cancer, but it does suggest chronic pancreatitis with beading of the side branches and an irregular main pancreatic duct.

With diagnosis in hand you see your patient once again in a follow-up visit. You present him with the test results and your diagnosis in a reassuring manner. You ask him again about any family history of pancreatitis, review his medication history, and inquire about prior operations or abdominal trauma. When none of this reveals a cause for chronic pancreatitis, you inquire again about his alcohol history in a nonthreatening manner. Ultimately, he admits that to deal with the pressures of his business he drinks an average of a fifth of scotch a week in addition to the wine and beer he previously admitted to. You encourage him to enter an alcohol treatment program, and after a few more visits with you he finally agrees. You treat him with pancreatic enzyme supplements containing exogenous lipase, protease, and amylase, and after 3 months the diarrhea is gone and he has begun to regain his weight.

SUMMARY

This chapter has sought to provide a moderately detailed overview of normal and abnormal pancreatic physiology and anatomy. Physiology has been used to illustrate why patients with pancreatic diseases present clinically as they do, and why we use certain tests to help define the nature of their problem. The ability to rationally approach patients with possible pancreatic disease requires a thorough understanding of pancreatic embryology, anatomy, and physiology as reviewed in this chapter. The reader with more interest is referred to the selected bibliography for additional reading.

SELECTED READING

Go Van Liang W, DiMagno EP, Gardner JB, Lebenthal E, Reber HA, Scheele GA, eds. The Pancreas: Biology, Pathobiology, and Disease, 2nd ed., New York: Raven Press, 1993.

Opie EL. The etiology of acute hemorrhagic pancreatitis. Bull Johns Hopkins Hosp 12:182, 1901.

Sleisinger MH, Fordtran JS, eds. Gastrointestinal Disease: Pathophysiology, Diagnosis, and Management, 5th ed. Philadelphia: WB Saunders, 1993.

Yamada T, Alpers DH, Owyang C, Powell DH, Silverstein FE, eds. Textbook of Gastroenterology, 2nd ed. Philadelphia: JB Lippincott, 1995.

Lippincott's Pathophysiology Series: Gastrointestinal Pathophysiology, edited by Joseph M. Henderson. Lippincott–Raven Publishers. Philadelphia © 1996.

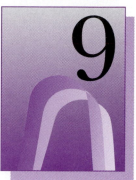

CHAPTER

9

Gastrointestinal Bleeding

Grace H. Elta

Gastrointestinal (GI) bleeding is a common clinical problem requiring over 300,000 hospitalizations annually in the United States. It varies in severity from life-threatening hemorrhage to slow, insidious bleeding that produces only iron deficiency. The overall mortality rate for acute upper gastrointestinal (UGI) bleeding is approximately 8% and has changed little over the past 40 years. In view of our aging population and the higher mortality from bleeding in the elderly, this may represent a slight improvement in mortality. The mortality from lower gastrointestinal (LGI) bleeding appears to have significantly improved, and this has been attributed to superior diagnostic techniques. The majority of bleeding episodes from both UGI and LGI sources resolve spontaneously. However, patients with severe and persistent bleeding have high mortality rates and may require invasive interventional techniques. Despite the increasing armamentarium of the therapeutic endoscopist and angiographer, it is important to remember that the cornerstone of management for GI hemorrhage remains rapid assessment of the patient and appropriate resuscitation. The patient must be hemodynamically stabilized before diagnosis, therapy, and prevention of rebleeding can begin.

CIRCULATORY ANATOMY

The major arteries supplying the stomach and intestines are the celiac, the superior mesenteric, and the inferior mesenteric arteries (Fig. 9-1). The celiac artery supplies the stomach, the first portion of the duodenum, a portion of the pancreas, and the liver. The short celiac trunk immediately branches into the common hepatic artery and the splenic artery. The superior mesenteric artery supplies the remainder of the pancreas and duodenum, the jejunum, the ileum, and the proximal two thirds of the colon. The inferior mesenteric artery supplies the remainder of the colon and rectum except for the distal rectum, which is supplied by

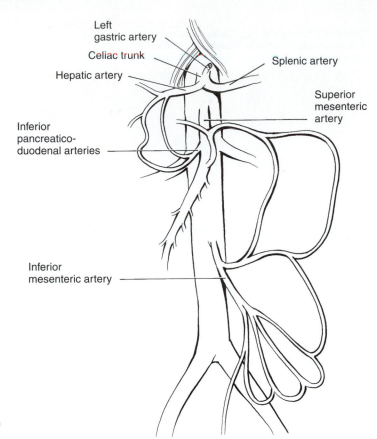

Figure 9-1. The arterial blood flow to the intestines is depicted.

way of rectal arteries arising from the internal iliac arteries. Venous drainage from the stomach, pancreas, and intestines is into the portal vein, except for the distal rectum, which drains into the internal iliac veins. There are multiple arterial and venous arcades along the mesenteric border of the intestine that anastomose together, forming a pathway for collateral flow. These arcades give rise to the vasa recta, which branch to encircle the intestine and ultimately pierce the circular muscle.

MICROCIRCULATION

In the stomach the submucosal arteries break up into capillaries at the base of gastric glands and pass to the luminal surface, where they form a capillary network that drains into mucosal venules in the laminal propria. These venules converge on mucosal collecting venules, which pass to the submucosal venous plexus.

In the small intestine, there is extensive self-anastomosis of both the arteries and veins in the deep submucosal plexus. The capillaries of the muscular, submucosal, and mucosal layers all branch from this plexus. Villous microvascular architecture consists of two arteriole systems (Fig. 9-2). One supplies the villus tip via an eccentrically placed arteriole, which breaks into a fountain-like pattern of capillaries. The second arteriole forms a tuft pattern of capillaries supplying the bottom

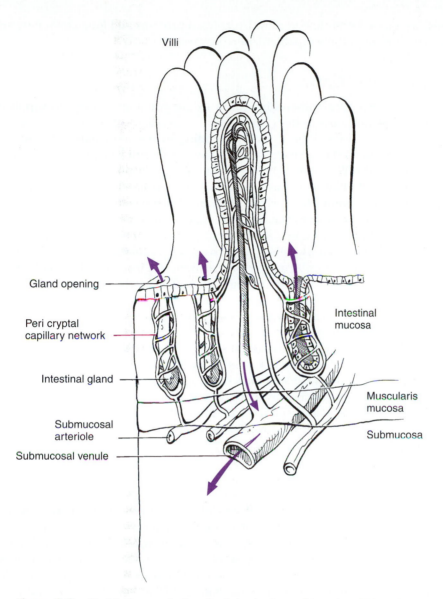

Villi

Gland opening

Peri cryptal
capillary network

Intestinal gland

Submucosal
arteriole

Submucosal venule

Intestinal
mucosa

Muscularis
mucosa

Submucosa

Figure 9-2. Model of mucosal microcirculation in the small intestine. (Adapted from Frasher WG Jr., Wayland H. Repeating modular organization of the microcirculation of cat mesentery. Microvas Res 4:62,1972.)

80% of the villus. Both of these capillary beds return to a venule that starts at about 20% of the villus height below the tip.

In the colon the arterioles and their capillary branches pass to the epithelial surface between they crypts to form a capillary plexus, which drains into venules passing to the submucosa.

Blood flow is normally maintained within narrow limits within the gastrointestinal tract. This autoregulation is maintained by myogenic, metabolic, and hormonal mechanisms to maintain arterial pressure and oxgenation of the tissues. Postprandial hyperemia, or an increase in blood flow after a meal, occurs in response to luminal stimuli, especially hydrolyzed proteins and long-chain fatty acids, and to activation of the sympathetic nervous system.

VISCERAL ISCHEMIA

GI ischemia occurs when blood flow to the gut is insufficient to supply oxygen and other nutrients to the cells. There is a gradient of sensitivity to ischemic injury beginning at the villus tip and extending to the muscularis. Mesenteric ischemia can be limited to characteristic mucosal lesions of subepithelial edema and loss of epithelial cells along the villus tip or can extend to transmural necrosis of the bowel wall. Marked increases in mucosal permeability occur in response to ischemia and reperfusion injury, which allow uptake of luminal toxins.

Reduced blood flow to the intestine may occur during generalized "nonocclusive" ischemia, as is seen in circulatory shock and congestive heart failure, or in occlusive disorders such as emboli, atherosclerosis, and thrombosis that involves the mesenteric circulation. Acute mesenteric ischemia involving the small intestine has an extremely high mortality owing to bowel necrosis and subsequent septic shock. Surgical treatment involves embolectomy when applicable and resection of the involved bowel. Local infusion of vasodilators, such as papaverine via angiographically placed catheters, is also used. Chronic mesenteric ischemia, which predominantly involves the large intestine, is a much more benign disorder that only rarely requires surgical intervention. The most common etiology is "low flow state," as seen in patients with cardiac failure or an episode of hypotension. This causes the clinical syndrome of ischemic colitis, which manifests with diarrhea, mild rectal bleeding, and abdominal discomfort. The mucosal damage that is evident endoscopically and histologically usually heals without sequelae, although it can lead to stricture formation.

ACUTE AND CHRONIC GI BLEEDING

GI bleeding has a multitude of possible etiologies. The pathogenesis of the bleeding episode is caused by one of two primary mechanisms. The first is damaged integrity of mucosa allowing exposure of deep vessels to lumen, i.e., erosion into a vessel from the luminal side. Examples of this include peptic ulcer bleeding, colonic bleeding in idiopathic or infectious inflammatory bowel disease, or bleeding from small bowel or colonic mucosa damaged by ischemia. The second mechanism for GI bleeding is rupture of a vessel into the lumen, which is presumably controlled by vascular pressure and wall tension rather than luminal factors. Examples of this type of bleeding include variceal hemorrhage, diverticular bleeding, and Dieulafoy's lesion (which is an unusually large ectatic gastric submucosal vessel that can rupture into lumen).

The presentation of GI bleeding depends on its acuity and the location of its source. Chronic GI blood loss may manifest with unsuspected iron deficiency anemia or occult blood in stools found on routine screening examinations. More severe cases of chronic or unrecognized GI bleeding may present with symptoms of anemia, such as pallor, dizziness, angina, or dyspnea. Acute GI bleeding usually has a much more obvious presentation. Bleeding from the UGI tract often is evidenced by hematemesis, or bloody vomitus. This may be recent bleeding, causing bright red vomitus, or previous bleeding, resulting in a coffee-ground appearance. Melena consists of black, tarry, loose, or sticky malodorous stools owing to degraded blood in the intestine and generally indicates an UGI source, although it may originate in the right side of the colon. Other causes of black stool, such as iron or bismuth ingestion, should be ruled out. Hematochezia is bright red blood from the rectum. It may be mixed with stool and generally indicates a lower GI lesion. When hematochezia is from an UGI source, it indicates that there is massive hemorrhage.

The first step in assessment of the bleeding patient is to determine the urgency of the situation. Agitation, pallor, hypotension, and tachycardia may indicate shock, requiring immediate volume replacement. Patients with severe blood loss may actually have bradycardia rather than tachycardia as a result of vagal slowing of the heart. Shock occurs when blood loss approaches 40% of blood volume. If there is no evidence of hypotension, orthostatic vital signs will help diagnose lesser degrees of intravascular volume depletion. Postural hypotension of 10 mmHg or more usually indicates at least a 20% reduction in blood volume. In the acutely bleeding patient, intravenous access should be established. If the patient has signs of shock or continued bleeding, a large-bore central intravenous line is useful. Blood samples for assessment of hematocrit, platelets, coagulation factors, and blood typing and cross-matching should be sent to the laboratory immediately. Intravascular volume should be replaced with normal saline until blood products are available, since it is the low perfusion pressure rather than the decreased oxygen-carrying capacity of blood that is primarily responsible for the life-threatening consequences of shock.

The initial hematocrit reading obtained in a patient with acute bleeding poorly reflects the degree of blood loss. Since the hematocrit is expressed in terms of red blood cell volume as a percent of total blood volume, it will not drop until blood volume has been restored. This repletion of blood volume from extravascular fluid begins immediately but takes 24 to 48 hours to equilibrate completely. Therefore in the acutely bleeding patient, close attention to blood pressure, pulse, and gross evidence of ongoing bleeding are better in evaluating blood loss than are laboratory tests. In contrast, the hematocrit accurately reflects the degree of anemia in patients with chronic blood loss, although the severity of iron deficiency, reflected by microcytic indices and low serum iron values, is a better indicator of the chronicity of bleeding.

The specific criteria that define when a patient requires transfusion vary with the age of the patient, the presence of concomitant cardiopulmonary disease, and the presence of continued bleeding. In general, the hematocrit should be maintained above 30% in elderly patients and above 20% in young, healthy patients. With continued evidence of bleeding, the decision to transfuse cannot be based on hematocrit readings alone. Unstable vital signs and gross evidence of active bleeding, e.g., hematemesis, bright red blood per nasogastric aspirate, or hematochezia, are better requisites for making a decision to give a transfusion. The hematocrit is a poor index for following the patient's need for additional transfusions. After acute GI bleeding the plasma volume is often overexpanded by intravenous fluids; thus the immediate posttransfusion hematocrit reading may underestimate the final value.

PORTAL HYPERTENSION

Portal hypertension usually presents as a manifestation of cirrhosis with one of three major symptoms: ascites, GI hemorrhage from either varices or portal gastropathy, or portosystemic encephalopathy. Portal pressure can be summarized by the equation DP = Q × R, i.e., changes in pressure across the portal system are equal to flow times resistance. Therefore, both increased flow and increased resistance can lead to higher pressures. If an increase in one factor on the right of the equation leads to a proportionate decrease in the other factor, pressure will remain constant.

Increased portal blood flow is an uncommon primary cause of portal hypertension. It is the principal pathophysiologic process in rare disorders such as arteriovenous fistulas within the liver, spleen, or splanchnic bed; idiopathic tropical splenomegaly; and the splenomegaly caused by various blood dyscrasias such as agnogenic myeloid metaplasia. Much more commonly, increased portal blood flow is a contributing factor to portal hypertension when the primary problem is increased resistance to flow.

Increased resistance to blood flow in the portal system is the most important cause of portal hypertension. Most of this resistance is determined by the radius of the vessels, since blood viscosity and length of vessels do not change much. Vascular resistance is increased by both physiologic and pathologic mechanisms. The physiologic factors include vascular smooth muscle contraction mediated by vasomotor nerves and hormones, passive contraction related to pressure changes, and contraction related to changes in metabolism. Pathologic changes include extravascular compression (i.e., from regenerating nodules), thrombosis of the vessels, and obstruction of flow due to collagen deposition. These pathologic factors may occur within the liver, within the portal vein or its tributaries (e.g., splenic vein thrombosis leading to partial portal hypertension), or within the vessels receiving hepatic drainage. The location of this increased resistance has led to a classification system for portal hypertension: prehepatic (portal vein thrombosis), intrahepatic, and posthepatic (inferior vena cava web). Intrahepatic portal hypertension can be further divided into presinusoidal (hepatic fibrosis), sinusoidal, and postsinusoidal (veno-occlusive disease) categories. Typical cirrhosis involves more than one of these intrahepatic sites.

Portal pressures can be measured by direct splenic puncture (not commonly done because of risk of bleeding) or by passing a catheter via the femoral vein into the hepatic vein and wedging it into a branch of the small intrahepatic veins. These measurements are generally done only if there is a plan for surgical decompression or for research purposes. Usually the presence of one of the consequences of portal hypertension, such as ascites or a variceal hemorrhage, is sufficient for diagnosis. Once portal hypertension is established and the wedge hepatic pressure is ≥12 mmHg, collateral vessels develop between the portal system and the systemic venous system. These collaterals attempt to divert portal blood flow from the liver and decompress the portal hypertension (Fig. 9-3). This somewhat dissipates elevated portal pressures, although never completely. These collateral vessels develop where branches of the systemic and portal systems exist in proximity, such as the esophageal submucosa where branches of the left gastric vein join branches of the azygos vein, in the rectal mucosa between the inferior and superior hemorrhoidal veins, and on the anterior abdominal wall where the umbilical vein meets the epigastric veins.

In approximately one third of patients with cirrhosis and portal hypertension, these collaterals, or varices, develop in a mucosal location, making them prone to luminal rupture presenting as rapid GI bleeding. Although portal pressure must be >12 mmHg in order for varices to form, the level of pressure elevation does not correlate with the risk of rupture. Indeed, similar portal pressures may exist in patients with no evidence of varices as well as in those with large

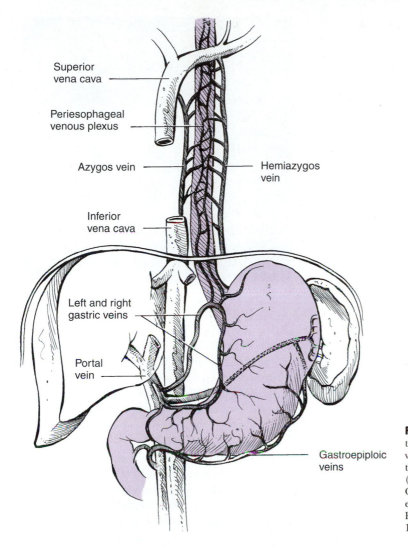

Superior
vena cava

Periesophageal
venous plexus

Azygos vein

Hemiazygos
vein

Inferior
vena cava

Left and right
gastric veins

Portal
vein

Gastroepiploic
veins

Figure 9-3. Schematic representation of the vessels of the portal venous system that are important in the formation of esophageal varices. (Adapted from Yamada T, Alpers DH, Owyang C, Powell DW, Silverstein FE, eds. Atlas of Gastroenterology. Philadelphia: JB Lippincott, 1992:646.)

varices. It appears that once a threshold portal pressure is present that permits varices, other factors control their formation and their risk of rupture. The best predictor of variceal hemorrhage is the size of the varices. Several studies have shown that large varices are more likely to bleed than small ones. Wall tension is a factor of diameter and wall thickness; therefore it is not surprising that larger varices are more likely to rupture. Another endoscopic finding of value in predicting variceal bleeding is the appearance of the vessel wall. Red marks on the varices that may look like whip marks or small red blisters and an overall bluish color of the varices are thought to be risk factors for bleeding (Fig. 9-4).

PRINCIPLES OF TREATMENT OF GI HEMORRHAGE IN PORTAL HYPERTENSION

Variceal bleeding is often the most rapid type of UGI hemorrhage. Therefore the emphasis in acute management is resuscitation. Over 90% of variceal bleeding episodes cause a drop in the hematocrit below 30% and require transfusions. How-

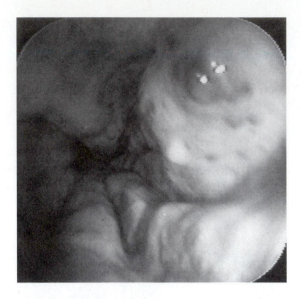

Figure 9-4.   Moderate sized (grades II-III) esophageal varices with multiple red marks.

ever, similar to other etiologies of UGI hemorrhage, 70 to 80% resolve without specific intervention. Urgent endoscopy is indicated in patients with a suspected variceal source because both the treatment of the acute bleeding episode and the prevention of recurrent bleeding differ from patients with bleeding from other UGI causes. One half to two thirds of patients with cirrhosis who present with bleeding have a nonvariceal source, and many of these patients have more than one lesion. This makes early endoscopic examination mandatory to determine the site and cause of bleeding.

Although a multitude of treatments are available for the management of bleeding from esophagogastric varices, all involve two general principles. One is to lower pressure in the variceal collaterals by either treatment with medicines or shunting of portal blood into the systemic circulation. The second is to obliterate the variceal collaterals. Each available treatment has varying utility, depending on whether one is attempting to arrest ongoing hemorrhage, prevent rebleeding, or prevent the first bleeding episode. All the treatments fail to treat the underlying liver disease and therefore have achieved little in improvement of survival. Patients with severe cirrhosis and successful treatment of bleeding tend to go on to die of other problems associated with liver disease, such as renal failure or infection, unless they undergo liver transplantation.

Lowering of portal pressure, thereby lowering pressure in the variceal collaterals, can be achieved by several medications. In the acutely bleeding patient both vasopressin and somatostatin analogue can be administered intravenously in an attempt to stop hemorrhage. Concomitant use of nitrates with vasopressin has been shown to improve efficacy and lower cardiovascular toxicity. Chronic use of propranolol has been clearly shown to be effective for prevention of a first variceal hemorrhage in high-risk patients in whom mortality from the first bleed is high. Propranolol has also been used for the prevention of rebleeding, although it may not be as effective as other available modalities.

Portal pressures can also be lowered by surgically shunting portal blood into the systemic circulation, namely, the inferior vena cava or one of its major tributaries. Although this is one of the most effective means of preventing rebleeding, the morbidity and mortality of the procedures are high in patients with advanced cirrhosis. Large medical centers with skilled angiographers now have a new percutaneous method for establishing a portosystemic shunt via a transjugular intrahepatic portosystemic shunt (TIPS). This essentially achieves the same type of shunt that is produced extrahepatically by surgeons without the morbidity and mortality of major surgery. One drawback of TIPS is its poor long-term patency (30% occlusion at 6 months), requiring periodic repeat angiographic procedures. However, in patients with advanced liver disease who are the worst candidates for major surgery and in whom medical or endoscopic treatment has failed, TIPS has become the procedure of choice. It is often used as a bridge to liver transplantation, the only truly lifesaving treatment available.

The second general method for the cessation or prevention of variceal bleeding is to try to obliterate the varices. The most common form of this treatment is endoscopic variceal sclerotherapy. Via a small needle that passes down the channel of an upper endoscope, a sclerosing substance is injected into or next to the varices, causing subsequent scarring and thrombosis of the vessels. Sclerotherapy is used effectively for both the cessation of ongoing bleeding and for the prevention of rebleeding. The risk of rebleeding remains high until all of the varices are obliterated, which usually takes several endoscopic sessions over a period of weeks to months. Most studies have not shown a benefit for sclerotherapy when used for prophylaxis of the first bleed. A newer alternative endoscopic treatment that appears to have a lower complication rate than sclerotherapy and achieves quicker obliteration of the varices is band ligation, which consists of placing small rubber bands on protuberant varices, causing local necrosis and scarring (Fig. 9-5). Finally, a technique that is used in the acutely bleeding patient when endoscopic therapy has failed or is not available is direct tamponade of the bleeding collaterals by inflation of balloons on a specialized nasogastric tube (Sengstaken-Blakemore tube). One balloon is positioned just below the gastroesophageal junction and the other is directly in the esophagus. One or both balloons can be inflated as needed. This method is usually used as a temporizing device in acute hemorrhage, since rebleeding once the balloon(s) is deflated is common.

LOCATION OF GI BLEEDING

In obvious UGI bleeding that presents with hematemesis, a nasogastric tube should be placed to further assess the rate of ongoing blood loss. When upper GI bleeding is only suspected, as in the patient with melena or with a history of previous epigastric symptoms or disease, a nasogastric tube aspirate demonstrating blood confirms the upper tract as the source. Not infrequently, however, there may be a negative nasogastric aspirate in duodenal bleeding manifesting with melena as a result of a competent pylorus that prevents duodenogastric reflux. Therefore, a negative nasogastric aspirate does not preclude the upper gut as the bleeding source. Melena usually indicates an UGI source (above the ligament of Treitz), although bleeding may be from the small bowel or proximal colon. Melena occurs when hemoglobin is converted to hematin or other hemochromes by bacterial degradation. This can be produced experimentally by ingestion of as little as 100 to 200 ml of blood. If the volume of a LGI hemorrhage is too small to cause hematochezia but large enough to supply enough hemoglobin for degradation, and if colonic motility is sufficiently slow, bleeding from either the small bowel or the proximal colon may cause melena. This is an uncommon occurrence because

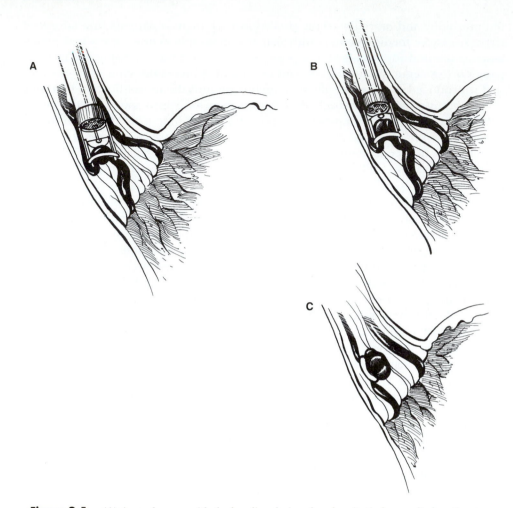

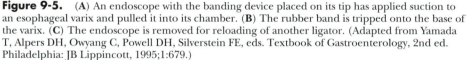

Figure 9-5. (**A**) An endoscope with the banding device placed on its tip has applied suction to an esophageal varix and pulled it into its chamber. (**B**) The rubber band is tripped onto the base of the varix. (**C**) The endoscope is removed for reloading of another ligator. (Adapted from Yamada T, Alpers DH, Owyang C, Powell DH, Silverstein FE, eds. Textbook of Gastroenterology, 2nd ed. Philadelphia: JB Lippincott, 1995;1:679.)

small bowel bleeding is rare and colonic sources either bleed slowly, causing Hemoccult-positive stools, or bleed rapidly enough to cause hematochezia. Another indication of an UGI source of bleeding is a mildly elevated blood urea nitrogen level. Some of this azotemia is caused by absorption of blood, but the experimental ingestion of blood results in elevations in blood urea nitrogen that are lower and of shorter duration that can be explained by absorption alone. This suggests that part of the azotemia is secondary to hypovolemia. Testing for occult blood in nasogastric aspirates is rarely necessary, since the blood is often obvious. The one occasion in which occult blood testing is helpful is when a coffee-ground aspirate appearance may be produced by some foods. In addition, a simple positive test for occult blood may merely indicate nasogastric tube trauma. When occult testing of gastric aspirates is utilized, it is important not to rely on standard stool kits, which may produce falsely negative results in acidic solutions.

Hematochezia usually indicates a LGI source. However, 11% of patients with rapid bleeding from an upper source pass bright red blood per rectum owing to rapid GI transit. Therefore, placement of a nasogastric tube and even performance of an endoscopic examination of the UGI tract should be considered if there is any clinical question of bleeding location in a patient with hematochezia.

PROGNOSTIC INDICATORS FOR UGI BLEEDING

Several factors that indicate a poor prognosis in UGI bleeding have been identified. The most important of these prognostic indicators is the cause of bleeding. Variceal hemorrhages have much higher rebleeding and mortality rates than other diagnoses. Mortality from variceal hemorrhage during the initial hospitalization is at least 30%, with rebleeding rates of 50 to 70%. Improvement in mortality rates from variceal bleeding would lower the overall mortality of UGI bleeding because varices account for approximately 10% of all bleeding episodes.

Endoscopic visualization of stigmata of recent bleeding at examination, such as active arterial spurting, oozing of blood, visible vessel, or fresh or old blood clot, is an important predictor of outcome in peptic ulcer bleeding (Table 9-1). Visible vessels are described endoscopically as elevated, dark red, blue or gray mounds that protrude from the ulcer crater and are resistant to washing. The endoscopic diagnosis of a visible vessel has been validated by pathologic correlation in a group of gastric ulcer patients who required surgical resection, although this "visible vessel" is often actually an organizing clot plugging a side hole in the bleeding artery located just below the ulcer base. The evolution of the endoscopic appearance of a visible vessel, or sentinal clot, has been described as an initial large red clot that becomes darker and smaller with time, eventually replaced by a white plug of fibrin and platelets that finally disappears. The dark small nonoozing sentinal clot and stigmata of older bleeding sites (flat black eschar or white clot) have lower rates of rebleeding. Despite the lack of uniform endoscopic descriptions and varying risks of rebleeding, depending upon the type of visible vessel, the presence of a visible vessel in an ulcer crater at endoscopic examination predicts an increased risk for surgical intervention and increased mortality. Ulcers with visible vessels have up to a 50% incidence of rebleeding compared with no observed rebleeding in patients with no stigmata of recent bleeding. When endoscopic examination is performed within 6 to 24 hours of patient admission, visible vessels are found in 20 to 50% of bleeding ulcers. The identification of predictors of recurrent hemorrhage may di-

TABLE 9-1. *STIGMATA OF HEMORRHAGE AND THE RISK OF REBLEEDING*

STIGMATA	INCIDENCE (%)	REBLEEDING (%)
Spurting arterial bleeding	8	85–100
Nonbleeding visible vessel (v.v.)	17–50	18–55 (mean=43%)
Adherent clot (no v.v.)	18–26	24–41
Older stigmata	12–18	5–9
No stigmata	10–36	0

Modified from Johnston JH. Endoscopic risk factors for bleeding peptic ulcer. Gastrointest Endosc 36:S16, 1990.

rect the need for therapeutic endoscopic techniques that are reported to lower mortality in patients with ulcers with stigmata of recent bleeding. Which stigmata require therapy in bleeding ulcer patients? Over 30 randomized trials have been reported, and although results have been variable, most authorities recommend treatment of actively bleeding visible vessels (either spurting or oozing) and of nonbleeding visible vessels that are raised and cannot be washed off. Adherent clot should be aggressively washed off to assess the possible underlying vessel if there is clinical evidence of major hemorrhage, e.g., hypotension, significant hematemesis, or >2 unit transfusion requirement.

Other important prognostic indicators include

1. The severity of the initial bleed as assessed by transfusion requirement, bright red blood in the nasogastric aspirate, or the presence of hypotension.
2. The age of the patient: elderly patients (>60 years) have been shown to have higher mortality rates than their younger counterparts, although this indicator may not be independent of concomitant disease.
3. The presence of concomitant disease, e.g., chronic renal failure.
4. Onset of bleeding during hospitalization has a mortality rate of 33 to 44% compared with only 7 to 12% in patients who start to bleed prior to admission.
5. Patients with giant ulcers (diameter >2.0 cm) have reported mortality rates as high as 40%.
6. Patients requiring emergency surgery have a surgical mortality rate as high as 30% compared with 10% for those undergoing elective surgery.

UGI BLEEDING EXAMPLE: PEPTIC ULCER DISEASE

Duodenal, gastric, and stomal ulcers account for about 50% of UGI bleeding episodes (Table 9-2). Although several effective therapies have been developed for peptic ulcer disease over the past 15 years, this has had little if any impact on hospitalization rates for bleeding ulcers. Perhaps the reason for this is that ulcers not infrequently bleed without prior history of peptic symptoms. Also there may actually be an increase in UGI bleeding in the elderly as a result of the widespread use of nonsteroidal anti-inflammatory drugs and aspirin. Anatomically, ulcers that are located high on the lesser curve of the stomach or on the posteroinferior wall of the duodenal bulb are more likely to rebleed. Bleeding tends to occur when an ulcer erodes into the lateral wall of a vessel. The vessel often loops up to the floor of the crater and commonly protrudes with an aneurysmal dilatation. An eccentric breach in a vessel is thought to be more likely associated with continued or recurrent bleeding than would occur with a transected vessel because retraction contraction of a severed vessel is an important mechanism of hemostasis. It is the patients with continued or recurrent ulcer bleeding who have increased mortality. Therapy is therefore directed at both cessation of bleeding and prevention of recurrent bleeding.

CESSATION OF PEPTIC ULCER BLEEDING

Gastric lavage with iced saline has been recommended as a method of treatment for UGI bleeding. Traditionally, this is performed through a nasogastric tube that has been placed to diagnose the location of bleeding. Cold solutions have a

TABLE 9-2. *FINAL DIAGNOSES OF CAUSE OF UGI BLEEDING IN 2225 PATIENTS*

DIAGNOSES	% OF TOTAL DIAGNOSES
Duodenal ulcer	24.3
Gastric erosions	23.4
Gastric ulcer	21.3
Varices	10.3
Mallory-Weiss tear	7.2
Esophagitis	6.3
Erosive duodenitis	5.8
Neoplasm	2.9
Stomal ulcer	1.8
Esophageal ulcer	1.7
Miscellaneous	6.8

Modified from Silverstein FE, Gilbert DA, Tedesco FA. The national ASGE survey on upper gastrointestinal bleeding. Gastointest Endosc 1981; 27:73, 1981.

theoretical advantage of slowing blood flow. However, it can also be argued that ice water may impair coagulation factors, and certainly it increases patient discomfort. Controlled trials have not shown any therapeutic benefit from cold lavage solutions. Therefore, one should simply lavage with room temperature tapwater for the important task of monitoring the rapidity of bleeding.

Multiple trials using various pharmacologic agents have failed to demonstrate any improvement in survival in patients with UGI bleeding. There have been over 25 randomized controlled studies using histamine H_2 antagonists in the management of UGI hemorrhage. An analysis of pooled results in over 2500 patients suggests that treatment may reduce rates of surgery and death by 20 and 30%, respectively, although these reductions were only marginally significant. Practically, since even a moderate reduction in mortality is still desirable and since H_2 blockers are without significant toxicity, these agents are commonly administered to patients with ulcer bleeding despite the lack of proven efficacy. Although it has been suggested that more potent acid suppression, with continuous intravenous H_2 antagonists or with high doses of omeprazole, may be more effective than standard doses of H_2 antagonists, two large trials failed to demonstrate this.

As a result of the failure of medical therapy, the emphasis in treating persistent ulcer hemorrhage is on endoscopic therapy or surgical intervention. Emergency surgery has an increased mortality rate; therefore, endoscopic methods are usually attempted prior to surgery. Endoscopic methods can be divided into two types, thermal and nonthermal. Nonthermal methods include injection of sclerosing agents such as alcohol or ethanolamine, injection of vasoconstrictors such as epinephrine, or simple injection of normal saline into the bleeding site. Comparisons between thermal and injection therapies suggest that they are equally effective. Thermal methods include the neodymium-yttrium aluminum garnet (Nd-YAG) laser, the heater probe, and electrocoagulation. The multipolar electrocoagulation probe (bicap) uses direct probe pressure to tamponade the bleeding vessel followed by raising the tissue temperature to coagulate and seal the vessel. A similar technique that uses pure thermal energy is the heater probe, which has also been shown to be efficacious in the treatment of bleeding ulcers and nonbleeding visible vessels. The major advantage of these two devices is that they are portable and relatively simple to use. The Nd-YAG laser is as effective as the heater probe and bicap; however, its immobility, requirement for trained support personnel, and the marked equipment expense reduce its attractiveness. If hemorrhage is not stopped or if it recurs, surgery should be considered early because mortality increases as the patient becomes more unstable. Peptic ulcer bleeding is effectively treated with surgery, and this is safer than other therapeutic alternatives such as angiographic embolization of the bleeding vessel, which is reserved for the patient who is too unstable to undergo surgery.

PREVENTION OF REBLEEDING FROM PEPTIC ULCER DISEASE

As is the case for cessation of bleeding, acid-reducing pharmacologic therapy remains of uncertain benefit in preventing ulcer rebleeding. The rationale is to prevent clot dissolution and allow healing of the underlying lesion. *In vitro* data show that coagulation and platelet function are better at a neutral pH. Although clot is not dissolved by acid alone, it is by gastric juice, suggesting that pepsin degradation may be important. Because the activity of pepsin is pH-dependent, it is reasonable to assume that the clot will not dissolve if gastric juice pH is high. The clinical importance of this *in vitro* data is unclear; there appears to be only slight, if any, reduction in rebleeding rates from gastric and duodenal ulcers with acid-reducing therapy. Either clot dissolution is not important in rebleeding or insufficient acid reduction is achieved with standard therapy. However, even the potent hydrogen-potassium adenosine triphosphatase inhibitor omeprazole and continuous intravenous H_2 antagonists, which are both capable of raising gastric pH to near neutral levels, have not been proved effective for prevention of rebleeding. Despite the lack of proven efficacy, acid suppression therapy is commonly used for prevention of recurrent bleeding because of its potential to benefit and its lack of toxicity.

The prevention of rebleeding by therapeutic endoscopic methods in high-risk ulcers with stigmata of bleeding is now widely accepted. However, some issues remain. First, the lack of standardized definitions of the various stigmata of recent hemorrhage and sufficient knowledge of each of their natural histories continue to be a problem. Second, therapeutic endoscopy adds to the risk of the endoscopic procedure, with the risk of precipitating bleeding being as high as 20% and with perforation occurring in up to 1%. Third, therapeutic endoscopy adds to the cost of treatment unless it successfully decreases the need for surgery or shortens the hospital stay, and therefore it must be applied judiciously.

GI BLEEDING EXAMPLE: DIVERTICULAR HEMORRHAGE

The two major causes of acute LGI bleeding are diverticulosis and angiodysplasia (Table 9-3). As is the case with UGI bleeding, 80% of bleeding episodes resolve spontaneously. In the patients in whom bleeding ceases, ~25% have recurrent bleeding. In contrast to UGI bleeding, most LGI bleeding is slow and intermittent and does not require hospitalization. The most common causes of chronic LGI bleeding are hemorrhoids and colonic neoplasia.

TABLE 9-3.	*FINAL DIAGNOSES OF MAJOR LGI BLEEDING*

DIAGNOSIS	% OF TOTAL DIAGNOSIS
Diverticulosis	43
Angiodysplasia	20
Undetermined	12
Neoplasia	9
Colitis:	
Radiation	6
Ischemic	2
Ulcerative	1
Other	7

Modified from Boley SJ, DiBiase A, Branett LJ, Sammantano RJ. Lower intestinal bleeding in the elderly. Am J Surg 137:57, 1979.

Diverticular bleeding occurs in only ~3% of patients with diverticulosis. However, it is the most common cause of major LGI hemorrhage because of the high prevalence of diverticulosis in the Western world. Prior to widespread availability of colonoscopy and angiography, the true incidence of diverticular bleeding was overestimated because this diagnosis is so frequently made by barium enema. Later angiographic studies have demonstrated that, despite the left-sided preponderance of diverticula, 70% of bleeding diverticula occur in the right side of the colon. Some of the decreased mortality from LGI hemorrhage that is reported in the last several decades is likely the result of better localization of the bleeding source, allowing directed surgical therapy and lower postsurgical rebleeding rates.

Diverticula are usually located in the colonic wall at the site of penetration of nutrient vessels. Bleeding presumably results from a colonic artery that penetrates into the dome of the diverticulum. The artery ruptures into the diverticular sac and causes copious bleeding. Clinical evidence of associated diverticulitis or inflammation is usually not present, so that vessel rupture is thought to be due to pressure erosion.

Diverticular bleeding manifests with acute painless maroon to bright red hematochezia, although melenic stools may occur. The degree of blood loss is often significant and may not be well tolerated in the elderly population at risk. Diverticulosis is not thought to be a cause of occult heme-positive stool or slow bleeding. If the initial bout of diverticular bleeding ceases spontaneously, no further therapy is indicated, since bleeding will not recur in the majority of patients. In the 80% of patients in whom bleeding ceases, 75% do not have a recurrence and 25% have repeated episodes of diverticular hemorrhage.

In the 20% of patients with persistent hemorrhage from diverticulosis, angiography is useful for both diagnosis and treatment. Selective catheterization with administration of intra-arterial vasopressin successfully controls the bleeding in the majority of patients. Any patient in whom angiographic control of diverticular bleeding is not successful should have urgent surgery to remove the portion of the colon bearing the bleeding site. In the event of failure to localize the bleeding site, emergency subtotal colectomy has been advocated. Patients with recurrent diverticular bleeding should have elective surgery if their general medical condition and anticipated lifespan warrant such aggressive therapy.

CHRONIC GI BLEEDING EXAMPLE: VASCULAR ECTASIA

Vascular ectasias, or angiodysplasias, are common causes of both major LGI hemorrhage and slow, intermittent blood loss. The majority of these are degenerative lesions associated with aging, in contrast to the congenital vascular lesions that occur throughout the GI tract in various age groups. Two thirds of patients with colonic angiodysplasia are over 70 years of age. Angiodysplastic lesions are usually multiple, less than 5 mm in diameter, and involve primarily the cecum and right side of the colon (Fig. 9-6). There appears to be some clinical association with aortic valve stenosis. The diagnosis of vascular ectasias can be made via either colonoscopy or angiography. Both diagnostic modalities frequently identify the lesions without demonstrating active bleeding. Despite this drawback, if no other source of GI bleeding is identified, the presence of angiodysplasia in a patient with recurrent or persistent GI bleeding is an indication for treatment.

The pathogenesis of angiodysplasias is unknown, but one theory is that repeated, partial intermittent obstruction of the submucosal veins where they pierce the muscle layers of the colon leads to dilatation and tortuosity of the veins. Eventually, the entire arteriole-capillary-venular unit dilates, creating a small arteriovenous communication. The predilection of these degenerative lesions for the right side of the colon may be caused by the greater tension in the cecal wall compared with wall tension in the rest of the colon.

There are always a few unfortunate patients with chronic bleeding or recurrent acute bleeding who elude diagnosis despite upper and lower GI x-ray films, endoscopic examination, and angiography. It has been estimated that as many as 5% of patients do not have an identifiable source of bleeding despite extensive examination. The etiology of GI bleeding in the majority of patients with bleeding

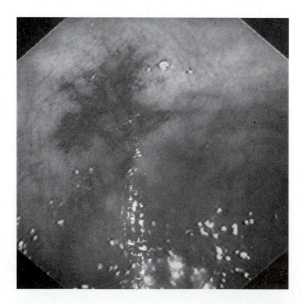

Figure 9-6. A typical angiodysplastic lesion in the colon.

from obscure origin is thought to be vascular ectasias. Unfortunately, many of these lesions are too small to be detected by angiography and can be missed or not reached by endoscopy.

Endoscopic thermal ablation of angiodysplasia is recommended when the lesions are accessible. If this is unsuccessful or not feasible because of multiple lesions, surgical resection of the involved segments may be necessary. When these vascular ectasias are associated with chronic renal failure and its attendant prolonged bleeding time as a result of platelet dysfunction, estrogen-progesterone therapy has been reported to be beneficial. Similar efficacy has been reported in patients with normal renal function and chronic GI blood loss from vascular ectasias, suggesting that the abnormal platelet function present in renal failure may not be a prerequisite for estrogen-progesterone treatment. A therapeutic trial of estrogen-progesterone therapy for the possible underlying diagnosis of vascular ectasias may be worthwhile even in some patients without a definite diagnosis. Unfortunately, there are a few patients with bleeding from an unknown source that eludes diagnosis or who are too ill for surgery. They are relegated to receive blood transfusions as needed.

DIAGNOSTIC EVALUATION OF GI BLEEDING

ENDOSCOPY

Barium contrast studies have been replaced by endoscopic study for diagnosis of UGI bleeding. The greater accuracy and therapeutic potential of endoscopy generally make it the diagnostic procedure of choice. Diagnostic endoscopy is viewed as a safe and simple procedure by both patient and physician, although morbidity rates of 1.0% and mortality rates of 0.1% have been reported. Endoscopy is contraindicated in uncooperative patients or in patients with a suspected perforated viscus. Endoscopy can locate precisely the site of bleeding when there is continued bleeding or when stigmata of bleeding persist. In patients with massive hemorrhage, the source of bleeding occasionally cannot be discerned by endoscopy. In patients whose bleeding has stopped and no stigmata of bleeding remain, a significant lesion seen on endoscopic examination, e.g., a clean ulcer base, is the presumed source. If either more than one lesion or no lesions are identified, no definitive diagnosis can be made, and these patients need to be restudied if the bleed recurs.

The timing of the diagnostic endoscopic examination depends on the severity and suspected cause of the hemorrhage. Patients who fail to stop bleeding with simple supportive care require urgent endoscopy to guide further therapeutic techniques. Also, patients with underlying cirrhosis should have endoscopic study as close to the bleeding episode as possible because they often have more than one source of potential hemorrhage, and the diagnosis of bleeding varices will alter future approaches to treatment. For the majority of patients whose bleeding ceases, diagnostic endoscopy can be postponed for 24 hours without seriously altering diagnostic accuracy or clinical outcome. When both the patient and physician are comfortable without a specific diagnosis in an uncomplicated patient, an empirical trial of treatment may be indicated. Barium x-ray studies may be used in this situation to rule out more serious or unexpected lesions, thereby avoiding the endoscopic examination altogether.

Colonoscopy has generally replaced barium enema for diagnostic evaluation of LGI bleeding. Several series have demonstrated the superior diagnostic sensitivity of colonoscopy, even when compared with double-contrast barium enema. In patients with LGI bleeding and normal barium enema results, 10 to 20% have abnormal findings at colonoscopy. When LGI bleeding is the clinical indication for colonoscopy, the diagnostic yield is very high (40 to 50%). In addition, if barium enema findings are abnormal, a colonoscopy is usually still indicated for biopsy or therapeutic maneuvers. Therefore, when the indication for diagnostic study is GI bleeding, a colonoscopic examination is usually called for regardless of the barium enema study results. For these reasons, most clinicians favor colonoscopy as the primary examination. In the occasional patient in whom full colonoscopy is not technically feasible or when the colonoscopy is nondiagnostic, a barium enema study is helpful.

Patients with rapid ongoing blood loss require either diagnostic angiography or urgent colonoscopy after purge. Although the traditional view is that colonoscopy in patients with severe hematochezia is impractical because of inadequate visualization, colonoscopy is used in some situations (e.g., bleeding from a prior polypectomy site that can be treated with electrocautery) after prior rapid cleansing. One advantage of angiography in the patient with ongoing bleeding is the potential for treatment in diverticular hemorrhage, the most common cause of major LGI bleeding.

RADIONUCLIDE SCANS

Localization of the site of GI bleeding can be accomplished by scanning for extravasation of intravascular radiolabeled blood. Technetium-99 sulfur colloid scans are obtained shortly after injection and demonstrate a localized collection of tracer at the site of bleeding. Technetium-99 pertechnetate-labeled red cells are technically more difficult to use, since they require removal and labeling of the patient's own red blood cells. However, they have the advantage of allowing repeated scans over 24 to 36 hours after injection to detect intermittent bleeding. These techniques can reveal bleeding when the rate of blood loss is as low as 0.5 ml/min, and they have no associated morbidity. The major disadvantage to radionuclide scans is that they merely localize the bleeding to an area of the abdomen but do not diagnose the specific location or the responsible lesion. For this reason, radionuclide studies are often used to screen patients to determine which ones have sufficient ongoing bleeding to warrant angiography, although their value as an angiography screen has recently been questioned. In addition, they may allow more selective angiographic studies, thereby decreasing the dye load to the patient. Radionuclide scans are more commonly used in the diagnosis of LGI bleeding than in the diagnosis of UGI bleeding. The accuracy and therapeutic alternatives of upper endoscopy make endoscopy the diagnostic method of choice in UGI bleeding, even in the rapidly bleeding patient. In the rare situation when massive hemorrhage makes endoscopy impossible, angiography should be obtained immediately and not delayed by prior radionuclide scans.

ANGIOGRAPHY

Angiography is used as a diagnostic examination in acute UGI bleeding only when endoscopy has failed. In LGI bleeding that is rapid and continuing, it is often the diagnostic examination of first choice. The bleeding must be arterial and at a rate of at least 0.5 to 0.6 ml/min to detect extravasation. Angiography represents a therapeutic alternative for delivery of intra-arterial vasopressin in stress gastritis or for embolization of bleeding ulcers or neoplasms in inoperable patients with UGI bleeding. In LGI bleeding intra-arterial vasopressin is effective in controlling 90% of hemorrhages from both diverticula and angiodysplasia. In addition, angiography may be utilized to diagnose difficult cases of recurrent GI bleeding from an unknown source. Angiographic demonstration of vascular ectasias may suggest the source of bleeding, although in patients who are not actively bleeding, the diagnosis is uncertain since these are common lesions. Angiography provides an accurate diagnosis in 50 to 75% of patients but is associated with a serious complication rate of about 2%. Complications from angiography are related either to catheter placement (dissection, thrombosis, false aneurysm) or to the contrast material (allergic reactions, renal failure). When embolic occlusion of vessels with Gelfoam or autologous clot is utilized, the complication rate increases because of the risks of ischemic necrosis and perforation.

CASE PRESENTATION

A 52-year-old man came to the emergency room with a 4-hour history of hematemesis. He was in his usual state of good health until he suddenly became nauseated while at work and proceeded to vomit a large quantity of bright red blood. He subsequently vomited blood two more times, and after arrival in the emergency room he passed a black tarry bowel movement. He also complained of lightheadedness but denied abdominal pain. He did not have a history of ulcers but admitted to rare use of antacids for heartburn in the past. He did not require any antacids in the past few weeks. He takes occasional aspirin for headaches but estimates that he has only taken two to four in the past couple of months and no other nonsteroidal anti-inflammatory drugs. He gave a history of alcoholism, during which time he drank a fifth of liquor daily for over 5 years, but he has been completely free of all alcohol for 3 years. He has smoked one pack of cigarettes per day for over 30 years. His past medical history is significant for a prior appendectomy and hemorrhoidectomy. He denies any other hospitalizations, although recalls having abdominal pain while drinking heavily, which he blamed on the "booze."

On physical examination he appeared to be pale and mildly agitated. His temperature was 37.7°C, pulse was 125 beats per minute, and respirations were 22 breaths per minute. His blood pressure in the supine position was 100/70 mmHg and dropped to 65 systolic while sitting. Examination of the skin revealed no spider angiomata or palmar erythema. The head and neck examination was normal. His lungs were clear on auscultation, and cardiac examination revealed tachycardia with a grade II/VI systolic murmur at the left sternal border. An abdominal examination revealed no organomegaly, masses, or tenderness. A rectal examination showed liquid black to maroon stool in the vault. The extremities showed no peripheral edema, and the neurologic exam was normal.

A nasogastric tube was placed, and bright red blood was suctioned from the patient's stomach. Two large-bore peripheral intravenous lines were started, and normal saline was infused as quickly as possible. Blood was sent to the blood bank for type and cross-matching. Initial laboratory results revealed a hematocrit of 30%, platelets of 66,000/mm^3, and a normal partial thromboplastin time and prothrombin time. The electrolytes were normal and the blood urea nitrogen concentration was 30 mg/dl with a creatinine level of 0.9 mg/dl. The serum transaminases, alkaline phosphatase, albumin, and total bilirubin values were normal. Despite the patient's initial fluid resuscitation, his blood pressure dropped to 80 mmHg systolic in the supine position, and a central line was placed for further fluid resuscitation. Bright red blood continued to be aspirated from the nasogastric tube. Packed red cells and platelets were ordered from the blood bank, and an intensive care unit bed was obtained for the patient. A diagnostic procedure was performed.

DIFFERENTIAL DIAGNOSIS

This patient had a marked orthostatic blood pressure drop that evolved into shock in the emergency room from an UGI hemorrhage that began only 4 hours prior to presentation. This type of rapid hemorrhage requires aggressive resuscitation. Blood and platelets need to be transfused as quickly as possible, with interim replacement of the blood volume with normal saline. A rapid hemorrhage such as this can be seen with variceal hemorrhage, although there is no history of liver disease and no physical findings of cirrhosis. In addition, the synthetic function of the liver is preserved with a normal prothrombin time and albumin levels. Ulcer disease can bleed this rapidly, although there is no significant history of dyspepsia and no prior nonsteroidal anti-inflammatory drug use. However, since 20% of bleeding peptic ulcers are asymptomatic and the patient was male and a smoker (both risks for peptic ulcer disease), a bleeding ulcer remains in the differential diagnosis. Other uncommon possible diagnoses include Dieulafoy's lesion, which is bleeding from a large mucosal arteriole in the proximal stomach, bleeding esophageal ulcers as hinted at by his history of occasional heartburn, or a Mallory-Weiss tear, a mucosal tear in the gastroesophageal mucosa most often caused by prior emesis although occasionally presenting on the first episode of emesis.

None of these diagnoses would explain the patient's low platelet count of 66,000/mm^3. Since the low count was obtained at the outset of his emergency room visit, it cannot be blamed on dilution. That leads to a consideration of isolated gastric varices, which often bleed massively and are caused by isolated portal hypertension and hypersplenism. This can occur when there is thrombosis of the splenic vein leading to splenic enlargement and gastric varices. The most common cause of splenic vein thrombosis is chronic pancreatitis, which causes contiguous inflammation and therefore thrombosis of the splenic vein as it courses along the upper posterior aspect of the pancreas. By far the most common cause of chronic pancreatitis is alcohol abuse. Although many patients with chronic alcoholic pancreatitis would have presented earlier with attacks of pancreatitis or abdominal pain, some come forward later, probably because they never sought medical care for symptoms of pain during alcohol binges.

The procedure performed was an upper endoscopic examination. The esophageal mucosa appeared normal to the gastroesophageal junction. A

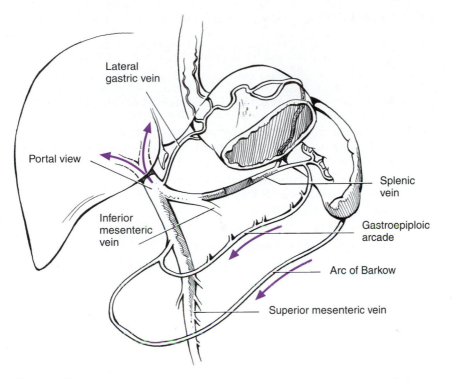

Figure 9-7. Diagram showing venous collateral pathways after splenic vein occlusion through the left gastric vein (LGV), gastroepiploic vein, an omental (arc of Barkow) vein. (Adapted from Yamada T, Alpers DH, Owyang C, Powell DW, Silverstein FE, eds. Atlas of Gastroenterology. Philadelphia: JB Lippincott, 1992:550.)

large amount of blood appeared to be pooling just below the gastroesophageal junction. The antrum and duodenum were blood-coated but appeared normal after washing. Upon retroflexion of the endoscope, blood could be seen to exit from a varix high in the fundus. Endoscopic band ligation was performed with successful cessation of hemorrhage. Several other varices were noted in the fundus but were not treated. A plain film of the abdomen was obtained on the following day, and diffuse small calcifications were seen in the area of the pancreas consistent with chronic pancreatitis. The patient was scheduled for a diagnostic mesenteric arteriogram and the general surgeons were consulted. The angiogram confirmed the presence of splenic vein thrombosis and isolated portal hypertension (Fig. 9-7). The patient was scheduled for splenectomy to decompress his gastric varices. His prognosis was quite good because his varices could be treated with relatively simple surgery and he had no evidence of liver disease.

SUMMARY

GI bleeding is a common clinical problem. Assessment of the severity of bleeding and resuscitation of the patient are the initial and most important parts of the medical intervention. Subsequently, diagnosis of the bleeding source will direct specific therapies, whether they are medical, endoscopic, angiographic, or surgical.

SELECTED READING

Allison MC, Howatson AG, Torrance CJ, et al. Gastrointestinal damage associated with the use of nonsteroidal anti-inflammatory drugs. N Engl J Med 327:749, 1992.

Cappell MS, Gupta A. Changing epidemiology of gastrointestinal angiodysplasia with increasing recognition of clinically milder cases. Angiodysplasia tends to produce mild chronic gastrointestinal bleeding in a study of 47 consecutive patients admitted from 1980–1989. Am J Gastroenterol 87:201, 1992.

Cello JP, Grendell JH, Crass RA, et al. Endoscopic sclerotherapy versus portacaval shunt in patients with severe cirrhosis and variceal hemorrhage. N Engl J Med 311:1589, 1984.

Collins R, Langman M. Treatment with histamine H_2 antagonists in acute upper gastrointestinal hemorrhage. N Engl J Med 131:660, 1985.

Cook DJ, Guyatt GH, Salena BJ, et al. Endoscopic therapy for acute nonvariceal upper gastrointestinal hemorrhage: A meta-analysis. Gastroenterology 102:139, 1992.

Graham DY, Smith JL. Aspirin and the stomach. Ann Int Med 104:390, 1986.

Hayes PC, Davis JM, Lewis JA, et al. Meta-analysis of value of propranolol in prevention of variceal hemorrhage. Lancet 336:153, 1990.

Silverstein FE, Gilbert DA, Tedesco FJ, et al. The national ASGE survey on upper gastrointestinal bleeding. II Clinical prognostic factors. Gastrointest Endosc 27:80, 1981.

Stiegmann GV, Goff JS, Michaletz-Onody PA, et al. Endoscopic sclerotherapy as compared with endoscopic ligation for bleeding esophageal varices. N Engl J Med 316:1527, 1992.

Swain CP, Storey DW, Bown SG. Nature of the bleeding vessel in recurrently bleeding gastric ulcers. Gastroenterology 90:595, 1986.

Van Cutsen E, Rutgeerts P, Vantrappen G. Treatment of bleeding gastrointestinal vascular malformations with oestrogen-progesterone. Lancet 335:953, 1990.

Vigneri S, Termini R, Piraino A, et al. The stomach in liver cirrhosis. Endoscopic, morphological, and clinical correlations. Gastroenterology 101:472, 1991.

Lippincott's Pathophysiology Series: Gastrointestinal Pathophysiology, edited by Joseph M. Henderson. Lippincott–Raven Publishers. Philadelphia © 1996.

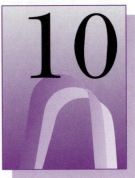
Neoplasia of the Gastrointestinal Tract

James M. Scheiman and C. Richard Boland

The gastrointestinal (GI) tract, including the hollow organs of the gut, pancreas, liver, and biliary tree, is the site of more cancers and cancer mortality than any other organ system in the body. However, there is no simple etiologic explanation to unify all gut tumors. Moreover, the most notable feature of international cancer epidemiology is the wide variability of tumor incidence from country to country by organ site. In the United States, three- to four-fold differences in incidence of esophageal cancer may be found simply based upon sex and race. In Japan, the incidence of gastric carcinoma is approximately 10 times higher than it is in the United States. Conversely, colorectal cancer occurs less commonly in Japan but is the most frequently occurring GI malignancy in North America, Western Europe, and much of the industrialized world. These marked differences in cancer risk are not based upon racial or genetic factors. When people migrate from a high incidence region to a low incidence region, the organ-specific rates of some cancers change to match those of the new region, usually within two generations. Collectively, the epidemiologic observations strongly indicate the importance of environmental factors in GI carcinogenesis.

Since our understanding of carcinogenesis in the gut is far from complete, it is necessary to consider the process of neoplastic progression in a general way and place the details into the scheme organ by organ. This chapter begins with a review of the broad issues involved in epithelial differentiation, proliferation, and tumor development and ends with details relevant to specific GI organs. The reading list emphasizes review articles to assist the reader interested in more reading in individual areas.

EPITHELIAL PROLIFERATION/DIFFERENTIATION

The esophagus is lined with squamous epithelium, unlike the remainder of the GI tract. Proliferation occurs in the basal layer, and daughter cells migrate to the surface where they flatten and differentiate and form an impermeable barrier. Most esophageal neoplasms are squamous cell carcinomas derived from the basal layers; adenocarcinomas arise from foci of metaplastic epithelium related to chronic injury from acid reflux. Gastric epithelium is more complex, made up of glands with specialized cell types, including mucus, parietal, chief, and endocrine cells. Cell turnover is dependent upon the region of the stomach, and the undifferentiated proliferating cells are found in the midportion of the gland. The specific cellular source of adenocarcinomas of the stomach is not known. The colonic epithelium is composed of glands containing absorptive cells and mucin-secreting goblet cells. The proliferative region is confined to the lower two thirds of the crypt, and daughter cells migrate toward the lumen.

Cancer is classically considered a disease of unregulated growth. Neoplastic cells give rise to cells that fail to differentiate properly, and a progressively larger proportion retain the capacity to proliferate. Cancer is thus a situation of accumulation of excessive numbers of incompletely differentiated cells that continue to proliferate.

An enhanced rate of cell turnover is characteristic of premalignant tissues; however, the signal for cellular proliferation in the gut is not known. Cell proliferation is regulated by peptide hormones such as gastrin, local growth factors such as epidermal growth factor (EGF) and transforming growth factor-alpha (TGFα), and by prostaglandins. Most hyperproliferative states in the GI tract are associated with cancer and also with chronic inflammation. In this chapter we discuss chronic atrophic gastritis and gastric carcinogenesis, epithelial metaplasia (Barret's esophagus) and adenocarcinoma of the esophagus, and inflammatory bowel disease and colorectal cancer.

CARCINOGENESIS

Our current concept of carcinogenesis in the GI tract begins with damage to normal cellular genes. This can occur through a variety of mechanisms. Mutations occur spontaneoulsy because of instability of the nucleotide bases themselves. The most common spontaneous mutation is depurination. Another spontaneous event, deamination, converts cytosine to uracil or 5-methylcytosine to thymine, which if not repaired leads to mispairing during the next round of replication. Both events are common and subject to revision by families of DNA repair enzymes. If they are not excised and corrected, single-base mutations may change the genetic code.

Several classes of environmental agents predictably damage DNA, including radiation injury, viral oncogenes, and chemical carcinogens. Chemical carcinogenesis is thought to be the most important exogenous mechanism involved in initiating adenocarcinoma of the GI tract because of its access, by ingestion, to the gut mucosa. This form of injury tends to produce single base mutations. Chemical carcinogens are ubiquitous in the human diet but may not reach all of the digestive organ mucosae in their active forms. The microbial flora of the GI tract and mucosal enzymes are important factors in the activation—and inactivation—of many carcinogens. For example, nitrosamines are produced from ingested dietary nitrites, which are then modified by the luminal flora, and are thought to be important in carcinogenesis in the esophagus and stomach.

Although cancer is best characterized as an acquired disease produced by environmental exposures, there are large individual differences in cancer susceptibility. The best known example of chemical carcinogenesis in humans is found in the relationship between tobacco use and lung cancer. But it is important to recognize that not all smokers are equally liable to develop cancer, even taking into account differences in numbers of cigarettes smoked. The enzyme cytochrome P450 IIE1 is responsible for the activation of many carcinogens (including those in tobacco smoke) and is expressed heterogeneously throughout the population. It is reasonable, therefore, to expect that individual differences exist in the ability to activate procarcinogens or inactivate proximate carcinogens and that these differences are important factors for cancer risk.

MECHANISMS BY WHICH GENES ARE DAMAGED

Single nucleotide base pair mutations may be characterized as "transitions" when they change one purine to another (or one pyrimidine to another), or "transversions" when they produce a change between classes. Losses or gains of one or more base pairs are called "deletions" or "insertions," respectively. Some single base pair changes are silent since they do not alter the amino acid code. Mutations that change the amino acid transcribed are termed "missense," and may be characterized as conservative if the amino acid change occurs within the same class (i.e., from one neutral amino acid to another, since it might not be expected to have a major impact on protein folding or charge) or as more serious if the change results in the appearance or removal of charge, cysteine residues, or other amino acids critical to the function of the protein. Changes that create a stop codon within an open reading frame are called "nonsense" mutations. Insertions and deletions that do not occur in groups of three create a "frameshift," which commonly produces a series of missense and nonsense changes downstream on the DNA strand.

Point Mutation. Chronic inflammation is a common setting in which cancer develops in the gut, such as in chronic esophagitis, chronic atrophic gastritis, and inflammatory bowel disease. Active forms of oxygen such as hydroxyl and superoxide radicals, hydrogen peroxide, and singlet oxygen arise as byproducts of chronic inflammation and oxygen stress. In fact, these reactive species also mediate damage induced by ionizing and some ultraviolet radiation. Reactive oxygen species create several forms of DNA damage, including strand breaks and single-base changes. Any genetic locus may be more or less likely to experience a specific mutation depending upon the mutagen involved. Some mutations are silent, but the appearance of others (by chance) can result in a growth advantage for the cell.

DNA Rearrangement. Gene expression may be modified by gross rearrangement of DNA sequences. For example, in chronic myelogeneous leukemia, a translocation occurs whereby sequences from chromosome 22 are accidentally spliced in frame with the cellular oncogene *ABL*. This translocation creates a chimeric messenger RNA, which translates into an abnormally large mutant *ABL* protein. At this time, it is not clear if this mechanism of gene disregulation is involved in the genesis of gastrointestinal cancers.

DNA Amplification. A normal cellular gene may become a transforming gene through DNA amplification. This mechanism has attracted attention because resistance to methotrexate, a chemotherapeutic drug, may be caused by amplification of the gene for dihydrofolate reductase. Amplification of the multidrug resistance gene (*MDR*) is common in gut neoplasms and confers resistance on many chemotherapeutic agents. Amplification of the oncogenes *ERBB2*, *MYC*, and *SRC* has been reported in certain GI cancers.

Altered Methylation of DNA. One mechanism to control gene expression is to silence genes through the stable, covalent methylation of the nucleotide base cytosine. DNA methylation is maintained by a specific methyltransferase, and the pattern of methylation is inherited in a stable way through successive generations of cells in a given tissue. A wide variety of genes are substantially hypomethylated in primary colorectal cancers when compared with the adjacent normal mucosa. Furthermore, hypomethylation was found in even the smallest polyps studied. The changes in methylation involved certain cellular oncogenes, raising the possibility that this may be one mechanism by which they are activated. Hypomethylation is seen in gastric and esophageal cancers as well as in tumors of the colon. Thus, perturbations in DNA methylation appear to be a general property of human cancers. Hypermethylation has been reported for other genetic loci in cancer, and in these instances it is thought that tumor suppressor genes may become inappropriately silenced (see below).

Gene Deletion. Cell proliferation is regulated by a family of genes known as tumor suppressor genes (TSGs). The function of these genes is to prevent inappropriate cell proliferation and to regulate the number of cells in a tissue. Unlike cellular oncogenes, these genes play a role in GI carcinogenesis through their inactivation or deletion from the nucleus. TSGs are discussed in detail in the following section.

CURRENT CONCEPTS OF TUMOR DEVELOPMENT

Oncogenes. It is clear that no single mutation or altered gene is sufficient to cause cancer in most cells. A number of oncogene mutations, genetic deletions, and chromosomal rearrangements have been found in cancers that have been studied carefully. However, the story began to unfold when single genes were found that, when "activated," could change the phenotype to become recognizably malignant. These initial cancer-causing genes were called "oncogenes" and were first discovered by studying oncogenic viruses that could transform chicken cells. The discovery of oncogenes then led to the astounding discovery that they were derived from normal cellular copies of the genes, or "proto-oncogenes." A growing number of these genes have been identified (over 20), and each is activated either by a point mutation that alters the activity of the gene product or a genetic rearrangement that results in an increase in gene expression (Table 10-1).

Several of the proto-oncogenes are involved in signal transduction between the plasma membrane and the nucleus. For example, some oncogenes are growth factors, and when production is not regulated, unremitting stimulation occurs. Similarly, other proto-oncogenes are growth factor receptors. The most intensively studied proto-oncogenes have been those such as *RAS* and related genes involved in signal transduction between the cell membrane receptor and the nucleus. These genes are activated by point mutations that maintain the protein in a perma-

TABLE 10-1.　FUNCTIONS OF CELL-DERIVED ONCOGENE PRODUCTS

Class 1—Growth Factors

sis	PDGF B-chain growth factor
int-2	FGF-related growth factor
hst (KS3)	FGF-related growth factor
FGF-5	FGF-related growth factor
int-1	Growth factor?

Class 2—Receptor and Nonreceptor Protein-Tyrosine Kinases

src	Membrane-associated nonreceptor protein-tyrosine kinase
yes	Membrane-associated nonreceptor protein-tyrosine kinase
fgr	Membrane-associated nonreceptor protein-tyrosine kinase
lck	Membrane-associated nonreceptor protein-tyrosine kinase
fps/fes	Nonreceptor protein-tyrosine kinase
abl/bcr–abl	Nonreceptor protein-tyrosine kinase
ros	Membrane-associated receptor-like protein-tyrosine kinase
erbB	Truncated EGF receptor protein-tyrosine kinase
neu	Receptor-like protein-tyrosine kinase
fms	Mutant CSF-1 receptor protein-tyrosine kinase
met	Soluble truncated receptor-like protein-tyrosine kinase
trk	Soluble truncated receptor-like protein-tyrosine kinase
kit (W locus)	Truncated stem-cell receptor protein-tyrosine kinase
sea	Membrane-associated truncated receptor-like protein-tyrosine kinase
ret	Truncated receptor-like protein-tyrosine kinase

Class 3—Receptors Lacking Protein Kinase Activity

mas	Angiotensin receptor

Class 4—Membrane-Associated G Proteins

H-ras	Membrane-associated GTP-binding/GTPase
K-ras	Membrane-associated GTP binding/GTPase
N-ras	Membrane-associated GTP-binding/GTPase
gsp	Mutant activated form of $G_s \alpha$
gip	Mutant activated form of $G_i \alpha$

Class 5—Cytoplasmic Protein-Serine Kinases

raf/mil	Cytoplasmic protein-serine kinase
pim-1	Cytoplasmic protein-serine kinase
mos	Cytoplasmic protein-serine kinase (cytostatic factor)
cot	Cytoplasmic protein-serine kinase?

Class 6—Cytoplasmic Regulators

crk	SH-2/3 protein that binds to (and regulates?) phosphotyrosine-containing proteins

Class 7—Nuclear Transcription Factors

myc	Sequence-specific DNA-binding protein
N-myc	Sequence-specific DNA-binding protein?
L-myc	Sequence-specific DNA-binding protein?
myb	Sequence-specific DNA-binding protein
lyl-1	Sequence-specific DNA-binding protein?
p53	Mutant form may sequester wild-type p53 growth suppressor
fos	Combines with c-jun product to form AP-1 transcription factor
jun	Sequence-specific DNA-binding protein; part of AP-1
erbA	Dominant negative mutant thyroxine receptor
rel	Dominant negative mutant NF-κB-related protein
vav	Transcription factor?
ets	Sequence-specific DNA-binding protein
ski	Transcription factor?
evi-1	Transcription factor?
gli-1	Transcription factor?
maf	Transcription factor?
pbx	Chimeric E2A–homeobox transcription factor
Hox2.4	Transcription factor?

Unclassified

dbl	Cytoplasmic truncated cytoskeletal protein?
bcl-2	Plasma membrane signal transducer?

From Hunter T. Cooperation between oncogenes. Cell 64:249, 1991.

nently activated configuration that ensures signal transduction, whether or not the appropriate ligand or receptor is in place. Finally, some of the proto-oncogenes are transcription factors that interact with DNA and regulate gene transcription.

Tumor Suppressor Genes. Widespread losses of genetic material are present in colorectal cancers. These identifiable "hot spots" for genetic loss are the locations of tumor suppressor genes relevant in the development of colorectal cancer. Perhaps the most important of these is the *p53* gene, which normally acts to prevent the cell from beginning new DNA synthesis or cell division. *p53* serves as a critical regulatory gene to prevent inappropriate proliferation and acts as a suppressor of potential tumor formation. A characteristic of tumor suppressor genes is that two events are required for their inactivation. There are two copies of every genetic locus in the nucleus, and tumor suppressor genes may be thought of as "dominantly acting" inasmuch as the presence of just a single intact copy of the gene is sufficient to suppress proliferation. The TSG concept has also accommodated the concept of familial predisposition to cancer. Inactivation of the first allele could be phenotypically silent if the activity of only one allele were sufficient to maintain the nonmalignant phenotype. However, such individuals would be at extremely high risk to develop cancer, since it would only require a single inactivation mutation in a single cell to produce a tumor. Table 10-2 includes TSGs important in human cancer.

Clonal Expansion. A variety of genetic techniques have demonstrated that neoplasms are derived from a single cell. The current concept of multistage carcinogenesis assumes that GI epithelium undergoes a constant barrage by environmental insults that threaten to damage DNA but that mutations probably occur one by one, at critical locations in genes related to the control of cell growth or survival. Many of these mutations may inhibit the function of genes essential for the life of the cell and would be lethal events. Other mutations provide the cell with a slight growth or survival advantage over the rest of the cells in the tissue. In these instances, the mutated cells proliferate faster than the surrounding cells and gradually represent a larger proportion of the tissue. In other instances, a mutated cell may be less capable of repairing DNA damage, which would facilitate the accumulation of mutations in succeeding generations. This expanded pool of cells continues to be susceptible to additional mutation.

Periodically, an individual cell within the expanding, mutated clone experiences another mutation that adds further to its growth or survival advantage, and the progeny of this cell will then overgrow the population from which it originated. Successive waves of clonal expansion occur by the chance accumulation of new mutational events, which add to the survival advantage of the cell in an evolutionary manner. Thus, when early stage neoplasms are examined, there is evidence for a small number of mutational events, and as lesions farther along in neoplastic progression are examined, a larger number of genetic lesions are found. Figure 10-1 demonstrates tumor progression as successive expansions of cellular clones emerge with new growth characteristics.

Multistep Carcinogenesis. Largely through the elegant work of the laboratories of Vogelstein and others, a concept of the genetic basis of colorectal cancer has been developed. This framework accommodated the growing evidence that colorectal cancers develop slowly and that multiple genes were involved in the process. By analyzing tumors along the neoplastic continuum, genetic alterations

TABLE 10-2. *EXAMPLES OF TUMOR-SUPPRESSOR GENES INVOLVED IN HUMAN CANCERS*

TUMOR-SUPPRESSOR GENE	CHROMO-SOMAL LOCUS	LOCATION/ PROPOSED FUNCTION	SOMATIC MUTATIONS		INHERITED MUTATIONS		
			MAJOR TYPES	EXAMPLES OF NEOPLASMS	SYNDROME	HETEROZYGOTE CARRIER RATE PER 10^5 BIRTHS	TYPICAL NEOPLASMS
p53	17p13.1	Nucleus/ transcription factor	Missense	Most types of human cancer	Li-Fraumeni syndrome	~2	Carcinomas of breast and adrenal cortex; sarcomas; leukemia; brain tumors
RB1	13q14	Nucleus/ transcription modifier	Deletion and nonsense	Retinoblastoma; osteosarcoma; carcinomas of the breast, prostate, bladder, and lung	Retinoblastoma	~2	Retinoblastoma; osteosarcoma
APC	5q21	Cytoplasm/ unknown	Deletion and nonsense	Carcinoma of the colon, stomach, and pancreas	Familial adenomatous polyposis coli	~10	Carcinomas of colon, thyroid, and stomach
WT1	11p13	Nucleus/ transcription factor	Missense	Wilms' tumor	Wilms' tumor	~0.5–1	Wilms' tumor
NF1	17q11	Cytoplasm/ guanosine triphosphatase–activating protein	Deletion	Schwannomas	Neurofibro-matosis type 1	~30	Neural tumors
NF2	22q	Cytoplasm/ cytoskeleton–membrane link	Deletion and nonsense	Schwannomas and meningiomas	Neurofibro-matosis type 2	~3	Central schwan-nomas and meningiomas
VHL	3p25	Unknown/ unknown	Deletion	Unknown	von Hippel-Lindau disease	~3	Hemangioblas-toma and renal-cell carcinoma

From Harris CC, Hollstein M. Clinical implications of the p53 tumor-suppressor gene. N Engl J Med 329:1318, 1993.

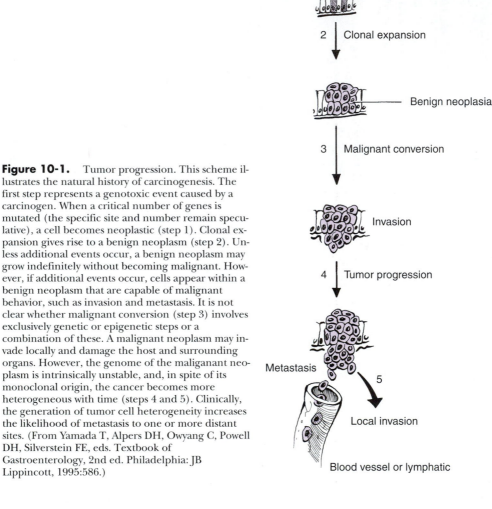

Figure 10-1. Tumor progression. This scheme illustrates the natural history of carcinogenesis. The first step represents a genotoxic event caused by a carcinogen. When a critical number of genes is mutated (the specific site and number remain speculative), a cell becomes neoplastic (step 1). Clonal expansion gives rise to a benign neoplasm (step 2). Unless additional events occur, a benign neoplasm may grow indefinitely without becoming malignant. However, if additional events occur, cells appear within a benign neoplasm that are capable of malignant behavior, such as invasion and metastasis. It is not clear whether malignant conversion (step 3) involves exclusively genetic or epigenetic steps or a combination of these. A malignant neoplasm may invade locally and damage the host and surrounding organs. However, the genome of the maliganant neoplasm is intrinsically unstable, and, in spite of its monoclonal origin, the cancer becomes more heterogeneous with time (steps 4 and 5). Clinically, the generation of tumor cell heterogeneity increases the likelihood of metastasis to one or more distant sites. (From Yamada T, Alpers DH, Owyang C, Powell DH, Silverstein FE, eds. Textbook of Gastroenterology, 2nd ed. Philadelphia: JB Lippincott, 1995:586.)

were found in the earliest tumors and progressively more genetic lesions were identified in more advanced tumors. Certain types of genetic damage tended to occur early and different types tended to occur later. It is not yet clear how strictly the sequence of events is followed in all neoplasms, but it has become evident that not all cancers have accumulated the same mutations or chromosomal deletions during their development. Because of the laboratory methods initially used to detect chromosomal segment loss, this loss of genetic information is referred to as loss of heterozygosity (LOH).

The following sequence of events appears to be relevant to typical tumor development in the human colon (Fig. 10-2). Hypomethylation of DNA occurs in the smallest adenomas and may be one of the early events in carcinogenesis. Mutations

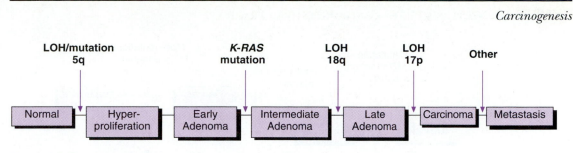

Figure 10-2. The concept of sequential genetic events mediating multistep carcinogenesis in the colon, as proposed by Fearon and Vogelstein with modifications based upon additional data. Above the sequence are mutational events and loss of heterozygosity (LOH), events found in colorectal cancer progression.

or loss of genetic information (LOH) on chromosome 5q in the adenomatous polyposis coli (APC) locus are also found in small adenomas. Mutations in the *K-RAS* and *p53* genes are both found in larger adenomatous polyps and are thought to play a mechanistic role in supporting neoplastic growth. Allelic deletion (LOH) at the TSGs located on 18q (also termed the deleted in colorectal cancer or "*DCC*") gene and at 17p (the *p53* gene locus) are later stage events, occurring at the point of malignant conversion. Although there are similarities between carcinogenesis in the colon and tumors elsewhere in the GI tract, the sequence of events and the genes involved are not identical to the situation in the colon. These details are just beginning to emerge.

Alternate Mechanisms for Tumor Progression. A second type of genomic instability may be involved in the genesis of colon cancers that does not result from the loss of TSGs. Microsatellites are repetitive DNA sequences that are used for gene mapping. Ordinarily these sequences are faithfully copied during cell replication, but in certain tumors, minor changes in their length have been noted. Microsatellite sequences are ubiquitous and may be present 10^5 times throughout the genome. It was noted, rather accidentally, that microsatellite sequences were not faithfully reproduced in certain colorectal cancers. Tumors that demonstrated *microsatellite instability* did so at multiple unrelated sites throughout the genome, suggesting that these tumors had lost their ability to copy these sequences faithfully. This failure of normal mutation repair appears to be an alternate mechanism for neoplastic progression. A proposed scheme for the alternative pathways for the progression of colorectal cancer is demonstrated in Figure 10-3.

TUMOR DEVELOPMENT

Loss of Proliferative Control. Proliferation is normally tightly regulated and confined to one portion of the epithelial unit within the GI tract. During periods of epithelial repair, as in the setting of trauma or inflammation, this regulation is relaxed, and the rate of proliferation increases. When a sufficient number of cells have been produced, the rate of proliferation slows to match the rate of cell loss.

It appears that loss of proliferative control is an early event in carcinogenesis of the colon. This conclusion is based upon the observation that some patients at high risk for cancer show an expansion of the proliferative pool of cells from its normally restricted site at the base of the crypt toward the top of the colonic crypt. The failure to suppress cell proliferation would not, in and of itself, be sufficient to

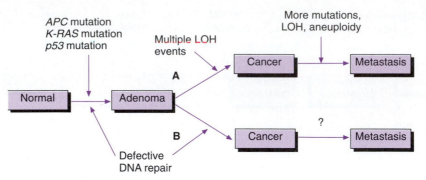

A – Multiple LOH events; more virulent tumor course, aneuploid tumor
B – Absence of LOH; microsatellite instability and the accumulation of multiple somatic
mutations; diploid tumors; more indolent course; seen in hereditary nonpolyposis
colorectal cancer + proximal colon cancers

Figure 10-3. An alternate genetic mechanism has been proposed for multistep
carcinogenesis in the colon. Colorectal cancers all accumulate mutations at the *APC,
K-RAS-2,* and *p53* loci that alter the functions of the gene products. However, some
tumors undergo a type of genomic instability that results in multiple LOH events, as illustrated on the upper arm. Other tumors, particularly those in the proximal colon and in
hereditary nonpolyposis colorectal cancer, do not show widespread LOH but instead
develop widespread errors in DNA replication, allowing mutations to accumulate or serving to disrupt gene expression randomly throughout the genome. This replicative defect
may be found in early stage lesions as well. (From Fearon ER, Vogelstein B. A genetic
model for colorectal tumorigenesis. Cell 61:759, 1990; Aaltonen LA, Peltomaki P, Leach
FS, et al. Clues to the pathogenesis of familial colorectal cancer. Science 260:812, 1993;
Thibodeau SN, Bren G, Schaid D. Microsatellite instability in cancer of the proximal
colon. Science 260:816, 1993; Ionov Y, Peinado MA, Malkhosyan S, et al. Ubiquitous
somatic mutations in simple repeated sequences reveal a new mechanism for colonic carcinogenesis. Nature 363:558, 1993.)

develop cancer. Additional genetic events, currently undefined, occur that interfere with normal epithelial cell differentiation, senescence, and detachment from
the crypt unit. The persistence of hyperproliferative, immature cells is what constitutes an adenoma. Since these cells continue to proliferate but are incapable of invasion, they tend to protrude above the mucosa and produce a polyp. This is a
common stage of development of neoplasia in the colon but is uncommon in the
natural history of neoplasia in the esophagus, stomach, and pancreas.

Growth of Benign Tumors. Small adenomatous polyps are common, and
in most individuals, they do not seem to grow. Over time, certain small adenomas
grow and undergo progressive changes in morphology. In the GI tract, the expanded pools of hyperproliferative cells undergo new DNA synthesis in the more
hazardous environment of the GI lumen. Ordinarily, cell proliferation takes place
at the base of the crypt and is relatively protected from luminal dietary content and
the products of bacterial metabolism. In addition, the unrestrained proliferation
permits the accumulation of mutated cells, hastening the appearance of alterations
that may provide a growth advantage.

It appears that the development of the adenoma in the colon is a reversible
biologic event. Evidence for this may be found in the spontaneous disappearance
of small adenomas from the rectums of patients with familial adenomatous polyposis (FAP) after subtotal colectomy. FAP is a genetic disorder wherein patients in-
herit a mutated gene, the *APC* locus, which leads to the development of many neo-

sis suppressor gene inasmuch as it is deleted in distant metastases from colorectal cancer. The cellular mechanism by which the NM23 locus confers metastatic capability is totally unknown. It is apparent that numerous genes participate in the metastatic phenotype, and the accumulation of them within malignant cells is responsible for the broad range of virulent behaviors seen in cancer.

SPECIFIC ORGAN INVOLVEMENT

The preceding sections have outlined the general framework by which GI carcinogenesis unfolds. However, each GI cancer is a distinct disease with a variety of unique aspects. Many of the details that have led to our current understanding of GI cancer have come from a study of colorectal cancer, and these principles may not necessarily pertain to cancers elsewhere in the gut. Therefore, this section highlights some of the information known about specific GI tumors to provide a framework for an understanding of future progress in GI cancers.

ESOPHAGEAL CANCER

Squamous cell carcinoma and adenocarcinoma of the esophagus are separate diseases with different etiologies and natural histories that should be considered independently. Squamous cell carcinoma has an extremely wide international incidence range that has puzzled tumor biologists for a long time. It is assumed that the variation in incidence is a reflection of the differential expression of one or more potent environmental carcinogens. First, severe chronic esophagitis is a precursor condition in young people who live in areas of the world at highest risk for squamous cell carcinoma of the esophagus. It is not known what causes this inflammation, but as described above, reactive oxygen species are powerful carcinogens. Second, human papillomavirus can be found in precancerous lesions and squamous cell carcinomas from China. Precursor lesions for squamous cell carcinoma have mutations in the p53 gene, and the lesions show accumulation of the abnormal p53 protein, similar to what is seen in colorectal cancer.

Barrett's esophagus is a condition in which the native squamous epithelium of the esophagus is replaced by a metaplastic columnar epithelium (intestinal type). It is believed that this change is a consequence of chronic gastroesophageal reflux, epithelial injury, and replacement by an epithelium more resistant to refluxed acid. Adenocarcinoma of the esophagus may arise in Barrett's epithelium. In Barrett's esophagus, aneuploidy is commonly seen early in the course of neoplastic progression. In fact aneuploidy, which reflects genomic instability, occurs in premalignant tissues and may be used to predict the risk of tumor progression. Thus, genomic instability occurs relatively early in this disease (compared to its later onset in the sporadic adenoma-to-carcinoma sequence in the colon), and a different sequence of events may be responsible for the virulent clinical course of cancer in the esophagus.

STOMACH CANCER

Carcinoma of the stomach occurs primarily in the setting of severe chronic gastritis. This again emphasizes the carcinogenic potential of reactive oxygen species formed during inflammation. Gastric carcinoma is associated with mutations in the APC gene, K-RAS gene, and p53 gene. LOH is seen at high frequency at

several chromosomal sites, including 17p (the locus of the p53 gene), 5q (the location of the APC gene), the DCC gene (18q), and other sites. Little is known about the sequence and time relationships of genomic instability in gastric cancer. RAS gene mutations appear to be relatively infrequent in this disease. The natural history of gastric cancer is that it occurs in the setting of chronic inflammation, is not frequently associated with obvious neoplastic polyps such as are found in the colon, and may be virulent and progress to a lethal stage quickly. This series of events suggests the possibility that the genetic events that trigger genomic instability may occur relatively early in gastric cancer, bypassing a prolonged premalignant phase, which has important implications for the clinical outcome in this disease. Less information is available for gastric carcinoma than colon cancer, but one would anticipate that differences in the responsible genetic lesions may account for the unique biologic and clinical behaviors of this cancer.

COLORECTAL CANCER

Many of the paradigms that are currently used to describe sequential carcinogenesis for solid tumors have been developed from the study of colorectal cancer, and this information has provided a general framework for much of the prior discussion. However, there are specific situations in which variations on this theme occur.

In the case of FAP, the affected individual has a germ line mutation in the APC gene, which results in the appearance of adenomatous polyps by a mean age of 16 years. The increased risk for cancer occurs because the colonic epithelium has a mutation built into its genetic program whereby the loss of proliferative control occurs very early. Furthermore, every colonic epithelial cell has this defect, which greatly expands the pool of hyperproliferative tissue. Perhaps a more important and subtle aspect of FAP can be found in the natural history of this disease. Without any early diagnosis or intervention, the average gene carrier dies of cancer at a mean age of 42 years. Furthermore, although many such patients have thousands of adenomatous polyps in the colon and have carried them for 25 years or more, most of these patients develop a relatively small number of cancers. Less than half have more than one malignant tumor, and the most found in one large series was seven cancers. This leads to the conclusion that the development of the adenoma is not the rate-limiting step in the development of cancer, indicating the necessity for additional genetic damage for neoplastic progression to occur.

Chronic ulcerative colitis is a condition in which an increased risk for colorectal cancer is seen. In general, many of the same genetic lesions are seen in ulcerative colitis cancers as in sporadically occurring tumors. However, there are three issues of particular interest with regard to cancers that occur in this condition. First, K-RAS gene mutations are reported to be relatively uncommon in colitic cancers. Thus, cancers in ulcerative colitis develop without activation of the gene that has been implicated as an important "middle event" in colorectal cancer and that may be responsible for the clonal expansion of premalignant tissue. Second, mutation in the p53 gene is found early and frequently in this disease. Third, aneuploidy is very common, occurs in extended clones of normal-appearing colonic tissue, and antedates the development of dysplasia and cancer. Thus, cancer in ulcerative colitis may tend to develop through a program that gives it a different "middle stage" that may be relatively abbreviated, resulting in the early onset of virulent, malignant disease. The mechanism to explain this different natural history is unknown;

colon cancer. However, countries with high fiber intake also tend to have lower intakes of fat and frequently lower life expectancies, which introduces confounding variables. If the entire body of data accumulated on the subject is considered, the majority of papers show a consistent protective effect of fiber, a small number of studies show no effect, and no study shows a deleterious effect of dietary fiber on colon cancer.

The intake on nonstarch polysaccharides (i.e., fiber) correlates directly with fecal weight in studies from diverse international populations, and the incidence of colorectal cancer shows a significant inverse correlation with fecal weight. Based on the observation that high-risk Western nations have fecal weights in the range of 80 to 120 g/day, investigators have suggested that an increase in fiber intake to >18 g/day would increase fecal weights to >150 g/day and might reduce cancer incidence. One trial has demonstrated that the addition of 13.5 g of bran fiber to the diet (which was a 1.5-ounce bowl of a commercially available bran cereal) resulted in a significant reduction in rectal epithelial proliferation in a group of high-risk patients with a past history of resected colorectal cancers.

A number of mechanisms have been proposed for the protective effect of fiber against colorectal cancer. Fiber increases the speed with which feces traverse the colon, and by virtue of its sheer presence in stool, tends to dilute the concentration of other colonic constituents. Both of these would tend to reduce contact between carcinogens and colonic epithelium. Second, fiber polymers may bind toxic substances and remove them from contact with epithelium. Third, fiber is neither digested nor absorbed in the small intestine but undergoes fermentation in the presence of the colonic flora, which reduces fecal pH and generates short-chain ("volatile") fatty acids. Certain of the short-chain organic acids derived from the fermentation of fiber can protect isolated colonic epithelial cells from deoxycholic acid–induced injury in culture. One of these, butyric acid, is present in high concentrations in the colonic lumen, is thought to be an important energy source for colonic epithelium, and has the ability to induce cellular differentiation in culture.

Nonsteroidal Anti-inflammatory Drugs. It has been appreciated by epidemiologists for some time that aspirin takers suffer less cancer than the rest of the population. In animal models of colorectal cancer, aspirin and nonsteroidal anti-inflammatory drugs (NSAIDs) inhibit the development of tumors. Furthermore, patients with FAP experience a regression of their adenomas after treatment with the NSAID sulindac.

In 1991, an American Cancer Society-sponsored survey of over 660,000 people revealed a significant reduction in colon cancer deaths in aspirin users, and among those who used aspirin ≥16 times per month, the relative risk was 0.60 for men and 0.58 for women. Reduction in risk was even seen in people who reported aspirin use as rarely as once per month, raising interesting speculation regarding the mechanism and dose effects of this intervention. Even more impressively, significant reductions of about 40% for deaths from cancer of the esophagus and stomach have been reported recently from the large American Cancer Society survey. The protection was greatest among long-time users (≥10 years), and protection was not found for tumors of nondigestive organs.

The mechanism of action by which aspirin and NSAIDs protect against tumor formation in the digestive tract remains an issue of speculation and includes many possibilities. It cannot be assumed that the antitumor effect is necessarily related to modifications in the production of prostaglandins in the gastrointestinal tract. Of interest, it has been demonstrated that cultured gastric cancer cells preferentially produce leukotrienes (whereas normal stomach tissue produces prostaglandins), that the leukotrienes act as stimulants of growth, and that prostaglandins inhibit the growth of the cancer cells. Thus, there may be a change in response to eicosanoids by tissues that undergo malignant transformation.

GASTRIC CANCER

The striking variation in regional stomach cancer incidence has prompted investigators to carefully scrutinize dietary practices in high- and low-risk areas. The situation appears to be very complex. There is no single factor that accounts for all the differences in cancer incidence, and there is no direct evidence that any specific food is important pathogenetically in the disease. The consumption of a carbohydrate-rich diet has been associated with an increased risk of gastric cancer; among the foods implicated are fava beans, potatoes, and "sour pancakes" in Shandong Province, China. Unfortunately, the implicated foods cannot be consistently found in all the high-risk regions. Moreover, carbohydrate-rich diets often overlap with high salt intake, contamination of grain supplies with mold, and reduced intake of fresh fruits and vegetables. The consumption of dried fish, soy sauce, and pickled foods correlates with stomach cancer risk in Japan, but ingestion of dried fish and pickled foods overlaps with diets that are saltier and lower in fresh fruits and vegetables. Moreover, preservation of foods by pickling or drying is common in areas where access to refrigeration is limited. It has been suggested that the widespread use of the home refrigerator and the growth of the frozen food industry have been key factors in the reduction of gastric cancer incidence in North America and Western Europe. It is not yet clear whether improved refrigeration is actually responsible for reducing the incidence of gastric cancer; not is it known whether this factor impacts upon carcinogenesis by reducing the intake of potential mutagens or alternatively by increasing the intake of anticarcinogens. Moreover, all of these observations were made before the role of *Helicobacter pylori* on the stomach was appreciated.

Some foods may serve to counteract the effects of certain carcinogens. For example, it has been suggested that there are *protective* effects conferred on persons consuming increased amounts of *Allium*-containing vegetables, such as garlic, onions, scallions, and others.

Tobacco and Alcohol. Increased use of tobacco and alcohol has been associated with an elevated risk of gastric cancer in the United States. However, tobacco use is an unlikely candidate as a gastric carcinogen because the incidence of this disease has fallen dramatically throughout the 20th century although tobacco use has increased markedly and has been associated with an epidemic of lung cancer. A prospective study found a relative risk of 2.7 for stomach cancer among smokers, but without a dose-response effect, suggesting that cigarette and alcohol use may be a marker of some other more relevant factor. That factor may ultimately be proved to be infection with the gram-negative organism *Helicobacter pylori,* the etiologic agent of chronic gastritis. Epidemiologic data to support this association and the pathogenesis of *H. pylori*–related gastric carcinogenesis are discussed in detail in the section on the Role of Inflammation in GI Cancer.

Sources of Water and Nitrate Ingestion. Gastric cancer is prevalent in Colombia and has been extensively studied in this South American country. High-

and low-risk regions have been identified within Colombia, and the population groups have been investigated for differences in dietary characteristics. High-risk groups tend to obtain their drinking water from wells with significantly higher nitrate concentrations than found in the low-risk regions and excrete higher amounts of nitrate in their urine. The high-risk groups have higher incidences of chronic atrophic gastritis and intestinal metaplasia. In the highest risk regions, three quarters of the population has developed chronic atrophic gastritis by age 45, whereas this change has occurred in less than half of the intermediate and lower risk populations by that age. Numerous other contaminants of water have been suspected to play a role in stomach cancer, including aflatoxin, pepper, vitamin or mineral deficiencies, and soft water. However, a compelling case has not emerged for any of these contaminants.

N-nitroso compounds are strong carcinogens suspected to play a role in upper GI carcinogenesis because of their spontaneous synthesis from dietary components and their ability to alkylate nucleic acids. Nitrosamides are a subset of the N-nitroso group formed in the stomach from nitrite and amides. Their spontaneous formation is favored by a low pH, and no enzymes are required for their synthesis. They are unstable and likely to react near the site of their formation. The actual compounds involved in human carcinogenesis may be more ephemeral reaction products generated locally in the stomach or compounds activated by mucosal enzymes from dietary procarcinogens.

The formation of nitrosamides in the stomach requires the presence of nitrites. Drinking water contains variable amounts of nitrate, which is readily absorbed from the gastrointestinal tract and actively secreted into saliva. Nitrate may be reduced to nitrite by the flora of the mouth or stomach. Human saliva typically contains 6 to 10 mg nitrite/L and 15 to 35 mg nitrate/L. Nitrite levels in gastric juice are substantially lower but increase with rising gastric pH in the presence of nitrate-reducing bacteria, which may be seen in the setting of atrophic gastritis or after acid-reducing surgery. Salivary nitrate and nitrite levels rise rapidly after an ingested dose of nitrate and are high in populations that have high rates of stomach cancer.

The sources of gastric nitrites have been estimated based upon current typical dietary practices in North America. Approximately 20% of gastric nitrite is derived directly from the diet. The most prominent source of dietary nitrate is vegetables, which account for 85% of the intake. It is estimated that 25% of dietary nitrate participates in the "enterosalivary circulation." Approximately 20% of the salivary nitrate is reduced to nitrite by the oral flora, and this accounts for the majority (80%) of gastric nitrite. In addition, the amine content of the diet is critical to the hypothesis that these compounds participate in gastric carcinogenesis. Nitrosamide precursor substances include a wide range of compounds, many of which are prominent in the diets of high-risk regions. Several compounds such as vitamins C and E have been found to inhibit the formation of nitrosamides from secondary amines and nitrites. The concentration of N-nitroso compounds has been measured in the gastric juice of patients with normal and diseased stomachs. An increase in the extractable N-nitrosamines occurred as the pH of the gastric juice rose from 1 to 7. The highest levels of these potentially carcinogenic compounds has been found in patients with gastric carcinoma, pernicious anemia, and partial gastrectomy. Thus, the nitrosamide theory provides a potential explanation for some geographical regions at very high risk for gastric cancer. This concept requires a dietary source of nitrate, a mechanism for its reduction to nitrite, and a dietary source of amines, and it is complicated by all those factors that inhibit the formation of these mutagens.

Other Factors. The cumulative effects of 20th century industrialization, including the introduction of plastics, solvents, and other novel substances into the food chain and general environment, have not been associated with an increase in gastric cancer. Furthermore, the use of the outdoor charcoal grill, which has increased dramatically in the United States over the past 30 to 40 years, also appears to have had no adverse impact on this disease.

THE ROLE OF INFLAMMATION IN GI CANCER

CHRONIC ATROPHIC GASTRITIS AND HELICOBACTER PYLORI

Intestinal metaplasia, the conversion of the native gastric epithelium to one with mature absorptive cells and goblet cells, occurs in association with more than 70% of gastric carcinomas but may also be seen in non-neoplastic disease. The intestinal type of gastric cancer is highly associated with the presence of intestinal metaplasia and frequently arises within it. Atrophic gastritis is present in 80 to 90% of patients with gastric carcinoma, and this close association has led to the assumption that it is etiologically related in this disease. In regions of the world at highest risk for gastric cancer, chronic atrophic gastritis is nearly universal among adults. Several studies from Scandinavia, Italy, and Great Britain indicate that approximately 10% of patients with chronic atrophic gastritis develop gastric carcinoma in approximately 15 years. A control group consisting of subjects with normal gastric mucosa or superficial gastritis developed no gastric carcinomas during the 15-year follow-up. Therefore, in any given population of patients, chronic atrophic gastritis and intestinal metaplasia are indices of the risk of gastric carcinoma in that group and are markers within individuals of the high risk of developing gastric cancer. It is usually difficult to date the onset of the process, and a relatively long period of time appears to be required for the development of neoplasia. Moreover, only 10% of patients with this preneoplastic condition might be expected to develop cancer, even when followed for 10 to 20 years, and the risk may be lower yet in low cancer incidence regions of the world such as the United States.

Atrophic gastritis is a complex entity in which mucosal atrophy and cellular hyperproliferation occur together. This process begins with superficial inflammation limited to the upper half of the gastric gland, typically starting in the antrum, and over time progresses in severity and distribution throughout the stomach. Eventually, inflammation may involve the entire gland, and in the later stages of the disease, a reduction in the inflammatory infiltrate and mucosal atrophy occur. The parietal cells do not disappear until relatively late in the disease process; therefore most patients continue to secrete acid and have normal levels of gastrin. This contrasts with the less common variety of chronic gastritis that begins in the fundus, is associated with parietal cell antibodies and destruction of the gastric glands that contain parietal and chief cells, and produces pernicious anemia. The variety of chronic atrophic gastritis that begins in the antrum is also referred to as type B gastritis and is epidemiologically linked to *H. pylori* infection. It is associated with a high incidence of antral ulcers and is very common in countries where carcinoma of the stomach is prevalent. Chronic atrophic gastritis that begins in the fundus, the type A variant, is a less common entity, is thought to have an autoimmune etiology, and is associated with gastric cancer in both high- and low-risk populations. In Denmark, where the incidence of pernicious anemia is relatively high, 2.2% of all new cases of gastric cancer occur in these patients.

Over a period of years, chronic atrophic gastritis may be complicated by the appearance of intestinal metaplasia and the subsequent development of gastric cancer. Population studies have confirmed that infection with *H. pylori* is endemic, particularly at an early age, in areas with high rates of stomach cancer such as Japan, China, and South America. The well-established association between gastric cancer and lower socioeconomic status has been linked similarly to early acquisition of *H. pylori* infection by studying the prevalence of antibodies to the organism. *H. pylori* infection is related to both the intestinal and diffuse types of cancer and is also related to the precursor lesion, intestinal metaplasia. *H. pylori*–induced persistent inflammation may lead to carcinogenesis by DNA damage from products of neutrophil metabolism, and the increased serum gastrin level present in this condition stimulates a hyperproliferative state that contributes to the risk for cancer.

However, *H. pylori* infection alone is not sufficient for cancer to develop. The infection occurs at an early age in Africa and Costa Rica, both of which have low-risk populations. Moreover, *H. pylori* infection occurs in as many as 50% of North American adults; yet gastric cancer develops in very few of those infected. Thus, additional environmental or genetic factors are necessary for cancer to develop.

INFLAMMATORY BOWEL DISEASE AND CANCER

Patients with chronic inflammatory bowel disease are at increased risk of developing GI cancer. The degree of risk, however, has been a subject of debate. A British study of 624 patients at a referral center indicated that 3.5% of the patients developed colorectal cancer, which was approximately sevenfold greater than expected from an age-matched control population. The diagnosis of cancer in this condition was made at an average age of 41 years, ranging from ages 20 to 74. Relatively fewer of these cancers occurred in the rectum (22%) compared with the expected rate in the general population (38%). Thus, there are important differences in clinical presentation in the setting of inflammatory bowel disease, the most important of these being age.

It has been recognized that the duration of ulcerative colitis is a critical factor in predicting the likelihood of developing adenocarcinoma of the colon. Cancer is more likely to occur among patients with pancolitis (13%) compared with those with only left-sided inflammatory bowel disease (5%), and the latter group tended to develop cancer a decade later than the former group. The incidence of colorectal cancer is less than 1% during the first decade of inflammatory bowel disease but progressively rises to 7% in the second decade, 16% in the third decade, and 53% in the fourth.

Patients with Crohn's disease are also at increased risk for colorectal cancer; however, the incidence is lower than that reported with ulcerative colitis. It is not yet possible to accurately estimate the risk of cancer in this setting; however, an excess of carcinomas of the colon, small intestine, stomach, and anus as well as an excess of lymphomas has been reported.

The survival of patients who develop cancers in the setting of ulcerative colitis is similar to that seen for noncolitic patients. To improve the early detection and survival from colon cancer in patients with colitis, attempts have been made to identify early neoplastic lesions. Dysplasia is currently the best marker for early cancer in this setting. Developing a standardized classification for dysplasia has been a major undertaking because inflammation and attendant repair can be easily confused with early neoplasia. True dysplasia is an early benign neoplastic lesion and biologically is analogous to adenomatous tissue. Just as it is difficult to predict the clinical behavior of a small adenoma, the behavior of low-grade dysplasia is also unpredictable. Low-grade dysplasia in a biopsy may have three interpretations. First, it may reflect inflammation and repairs and be a transient change. Second, it may reflect the presence of a higher grade lesion (such as carcinoma) immediately adjacent to the biopsy site. Third, it may be a harbinger of a generalized problem in the colon, with additional neoplastic lesions elsewhere. Dysplasia in a plaque or elevated mass is especially worrisome and suggests the need to consider colectomy. When low grades of dysplasia are found in random biopsies of flat mucosa, this is less likely to be associated with a nearby cancer, but it is still a worrisome lesion. At this time, the management of low-grade dysplasia in ulcerative colitis is as troublesome as the management of small adenomatous polyps in the noncolitic colon. High-grade dysplasia is somewhat less ambiguous and is also a very worrisome finding; when found in a colonic mass, total colectomy should be offered to the patient. When the surgical specimen is examined, most of these patients have confirmation of the high-grade dysplasia (which is the equivalent of carcinoma-in-situ) or have a frank, invasive cancer.

BARRETT'S ESOPHAGUS AND ESOPHAGEAL ADENOCARCINOMA

Although the incidence of adenocarcinoma in Barrett's esophagus is not known, the risk is estimated to be 20- to 40-fold higher than in patients with squamous epithelium. Presumably the mechanism of carcinogenesis is similar to that in the conditions described above, in which chronic epithelial injury and proliferation lead to genetic alterations and ultimately to tumorigenesis. Progression to neoplasia appears stepwise as in ulcerative colitis, and dysplasia is believed to be an important high-risk situation and is the "intermediate target" for screening programs. The presence of dysplasia, particularly high-grade dysplasia, is considered an indication for esophagectomy because of the high incidence of subsequent progression to cancer.

CLINICAL TESTING—SCREENING FOR COLON CANCER

Screening refers to testing apparently healthy people for asymptomatic disease. A good screening test must in some way improve the lives of those screened, either by prolonging life or improving its quality. To be effective, the test must be sensitive (optimally detect all diseased individuals), specific (not subject nondiseased individuals to excessive anxiety or extra testing), and acceptable to and affordable by those tested. At present, two modalities have been evaluated for efficacy as screening tests for colorectal cancer: testing feces for occult blood and endoscopic examination of the bowel. Both modalities are effective in reducing cancer mortality, but each has its limitations.

FECAL OCCULT BLOOD TESTS

It has long been appreciated that colorectal neoplasms bleed early in their natural history. Hemoglobin contains peroxidase activity, which may be detected using the guaiac test. Gum guaiac is a colorless indicator that may be oxidized to a pigmented quinone in the presence of peroxidase and hydrogen peroxide. The traditional bench guaiac test required the application of feces to filter paper, followed by the application of the guaiac reagent, acetic acid, and hydrogen peroxide. This was a very sensitive means of detecting fecal peroxidase activity but it was poorly standardized and overly sensitive. Therefore, guaiac-impregnated "slide" tests have been developed that were slightly less sensitive but more highly standardized. The guaiac slide test can detect hemoglobin concentrations as low as 0.12 mg/ml. In a typical 150-g stool, the following rule of thumb may be used: each 1 ml of blood results in approximately 1 mg of hemoglobin per gram of stool. Thus, the detection of tiny blood losses into the GI tract should be a simple task. In fact, however, this test is fraught with complexities.

The normal GI losses of blood are approximately 0.5 to 1.0 ml/day. During its transit in the GI tract, the blood is dispersed throughout the stool and undergoes degradation because of the presence of digestive and bacterial enzymes. Moreover, there are natural inhibitors of peroxidase activity in feces. The standardized guaiac test is reliably negative in control subjects on restricted diets, and less than 1% of tests are falsely positive on a low peroxidase diet. However, the test becomes unreliable when performed with rehydration (which increases the sensitivity of the test on samples that have dried out during transit or storage) unless the diet is strictly regulated, diminishing the value of this maneuver.

A critical issue in the development of fetal occult blood tests is to understand how much colorectal neoplasms bleed. The mean blood loss from a cohort of symptomatic tumors of the cecum and ascending colon was 9.3 ml/day (ranging from 2 to 28 ml/day) but was much less for lesions located distal to the hepatic flexure, where the mean blood loss was typically less than 2 ml/day. This difference may have been owing to the presence of larger lesions in the proximal colon. The proportion of positive guaiac tests is closely related to the amount of blood in the stool. The test results are usually negative when the stool hemoglobin concentration is less than 2 ml/g of stool and are more likely to be positive with increasing fecal hemoglobin. Colonic polyps may also be detected by the tests for occult bleeding, but benign lesions lose less blood and the sensitivity of the test is much lower. The mean blood loss from an adenomatous polyp is approximately 1.3 ml of blood per day, regardless of its location. However, polyps in the distal colon (descending colon, sigmoid colon, and rectum) produce positive tests only 54% of the time, whereas those in the proximal colon produce positive tests more infrequently, only 17% of the time.

Colorectal neoplasms usually add a very small amount of blood to the feces, which can make them difficult to detect using tests for fecal occult blood. Blood deposited in the stool is mixed throughout the stool and undergoes degradation, making it more difficult to detect with a guaiac test. Lesions located in the distal colon are generally easier to detect because the blood is deposited on the surface of the stool, where the mixing and dilution are limited. The fecal hemoglobin concentration on the surface of a solid stool may be high enough to produce a positive test, even considering the rigors of dehydration and degradation during the time the guaiac cards are mailed back to the physician. In general, maneuvers designed to increase the sensitivity of the guaiac test, such as rehydration, may increase the rate of false-positive results faster than the rate of true-positive results. Thus, the guaiac-impregnated cards can be used to detect approximately two thirds of colorectal cancers and a smaller proportion of adenomatous polyps, based upon both their size and location in the colon. Finally, because the basis of the guaiac test is the oxidation of an indicator substance (guaiac), the presence of strong *antioxidants* could interfere with the reaction. For example, ingestion of 1 to 2 g/day of ascorbic acid (vitamin C) has been reported to produce a spuriously negative guaiac test.

Numerous attempts have been made to develop a better fecal occult bleeding test. The manufacturers of Hemoccult II have developed a more sensitive slide test, called Hemoccult SENSA (SmithKline Diagnostics, San Jose, CA), which seems to provide sensitivity similar to that seen with rehydrated Hemoccult slides. The same manufacturer has also developed an immunochemical test for fecal hemoglobin called HemeSelect. This test uses a specific antibody for human hemoglobin but must be performed in the laboratory and is not a bedside test, as are the guaiac-based slide tests. The antibody-based test has the theoretical advantage of not cross-reacting with nonhuman hemoglobin (such as that found in ingested meat) and should also not detect bleeding from an upper GI site because of degradation of the intact molecule. Both Hemoccult SENSA and HemeSelect tests are significantly more sensitive than Hemoccult II, and it was reported that they detected 94% and 97%, respectively, of the symptomatic colorectal cancers in the one study compared with 89% for Hemoccult II; however, the sensitivity for silent cancers (which are obviously more difficult to detect and are the true target lesions) was uncertain. The newer tests were also sensitive for adenomatous polyps ≥1 cm; Hemoccult SENSA and HemeSelect were positive in 76% and 60% of cases, respectively, versus 42% for Hemoccult II. These two new tests were positive in 5.0% and 3.0% of screened individuals, respectively, and most of these positive test results were not associated with colorectal neoplasia. Therefore, the price of increased sensitivity is the need to perform a larger number of definitive work-ups (i.e., colonoscopy) in response to false-positive tests.

A quantitative test for fecal heme has been developed in the HemoQuant test. This assay provides a quantitative measurement of occult gastrointestinal bleeding and can detect the tiny increments of bleeding that occur in the setting of colorectal neoplasia. The test is not influenced by dietary peroxidase and should be superior to Hemoccult as a diagnostic test. Unfortunately, the amount of bleeding from a variety of different lesions overlaps with that seen in colon cancer. Stool samples must be sent to the laboratory for analysis, so this is neither a simple nor a bedside test. Furthermore, it may not be as sensitive as the tests described above. Several studies are available that illustrate the benefits and limitations of screening for colon cancer. Controlled trials indicate that fecal occult blood tests provide an effective means for screening asymptomatic, average risk patients for colorectal cancer. Asymptomatic populations will have approximately 1.0 to 2.4% positive tests. Generally, when more than 1 to 2% of tests are positive, it suggests that dietary restrictions have not been adequately followed or that clinicians have used rehydration of the guaiac test or a more sensitive version of the test. It is recommended that beef be eliminated from the diet during the lead-in period and during the testing of feces. In addition, anti-inflammatory agents and antioxidants such as vitamin C should be avoided. Furthermore, the physician or technician should develop the slides as soon as possible, not rehydrate the slides, and should be aware of the potential for misinterpretation of the slides in patients taking iron supplements. This will minimize the number of false-positive fecal occult blood tests, which increase the cost of a surveillance program. However, by limiting the sensitivity of the test, at least one third of colorectal cancers will be missed.

Early stage cancers can be detected using fecal occult blood tests, and recent data make the important confirmation that colorectal cancer mortality is reduced by finding these tumors. First, a case-control study published from the Oakland Kaiser-Permanente health maintenance organization suggested a 25% reduction in colorectal cancer mortality for those individuals who had had their stools screened for occult fecal blood within the past 5 years. The most important study of fecal occult blood tests was reported from the University of Minnesota and involved the use of mainly (83%) rehydrated Hemoccult cards on >46,000 patients studied prospectively for an average of 13 years. In this study, annual fecal occult blood tests resulted in a 33% reduction of colorectal cancer mortality. This was largely achieved through "stage shift" in which there was a 50% reduction in advanced (Dukes' D Stage) tumors in the screened group, which had a profound effect on survival. It appears that annual testing is necessary to reduce colorectal cancer mortality and that the benefit is diminished as the interval between tests is increased.

ENDOSCOPIC SCREENING FOR COLON CANCER

Screening with fecal occult blood tests has its limitations, and since approximately two thirds of colorectal neoplasms are within reach of the flexible sigmoidoscope, screening with this instrument has been recommended. The development of flexible instruments that can reach from the anus to the cecum has raised the obvious issue of how far to take the examinations.

There are currently two studies that suggest a significant reduction in mortality from screening sigmoidoscopic examination. A case-control study from the Oakland Kaiser-Permanente Program examined the use of screening sigmoidoscopy among 261 patients who died of cancer of the rectum or distal colon compared with case-matched controls. Only 8.8% of the cancer patients had undergone screening sigmoidoscopy compared with 24.2% of the controls. The authors estimated from this outcome that screened subjects had only 30% of the risk for fatal cancers of the rectum and distal colon compared with the unscreened cohort. Furthermore, the data suggested that screening sigmoidoscopic examination may have provided risk reduction for as long as 10 years. There was a similar number of fatal colon cancers above the reach of a sigmoidoscopic examination in both the screened and unscreened groups, which supported the contention that the two groups were evenly matched for colorectal cancer risk. This observation was confirmed by another retrospective case-control study from Wisconsin. A history of at least a single screening sigmoidoscopic examination over the 10-year period of study was present in 10% of those who died of colorectal cancer versus 30% of case-controls. This group estimated that the risk of death from colorectal cancer was reduced by 79% after a single examination, whereas no benefits were observed among patients who had undergone digital examinations of the rectum or fecal occult blood test.

At the time of this writing, no controlled prospective trial has been published that tests the efficacy of endoscopic screening using either sigmoidoscopy or colonoscopy. Nonetheless, there is strong and compelling evidence for a protective effect of sigmoidoscopy and by inference, the removal of premalignant lesions. Endoscopic screening appears to bring with it a protective effect that lasts substantially longer than the 1-year protection provided by fecal occult blood tests. Furthermore, the magnitude of reduced cancer mortality is substantially greater than that derived from fecal occult blood tests presumably since one can detect not only early stage lesions but also remove premalignant lesions and interrupt neoplastic progression early in its long natural history.

The American Cancer Society, the National Cancer Institute, and several other advisory panels have recommended that screening for colorectal cancer in average risk individuals should begin at age 50 and consist of annual fecal occult blood tests and flexible sigmoidoscopy every 3 to 5 years. Screened patients are significantly less likely to die of colorectal cancer or suffer morbidity related to cancer or surgery. Patients screened by endoscopic procedures appear to have even greater protection than those screened with fecal occult blood tests, both in terms of the magnitude of reduced mortality and the duration of protection provided by the examination. More screening will prevent more cancer deaths, but it also costs more. Therefore, the real controversy surrounds how much screening can be afforded.

SCREENING FOR COLON CANCER IN THE 21ST CENTURY— GENETIC APPROACHES

A better understanding of the genetic pathogenesis of GI cancer will provide the physician with new tools with which to anticipate the diagnosis of cancer. Progress has been made already in the area of colorectal cancer, and it is anticipated that the same will occur for other GI organs in the near future.

Germline Mutations. It will be possible to test for familial colorectal cancer syndromes using a blood test to detect germline mutations in the *APC* gene (which cause FAP) or in the genes responsible for hereditary nonpolyposis colorectal cancer (HNPCC), which include the *hMSH2, hMLH1,* and other genes. This will be of particular importance because each unrelated family affected by these genetic abnormalities will usually have a unique mutation. All those affected within that specific family will carry the same mutation, which may permit rapid screening. Each family's mutation may carry with it unique phenotypic variations that may include different ages for onset of disease, different degrees of virulence of the colorectal cancer, and a different constellation of associated noncolonic cancers. By defining the lesion in a family and by understanding the risks associated with each individual mutation, the physician can anticipate more rationally the associated tumor spectrum within each family. For example, at present, it is known that mutations at the 5′ end of the *APC* gene (i.e., the first three or four exons) are associated with "attenuated" forms of FAP (called AAPC) and that mutations occurring in one isolated region of the *APC* gene (consisting of approximately 150 codons of the gene) are associated with an early-onset, more virulent form of FAP. The genetic locus of some families with HNPCC has been located on chromosomes 2p and 3p, and it is known that additional families have the same clinical features of HNPCC but the disease is not caused by the gene on either of these chromosomes. Rapid screening tests are under development for the diagnosis of FAP but remain an area for development in HNPCC.

Oncogene Detection in the Stool. Mutations in the *K-RAS 2* gene are not seen in premalignant tissue or in very small adenomas but occur in approximately 50% of larger adenomas and carcinomas of the colon and rectum. It has been demonstrated that the mutated *RAS* gene may be identified in fecal extracts using the polymerase chain reaction, even though the mutated gene makes up only a tiny fraction of the host DNA present in stool. Thus, it has been suggested that this might be utilized as a test to screen for the appearance of sporadic cancer of the colon or rectum. This has only been tested in a small pilot study, and it is not yet known whether it is technically feasible to screen asymptomatic populations for the presence of this gene. Nonetheless, the limitations of fecal occult blood testing and endoscopic screening tests for colorectal cancer suggest the possibility that searching for the presence of a cancer-related gene in stool may be an area for future investigation.

CASE PRESENTATION

A 60-year-old man is referred to a gastroenterologist for evaluation of weight loss, epigastric pain, and anemia. The pain is worse postprandially, and even small amounts of food lead to a feeling of fullness. His past medical history is notable for appendectomy and a bleeding ulcer treated by partial gastrectomy 25 years ago. He takes no medications, avoiding over-the-counter analgesics because of his prior history of ulcer disease. Family history is notable for peptic ulcer disease in his father. Review of systems reveals bloating and occasional diarrhea after large meals, which has been present since his stomach surgery.

Physical examination revealed a thin male in no distress. Vital signs were normal. The head, eyes, ears, nose, and throat examination noted pallor of the bulbar conjunctiva and oral mucosa. The heart and lungs were normal. The abdomen was scaphoid with a normal liver and spleen. Rectal examination revealed brown, Hemoccult-positive stool. Laboratory examination revealed a hemoglobin of 11 g/dl with a mean corpuscular volume of 70 fl. The serum chemistry profile was normal. The patient underwent an upper GI barium study that was consistent with previous partial gastrectomy and gastrojejunostomy and showed an ulcer at the surgical anastomosis (Fig. 10-4).

Weight loss and epigastric pain in a postgastrectomy patient should immediately raise the question of a late postoperative complication such as gastric carcinoma. Although poor gastric emptying (gastroparesis) can occur postoperatively owing to the vagotomy typically performed in ulcer surgery, symptoms usually arise closer to the operative procedure than was reported by this patient. Our patient's symptoms are those of poor gastric distensibility and emptying with early satiety (excessive feeling of fullness postprandially). An ulcer at the anastomosis could also cause our patient's symptoms, and endoscopic examination is necessary to make this diagnosis. The patient's bloating and occasional diarrhea after large meals are consistent with mild dysmotility symptoms of dumping syndrome for many years. However, the symptom of early satiety points to a new, worrisome process. An upper GI barium study is a reasonable starting point for investigation. However, the test can be quite insensitive in the deformed postoperative stomach, and direct endoscopic examination is necessary to exclude a tumor or ulcer.

The patient exhibited pallor on physical examination, and laboratory studies revealed anemia. The development of microcytic anemia, as suggested by the mean corpuscular volume, also raised the question of GI blood loss, particularly when complicated by iron deficiency. In patients such as

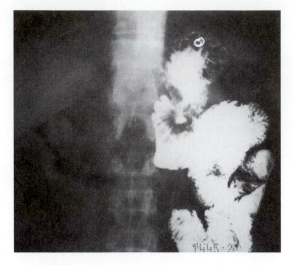

Figure 10-4. Upper GI barium study. The stomach has been partially resected and a gastrojejunostomy performed. There is a constant 12-mm collection of barium with radiating folds on the jejunal side of the anastomosis consistent with an ulcer. (Coutesy of the Radiology Teaching File of the American College of Radiology, developed in conjunction with the Bureau of Radiological Health, Food and Drug Administration.)

this, iron deficiency may occur owing to the postgastrectomy state, wherein hypochlorhydria leads to poor iron absorption in combination with chronic blood loss caused by bile reflux gastritis. The Hemoccult test, which was designed to screen for colonic bleeding, revealed occult blood loss. In most clinical situations, unless the symptoms suggest an upper GI source of the bleeding, colonscopy is required to exclude colorectal neoplasia.

The diagnostic test of choice in this patient is upper GI endoscopy. It revealed a 1.5-cm flat ulcerated mass at the gastrojejunal anastomosis. Biopsy results were positive for adenocarcinoma, with intestinal metaplasia in the surrounding epithelium. An abdominal CT scan was then ordered and was negative for liver metastases. The patient was scheduled for resective surgery.

Chronic gastric inflammation (commonly due to *H. pylori*) predisposed this patient to peptic ulcer disease, and gastric surgery became necessary when the patient developed a complicated ulcer before the days of effective therapeutic endoscopy, potent antisecretory therapy, and the recognition of the role of the bacteria in ulcer disease. Positive family histories of ulcer disease are frequently present because of common environmental exposures and "familial" infection with *H. pylori*. The presence of intestinal metaplasia indicated the effect of longstanding chronic gastritis. The partial gastrectomy did not eradicate the organism, allowing continued inflammation and the development of metaplasia. Performing a partial gastrectomy only exacerbated the chronic inflammation by exposing the stomach to bile reflux. The vagotomy reduced acid secretion, leading to an increase in gastrin serum and facilitating bacterial overgrowth. Mutagens formed in the gastric lumen from bacterial overgrowth, and the chronic inflammation resulted in the release of a variety of cytokines. All these factors conspired to produce a hyperproliferative epithelium. The result was progression to dysplasia and the ultimate development of adenocarcinoma.

261

Selected Reading

SELECTED READING

Choi PM, Nugent FW, Schoetz DJ, et al. Colonoscopic surveillance reduces mortality from colorectal cancer in ulcerative colitis. Gastroenterology 105:418, 1993.

Correa P. Human gastric carcinogenesis: A multistep and multifactorial process—first American Cancer Society Award lecture on cancer epidemiology and prevention. Cancer Res 52:6735, 1992.

Correa P, Cuello C, Fajardo LF, et al. Diet and gastric cancer: Nutrition survey in a high-risk area. J Natl Cancer Inst 70:673, 1973.

Fearon ER, Vogelstein B. A genetic model for colorectal tumorigenesis. Cell 61:759, 1990.

Fennerty MB, Sampliner RE, Garewal HS. Review Article: Barrett's oesophagus—cancer risk, biology and therapeutic management. Aliment Pharmacol Ther 7:339, 1993.

Harris CC. Chemical and physical carcinogenesis: Advances and perspectives for the 1990s. Cancer Res 55:50235, 1991.

Harris CC, Hollstein M. Clinical implications of the p53 tumor-suppressor gene. N Engl J Med 329:1318, 1993.

Labayle D, Fischer D, Vielh P, et al. Sulindac causes regression of rectal polyps in familial adenomatous polyposis. Gastroenterology 101:635, 1991.

Mandel JS, Bond JH, Church TR, et al. Reducing mortality from colorectal cancer by screening for fecal occult blood. N Engl J Med 328:1365, 1993.

Marshall CJ. Tumor suppressor genes. Cell 64:313, 1991.

Parsonett J. *Helicobacter pylori* and gastric cancer. Gastroenterol Clin North Am 22:89, 1993.

Peltomaki P, Aaltonen LA, Sistonen P, et al. Genetic mapping of a locus predisposing to human colorectal cancer. Science 260:810, 1993.

Powell SM, Zilz N, Beazer-Barclay Y, et al. *APC* mutations occur early during colorectal tumorigenesis. Nature 359:235, 1992.

Selby JV, Friedman GD, Quesenberry CP Jr, et al. A case-control study of screening sigmoidoscopy and mortality from colorectal cancer. N Engl J Med 326:653, 1992.

Shields PG, Harris CC. Molecular epidemiology and the genetics of environmental cancer. JAMA 266:681, 1991.

Thibodeau SN, Bren G, Schaid D. Microsatellite instability in cancer of the proximal colon. Science 260:816, 1993.

Thun MJ, Namboodiri MM, Heath Jr. CW. Aspirin use and reduced risk of fatal colon cancer. N Engl J Med 325:1593, 1991.

Wright PA, Williams GT. Molecular biology and gastric carcinoma. Gut 34:145, 1993.

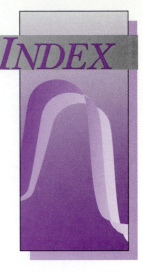

INDEX

Page numbers followed by a *t* refer to tables; those followed by an *f* refer to figures.

salt, 79–81
of vasoactive intestinal polypeptide, 199
water, 74–75, 75f
Secretory cells, sodium transport in, 79–80
Segmentation, small intestinal, 121
Shigella, enterotoxin of, 93
Short bowel syndrome, malabsorption in, 144
Sigmoidoscopy, cancer screening with, 257–258
Sinusoidal membrane, 153–154, 154f
Sitophobia, 53
Small intestine
absorption in, 120–135. *See also* Absorption
biopsy of, 148
in malabsorption, 150, 151f
brush border of, 195
crypts in, 95, 97f, 120, 122f
follow-through radiography of, 148
in malabsorption, 150, 150f, 151f
ischemia of, 216
in lipid digestion, 130
mechanical obstruction of, 60
microcirculation in, 214–215, 215f
motility disorders of, 62
mucosa of
in celiac sprue, 140, 142f
diarrhea and, 87, 95, 97, 98t, 136
malabsorption and, 140–143, 142f
in tropical sprue, 142
perfusion study of, 103–104
peristalsis in, 121–122
pseudo-obstruction syndromes of, 62
segmentation in, 121
surface area of, 72, 73f
villi in, 120, 120f
villi in, 95, 97f, 120–121, 120–122f
water absorption in, 72, 73f
water transport in
active, 77–78
passive, 75–76
permeability and, 76–77, 77f
salt transport in, 77–78
Sodium. *See also* Electrolytes; Salt
absorption of, 123–124, 124f
glucose in, 79, 85
active transport of, 78
malabsorption of, 136
transport of
membrane proteins in, 78, 79f
in secretory cells, 79–80
Solutes
concentration of, 76
osmotic, and diarrhea, 75, 97
Somatosensory cortex, in visceral pain, 3, 4f
Somatostatin
in gastric acid secretion, 34, 35f
pancreatic secretion inhibition by, 118–119, 201
for Zollinger-Ellison syndrome, 42
Sorbitol, diarrhea from, 97
Sphincter of Oddi, 189, 189f
Spinal cord, pain transmission modulation at, 5, 5f
Spinal nerve fibers, in visceral pain, 2–3, 4f
Spinoreticular tract, in visceral pain, 3, 4f
Spinothalamic tract, in visceral pain, 3, 4f
Splanchnic nerve, in vomiting, 54–55, 55f

Splenic vein, 192, 192f
thrombosis of, 231–233, 233f
Sprue
celiac, 140–141, 142f, 151
tropical, 141–143
Squamous cell carcinoma, esophageal, 246
Starch, digestion of, 196
Steatorrhea
in diabetes mellitus, 145
diarrhea from, 95
in lipid malabsorption, 135–136
in pancreatic exocrine deficiency, 137
in Zollinger-Ellison syndrome, 40
Stomach
adenocarcinoma of, 30
arterial supply of, 213–214, 214f
atrophy of, 41, 42t
carcinoma of, 246–247
alcohol use and, 250
chronic atrophic gastritis in, 252–253
diet and, 250–252
epidemiology of, 235
nitrate ingestion and, 251
tobacco use and, 250
water source and, 250–251
digestive functions of, 115–117
disorders of, 139f, 139–140, 141f
emptying of
disorders of, 61
nutrient type and, 116–117
studies of, 65–66
epithelial cells of, 32–33
epithelial proliferation in, 236
food-handling functions of, 115–117
grinding by, 116
hydrochloric acid secretion in, 113–115, 114–116f. *See also* Gastric acid, secretion of
in lipid digestion, 130
microcirculation in, 214
motility in, and vomiting, 56
mucosa of
barrier function of, 32–34, 33f
Helicobacter pylori–mediated damage of, 35–36, 36f
nonsteroidal anti-inflammatory drug damage to, 36
oxyntic gland in, 32, 32f
in peptic ulcer disease, 32f, 32–36, 33f, 35f, 36f
prostaglandins in, 33–34
reconstitution of, 33–34
mucus cells of, 32, 32f
musculature of, 115–116
pacemaker disturbances of, 61
pH of, 32–33
receptive relaxation of, 116
sieving by, 116
smooth muscle dysfunction in, 61
Stroke, upper esophageal sphincter dysfunction after, 19, 20f
Submandibular salivary gland, 112, 112f
Sucralfate, for peptic ulcer disease, 38
Sucrase-isomaltase complex, 128–129
Surgery
diarrhea after, 99
pancreatitis after, 203–204

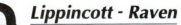

plastic polyps (adenomas) and eventual carcinoma at an early age. Similarly, FAP patients who have hundreds of colonic adenomas may undergo regression of these lesions after the administration of a nonsteroidal anti-inflammatory drug such as sulindac. The mechanism underlying adenoma involution in response to sulindac is unknown. It has long been known that small, sporadic adenomatous polyps may disappear without therapy when evaluated by serial colonoscopic examinations, further underscoring the dynamic nature of early colorectal neoplasia. Clonal expansion is probably mediated in part by the abnormal expression of growth factors, excess expression of their receptors, or disregulation of the signal transduction mechanism between membrane receptors and the nucleus. It is not known to what degree this process of neoplastic progression may be inhibited or reversed or how it takes place.

Malignant Conversion. The clonal expansion of a hyperproliferative pool of cells exposed to an environment rich in carcinogens provides the substrate for a catalclysmic biologic event. In certain premalignant tissues, additional genetic events occur that give rise to the malignant phenotype. As described above, there are at least two genetic mechanisms that seem to permit the appearance of cancer. Both of these involve the breakdown of a homeostatic mechanism whereby DNA sequences or chromosomes are faithfully replicated.

Malignant cells are capable of continued growth, invasion, and the formation of distant metastases, and unlike benign neoplasms, they do not spontaneously regress. Malignant tumors are dynamic, by virtue of their genomic instability. Many of the newly created cells have lost proteins essential for survival, and cells die. Cell necrosis is commonly observed in tumors. Other rearrangements or genetic damage results in the generation of more virulent clones that overgrow and replace the parent tumor. Thus, the malignant phenotype is an unstable, dynamic state in which the ability to grow, invade, and spread is under strong selective pressures.

Metastasis. The metastasis of tumor cells is not a random or accidental process. For a tumor to metastasize, it must degrade the basement membrane and associated matrix components, migrate through the subtending connective tissue, enter into a lymphatic or blood vessel, migrate away from the parent tumor, avoid a gauntlet of naturally occurring defensive mechanisms, lodge at a distant site, emigrate from the vessel, and effectively colonize elsewhere. Metastasis generally occurs as a late event in the natural history of a tumor, because time is required for the gradual evolution of cells that have accumulated additional genetic changes to make them capable of all of the above behaviors.

Tumor cells require a blood supply to survive. Oxygen can normally diffuse approximately 100 to 200 μm from a blood vessel, or roughly only 4 to 10 cell diameters, depending upon the cell type. Tumors can stimulate the growth of capillaries (i.e., neovascularization) to facilitate their egress from the primary mass and their growth at metastatic sites. Tumor-associated angiogenesis appears to be mediated by a variety of different tumor growth factors, including an "angiogenesis factor." The sites to which malignant cells metastasize may appear to be random, based purely on the blood supply of an organ, but the process is more complicated, and tumor cell targeting to distant organs may be mediated by specific cell membrane receptors.

The genetic basis of metastasis is undoubtedly complex and is currently incompletely understood. One gene has been identified that is associated with distant metastasis in certain cancers. The *NM23* gene seems to function as a metastasis suppressor gene inasmuch as it is deleted in distant metastases from colorectal cancer. The cellular mechanism by which the *NM23* locus confers metastatic capability is totally unknown. It is apparent that numerous genes participate in the metastatic phenotype, and the accumulation of them within malignant cells is responsible for the broad range of virulent behaviors seen in cancer.

SPECIFIC ORGAN INVOLVEMENT

The preceding sections have outlined the general framework by which GI carcinogenesis unfolds. However, each GI cancer is a distinct disease with a variety of unique aspects. Many of the details that have led to our current understanding of GI cancer have come from a study of colorectal cancer, and these principles may not necessarily pertain to cancers elsewhere in the gut. Therefore, this section highlights some of the information known about specific GI tumors to provide a framework for an understanding of future progress in GI cancers.

ESOPHAGEAL CANCER

Squamous cell carcinoma and adenocarcinoma of the esophagus are separate diseases with different etiologies and natural histories that should be considered independently. Squamous cell carcinoma has an extremely wide international incidence range that has puzzled tumor biologists for a long time. It is assumed that the variation in incidence is a reflection of the differential expression of one or more potent environmental carcinogens. First, severe chronic esophagitis is a precursor condition in young people who live in areas of the world at highest risk for squamous cell carcinoma of the esophagus. It is not known what causes this inflammation, but as described above, reactive oxygen species are powerful carcinogens. Second, human papillomavirus can be found in precancerous lesions and squamous cell carcinomas from China. Precursor lesions for squamous cell carcinoma have mutations in the *p53* gene, and the lesions show accumulation of the abnormal *p53* protein, similar to what is seen in colorectal cancer.

Barrett's esophagus is a condition in which the native squamous epithelium of the esophagus is replaced by a metaplastic columnar epithelium (intestinal type). It is believed that this change is a consequence of chronic gastroesophageal reflux, epithelial injury, and replacement by an epithelium more resistant to refluxed acid. Adenocarcinoma of the esophagus may arise in Barrett's epithelium. In Barrett's esophagus, aneuploidy is commonly seen early in the course of neoplastic progression. In fact aneuploidy, which reflects genomic instability, occurs in premalignant tissues and may be used to predict the risk of tumor progression. Thus, genomic instability occurs relatively early in this disease (compared to its later onset in the sporadic adenoma-to-carcinoma sequence in the colon), and a different sequence of events may be responsible for the virulent clinical course of cancer in the esophagus.

STOMACH CANCER

Carcinoma of the stomach occurs primarily in the setting of severe chronic gastritis. This again emphasizes the carcinogenic potential of reactive oxygen species formed during inflammation. Gastric carcinoma is associated with mutations in the *APC* gene, *K-RAS* gene, and *p53* gene. LOH is seen at high frequency at several chromosomal sites, including 17p (the locus of the *p53* gene), 5q (the location of the *APC* gene), the *DCC* gene (18q), and other sites. Little is known about the sequence and time relationships of genomic instability in gastric cancer. *RAS* gene mutations appear to be relatively infrequent in this disease. The natural history of gastric cancer is that it occurs in the setting of chronic inflammation, is not frequently associated with obvious neoplastic polyps such as are found in the colon, and may be virulent and progress to a lethal stage quickly. This series of events suggests the possibility that the genetic events that trigger genomic instability may occur relatively early in gastric cancer, bypassing a prolonged premalignant phase, which has important implications for the clinical outcome in this disease. Less information is available for gastric carcinoma than colon cancer, but one would anticipate that differences in the responsible genetic lesions may account for the unique biologic and clinical behaviors of this cancer.

COLORECTAL CANCER

Many of the paradigms that are currently used to describe sequential carcinogenesis for solid tumors have been developed from the study of colorectal cancer, and this information has provided a general framework for much of the prior discussion. However, there are specific situations in which variations on this theme occur.

In the case of FAP, the affected individual has a germ line mutation in the *APC* gene, which results in the appearance of adenomatous polyps by a mean age of 16 years. The increased risk for cancer occurs because the colonic epithelium has a mutation built into its genetic program whereby the loss of proliferative control occurs very early. Furthermore, every colonic epithelial cell has this defect, which greatly expands the pool of hyperproliferative tissue. Perhaps a more important and subtle aspect of FAP can be found in the natural history of this disease. Without any early diagnosis or intervention, the average gene carrier dies of cancer at a mean age of 42 years. Furthermore, although many such patients have thousands of adenomatous polyps in the colon and have carried them for 25 years or more, most of these patients develop a relatively small number of cancers. Less than half have more than one malignant tumor, and the most found in one large series was seven cancers. This leads to the conclusion that the development of the adenoma is not the rate-limiting step in the development of cancer, indicating the necessity for additional genetic damage for neoplastic progression to occur.

Chronic ulcerative colitis is a condition in which an increased risk for colorectal cancer is seen. In general, many of the same genetic lesions are seen in ulcerative colitis cancers as in sporadically occurring tumors. However, there are three issues of particular interest with regard to cancers that occur in this condition. First, *K-RAS* gene mutations are reported to be relatively uncommon in colitic cancers. Thus, cancers in ulcerative colitis develop without activation of the gene that has been implicated as an important "middle event" in colorectal cancer and that may be responsible for the clonal expansion of premalignant tissue. Second, mutation in the *p53* gene is found early and frequently in this disease. Third, aneuploidy is very common, occurs in extended clones of normal-appearing colonic tissue, and antedates the development of dysplasia and cancer. Thus, cancer in ulcerative colitis may tend to develop through a program that gives it a different "middle stage" that may be relatively abbreviated, resulting in the early onset of virulent, malignant disease. The mechanism to explain this different natural history is unknown;

however, colitic cancers occur in the setting of chronic inflammation, unlike the sporadically occurring variety.

DIET AND GI CANCER

COLORECTAL CANCER

Investigators have been suspicious of the role of diet in the causation of colorectal cancer. But studying the diet to identify colonic carcinogens is a complicated undertaking. The human diet contains a great variety of naturally occurring mutagens and carcinogens—not to mention blockers and antagonists of each. Furthermore, since proximate carcinogens are by their very nature highly reactive and short-lived molecules, the procarcinogens in the diet are probably a more appropriate target to study but are difficult to identify out of the context of the fecal contents and activating enzymes present in the mucosa.

It is difficult to dissect the components of the diet that are most important in conferring cancer risk. To begin with, the estimated risk of colon cancer increases by 2.3% for each 100 calories ingested per day, and the total energy intake may be powerful enough to overwhelm the analysis of individual dietary components. Compelling epidemiologic leads have come from studies of the dietary intakes of fat, meat, and fiber, and there is a very strong, dose-related associated between the per capita intake of total dietary fat or meat and the incidence of colorectal cancer.

The mechanism by which a high-fat diet enhances tumor production appears to be related to the role of bile acids on colonic epithelial proliferation. Increasing the intake of animal fat from 62 to 152 g per day produced a significant increase in total fecal bile acid and fatty acid excretion in humans, without affecting fecal weight, number of stools, transit time, fecal-β-glucuronidase, or fecal steroid degradation. The intracolonic instillation of the bile acid deoxycholic acid increases cellular proliferation. It has been shown that deoxycholic acid produces reactive oxygen radicals in the colon and that the generation of such molecular species can independently stimulate mucosal proliferation. The proliferative response to deoxycholic acid may be abolished by agents that destroy superoxide (such as superoxide dismutase) or inhibit lipoxygenase activity. Therefore, the generation of reactive oxygen may be the mechanism by which oxidized fatty acid residues are produced in the colon, which then stimulate colonic cell proliferation. The oxidation of unsaturated fatty acids may produce compounds that stimulate cell proliferation. This could explain why unsaturated fatty acids are more effective in supporting tumor production in animal models and also explain the coordinate role of bile acids and fat in the pathogenesis of colorectal cancer.

Certain fats can induce mitogenesis in neoplastic colonic epithelial cells but not in the normal colon. Diglycerides containing stearic, oleic, palmitic, and myristic acid side chains have been found in human fecal extracts in concentrations that stimulate mitogenesis in cultured explants of human adenomas and carcinomas. A high-fat diet, even administered as a bolus, can lead to an increase in the proliferation of human colonic epithelium. Therefore, fats may play a critical role in regulating proliferation of both normal and transformed epithelium; however, the specific lipids involved may depend upon the maturational status of the epithelial cell.

Fiber. The Western diet is relatively deficient in fiber compared to the diet of non-Western populations, and this may be important in the pathogenesis of